International
REVIEW OF
Neurobiology
Volume 61

International

REVIEW OF

Neurobiology

Volume 61

SERIES EDITORS

RONALD J. BRADLEY
Department of Psychiatry, School of Medicine
Louisiana State University Medical Center
Shreveport, Louisiana, USA

R. ADRON HARRIS
Waggoner Center for Alcohol and Drug Addiction Research
The University of Texas at Austin
Austin, Texas, USA

PETER JENNER
Division of Pharmacology and Therapeutics
GKT School of Biomedical Sciences
King's College, London, UK

EDITORIAL BOARD

CONTENTS

SECTION I
HIGH-THROUGHPUT TECHNOLOGIES

Biomarker Discovery Using Molecular Profiling Approaches
STEPHEN J. WALKER AND ARRON XU

Proteomic Analysis of Mitochondrial Proteins
MARY F. LOPEZ, SIMON MELOV, FELICITY JOHNSON,
NICOLE NAGULKO, EVA GOLENKO, SCOTT KUZDZAL,
SUZANNE ACKLOO, AND ALVYDAS MIKULSKIS

SECTION II
PROTEOMIC APPLICATIONS

NMDA Receptors, Neural Pathways, and Protein Interaction Databases

HOLGER HUSI

Dopamine Transporter Network and Pathways

RAJANI MAIYA AND R. DAYNE MAYFIELD

Proteomic Approaches in Drug Discovery and Development

HOLLY D. SOARES, STEPHEN A. WILLIAMS, PETER J. SNYDER, FENG GAO, TOM STIGER, CHRISTIAN ROHLFF, ATHULA HERATH, TREY SUNDERLAND, KAREN PUTNAM, AND W. FROST WHITE

SECTION III
INFORMATICS

Proteomic Informatics

STEVEN A. RUSSELL, WILLIAM OLD, KATHERYN A. RESING,
AND LAWRENCE HUNTER

SECTION IV
CHANGES IN THE PROTEOME BY DISEASE

Proteomics Analysis in Alzheimer's Disease: New Insights into Mechanisms of Neurodegeneration

D. ALLAN BUTTERFIELD AND DEBRA BOYD-KIMBALL

Proteomics and Alcoholism

FRANK A. WITZMANN AND WENDY N. STROTHER

Proteomics Studies of Traumatic Brain Injury

Kevin K. W. Wang, Andrew Ottens, William Haskins, Ming Cheng Liu, Firas Kobeissy, Nancy Denslow, SuShing Chen, and Ronald L. Hayes

Influence of Huntington's Disease on the Human and Mouse Proteome

Claus Zabel and Joachim Klose

SECTION V
OVERVIEW OF THE NEUROPROTEOME

Proteomics—Application to the Brain

Katrin Marcus, Oliver Schmidt, Heike Schaefer, Michael Hamacher, André van Hall, and Helmut E. Meyer

CONTRIBUTORS

Numbers in parentheses indicate the pages on which the authors' contributions begin.

Suzanne Ackloo (31), MDS Sciex, Concord, Ontario, Canada L4K 4V8

Debra Boyd-Kimball (161), Department of Chemistry, Center of Membrane Sciences, University of Kentucky, Lexington, Kentucky 40506

D. Allan Butterfield (161), Department of Chemistry, Center of Membrane Sciences, and Sanders-Brown Center on Aging, University of Kentucky, Lexington, Kentucky 40506

SuShing Chen (215), Center of Neuroproteomics and Biomarkers Research and computing and Information Science Engineering, University of Florida, Gainesville, Florida 32610

Ming Cheng Liu (215), Center of Neuroproteomics and Biomarkers Research, Center for Traumatic Brain Injury Studies, and Department of Neuroscience, University of Florida, Gainesville, Florida 32610

Nancy Denslow (215), Center of Neuroproteomics and Biomarkers Research, and Interdisciplinary Center of Biomedical Research, University of Florida, Gainesville, Florida 32610

Feng Gao (97), Nonclinical Statistics, Pfizer Global Research and Development, Groton, Connecticut 06340

Eva Golenko (31), PerkinElmer Life and Analytical Sciences, Boston, Massachusetts 02118

Michael Hamacher (287), Medical Proteom-Center, Ruhr University of Bochum, Bochum, Germany 44780

William Haskins (215), Center of Neuroproteomics and Biomarkers Research, Center for Traumatic Brain Injury Studies, and Department of Neuroscience, University of Florida, Gainesville, Florida 32610

Ronald L. Hayes (215), Center for Traumatic Brain Injury Studies, Department of Psychiatry, and Department of Neuroscience, University of Florida, Gainesville, Florida 32610

Athula Herath (97), Oxford Glycosciences, Abingdon OX3 3YS, United Kingdom

Holger Husi (51), Division of Neuroscience, University of Edinburgh, Edinburgh EH8 9JZ, United Kingdom

Lawrence Hunter (129), Center for Computational Pharmacology, University of Colorado Health Sciences Center, Aurora, Colorado 80045

Felicity Johnson (31), Buck Institute for Age Research, Novato, California 94945

Joachim Klose (241), Institute for Human Genetics, Charité—University Medicine Berlin, 13353 Berlin, Germany

Firas Kobeissy (215), Center of Neuroproteomics and Biomarkers Research, Center for Traumatic Brain Injury Studies, Department of Psychiatry, and Department of Neuroscience, University of Florida, Gainesville, Florida 32610

Scott Kuzdzal (31), PerkinElmer Life and Analytical Sciences, Shelton, Connecticut 06484

Mary F. Lopez (31), PerkinElmer Life and Analytical Sciences, Boston, Massachusetts 02118

Rajani Maiya (79), Institute for Cellular and Molecular Biology, University of Texas at Austin, Austin, Texas 78712

Katrin Marcus (287), Medical Proteom-Center, Ruhr University of Bochum, Bochum, Germany 44780

R. Dayne Mayfield (79), Waggoner Center for Alcohol and Addiction Research, University of Texas at Austin, Austin, Texas 78712

Simon Melov (31), Buck Institute for Age Research, Novato, California 94945

Helmut E. Meyer (287), Medical Proteom-Center, Ruhr University of Bochum, Bochum, Germany 44780

Alvydas Mikulskis (31), PerkinElmer Life and Analytical Sciences, Boston, Massachusetts 02118

Nicole Nagulko (31), Buck Institute for Age Research, Novato, California 94945

William Old (129), Department of Chemistry and Biochemistry, University of Colorado, Boulder, Colorado 80309

Andrew Ottens (215), Center of Neuroproteomics and Biomarkers Research, Center for Traumatic Brain Injury Studies, and Department of Neuroscience, University of Florida, Gainesville, Florida 32610

Karen Putnam (97), Geriatric Psychiatry Branch, National Institute of Mental Health, Bethesda, Maryland 20892

Katheryn A. Resing (129), Department of Chemistry and Biochemistry, University of Colorado, Boulder, Colorado 80309

Christian Rohlff (97), Oxford Genome Sciences UK Ltd., Oxford Centre for Gene Function, Oxford OX1 3QX, United Kingdom

Steven A. Russell (129), Center for Computational Pharmacology, University of Colorado Health Sciences Center, Aurora, Colorado 80045

Heike Schaefer (287), Medical Proteom-Center, Ruhr University of Bochum, Bochum, Germany 44780

Oliver Schmidt (287), Medical Proteom-Center, Ruhr University of Bochum, Bochum, Germany 44780

Peter J. Snyder (97), Exploratory Development, Pfizer Global Research and Development, Groton, Connecticut 06340

Holly D. Soares (97), Clinical Biochemical Measurements, Pfizer Global Research and Development, Groton, Connecticut 06340

Tom Stiger (97), Clinical Statistics, Pfizer Global Research and Development, Groton, Connecticut 06340

Wendy N. Strother (189), Department of Psychiatry, Institute of Psychiatric Research, Indiana University School of Medicine, Indianapolis, Indiana 46202

Trey Sunderland (97), Geriatric Psychiatry Branch, National Institute of Mental Health, Bethesda, Maryland 20892

André van Hall (287), Medical Proteom-Center, Ruhr University of Bochum, Bochum, Germany 44780

Stephen J. Walker (3), Wake Forest University School of Medicine, Department of Physiology and Pharmacology, Winston-Salem, North Carolina 27101

Kevin K. W. Wang (215), Center of Neuroproteomics and Biomarkers Research, Center for Traumatic Brain Injury Studies, Department of Psychiatry, and Department of Neuroscience, University of Florida, Gainesville, Florida 32610

W. Frost White (97), CNS Discovery Biology, Pfizer Global Research and Development, Groton, Connecticut 06340

Stephen A. Williams (97), Clinical Technology, Pfizer Global Research and Development, Groton, Connecticut 06340

Frank A. Witzmann (189), Department of Cellular and Integrative Physiology, Indiana University School of Medicine, Indianapolis, Indiana 46202

Arron Xu (3), Ciphergen Biosystems, Fremont, California 94555

Claus Zabel (241), Institute for Human Genetics, Charité—University Medicine Berlin, 13353 Berlin, Germany

SECTION I

HIGH-THROUGHPUT TECHNOLOGIES

BIOMARKER DISCOVERY USING MOLECULAR PROFILING APPROACHES

Stephen J. Walker* and Arron Xu[†]

*Wake Forest University School of Medicine
Department of Physiology and Pharmacology
Winston-Salem, North Carolina 27101
[†]Ciphergen Biosystems
Fremont, California 94555

I. Introduction

A *biomarker* may be defined as any parameter that can be used to measure an interaction between a biological system and an environmental agent, be it chemical (e.g., toxins), physical (e.g., administration of a drug), or biological (e.g., genetic polymorphism; World Health Organization, 1993). There is an enormous interest in the identification of biological markers relevant to neurological (and other) disease processes. The potential now exists to capture unique fingerprints composed of molecular changes and to subject them to interpretation, with the goal of class discovery, comparison, or prediction (Bailey and Ulrich, 2004). Evaluating cellular responses to perturbations caused by disease and/or the administration of drugs, or environmental insult (e.g., toxins), can be achieved through a systems approach using an arsenal of molecular tools. A vast supply of molecular tools and methods for tasks such as gene expression profiling (functional genomics), protein profiling (proteomics), and integrative biochemical profiling (metabolomics and metabonomics) are either currently available for routine use or are being developed and enhanced on an ongoing basis. Perhaps the greatest challenges today are in the areas of data management and data analysis. The task of interpretation and integration of the unprecedented volumes of data being generated to yield clinically useful information, although not impossible, is daunting.

This chapter should serve as an introduction to some of the methodologies currently used to uncover unique molecular profiles that describe a particular cellular "state," whether it be caused by disease, environment, genetic predisposition, or some combination of factors. Although we will spend some time discussing gene expression profiling and metabolomics, the majority of this chapter will focus on protein profiling technology, specifically the use of surface-enhanced laser desorption ionization time-of-flight (SELDI-TOF) mass spectrometry technology for biomarker identification. Moreover, although the focus of this book is the brain proteome, we will also discuss biomarker profiling in other tissues (e.g., blood, cerebrospinal fluid) that, in combination with data from brain tissues, may be useful in understanding neurological deficits and disease.

II. Transcriptomics

To begin to answer complex biological questions, it has become imperative to develop new experimental approaches that permit the examination of, for example, the entire repertoire of genes being expressed at a given point in time. For example, we may know that at the blood-brain barrier (bbb) there are tumor necrosis factor-α (TNF-α) responsive cells, and that the bbb, under some disease conditions, is "leaky." In this instance it is unclear whether a breach of the blood-brain barrier is a direct result of TNF-α affecting cytokine-responsive genes, or whether the observed changes occur through transcription factor mediation or through second messenger systems that initiate gene expression cascades. Given the complex nature of the potential interactions that may be occurring, it is not possible for any approach that studies only one or a few genes at a time to provide the magnitude of data typically generated with array studies. Complex expression patterns are difficult to untangle by traditional measurements of a few messenger RNAs (mRNAs) but are well suited to microarray analysis. Coupled with the fact that the enabling technology is now readily available for large-scale gene expression profiling (hundreds to thousands of genes can be assayed simultaneously), many laboratories have begun to perform more comprehensive expression profiling.

A. The Technology

The current method of choice for functional genomic studies is the hybridization array. Using this technology, mRNA from experimental and control samples is reverse-transcribed, labeled, and used to query gene-specific DNA fragments situated on a matrix of some sort (e.g., nitrocellulose, glass slides, or microchip wafers). Numerous platforms are commercially available that allow one to screen from as few as 100 genes (e.g., SuperArray), up to the entire genome (e.g., GeneChips [Affymetrix]), and in a single experiment (Freeman *et al.*, 2000). Analysis of the differences in patterns of gene expression between the experimental and control samples often provides novel insight into underlying biological pathways and systems that are affected by the experimental condition(s) being tested. The technology necessary to generate and analyze these global "snapshots" of the entire transcriptome has only recently become widely available.

B. Specific Example—Alcoholism

The most commonly acquired degenerative condition affecting the cerebellum is chronic alcoholism (Baker *et al.*, 1999). Patients with alcoholism provide a human model of cerebellar pathology with well-documented *in vivo* brain structural volume deficits and associated functional sequelae (Sullivan *et al.*, 2000a), along with convergent findings from neuropathological studies (Torvik and Torp, 1986; Victor *et al.*, 1959). Ataxia of stance and gait are the most frequently observed clinical signs of cerebellar dysfunction in alcoholics (Victor *et al.*, 1989). Studies of neuropathology associated with certain psychiatric disorders also suggest a cerebellar role in cognition and emotion. What is currently lacking in the literature is a detailed examination of gene expression changes in this important brain region, and a look at how these alterations may be functionally related to alcohol-induced pathology.

Several studies have looked specifically at cerebellar gene expression. We have performed hybridization array studies in rat cerebellar granular neurons exposed to ethanol. These studies revealed changes in mRNA levels for genes coding for vesicular sequestration and docking proteins, including synapsin II, synaptasomal associated protein of 25 kilodaltons (SNAP-25), synaptotagmin XI, syntaxin 1B, and synaptobrevin 2 (Worst *et al.*, 2004). In addition, Schafer *et al.* (2001) found a cerebellum-specific pattern of ethanol-induced regulation of RTN1 (neuroendocrine specific protein or reticulon 1) genes in mouse brains. The exact function of these reticulons is not currently known; however, they are postulated to play a role in vesicular formation, packaging of secretory products, and perhaps regulation of intracellular Ca^{2+} levels.

Alcohol-responsive changes in gene expression have also been identified in other brain regions, both in individual genes and in groups of genes related by function (pathways). For example, chronic exposure to ethanol results in changes in the expression of selected genes coding for neurotransmitter receptors, hormones and their receptors, signaling molecules, molecular chaperones, transcription factors, and cytokines (Miles, 1995). Studies examining tissue derived from human brains reveal that alcoholism results in changes in the expression of mitochondrial genes in selected brain regions (Fan *et al.*, 1999) and in γ-aminobutyric acid type A (GABA$_A$) receptor subunit genes (Lewohl *et al.*, 1997). Moreover, alcohol has been shown to produce changes in 5-HT3, G-proteins, protein kinase C (PKC), pro-opiomelanocortin, glial fibrillary acid protein, GABA$_A$, tyrosine hydroxylase, opioid receptors, calcium channels, and other genes (reviewed in Diamond and Gordon, 1997). Finally, Mayfield *et al.* (2002) used complementary DNA (cDNA) arrays to examine expression of nearly 10,000 genes in the frontal and motor cortices of three groups of chronic alcoholic and matched control cases. Their data revealed a selective reprogramming of gene expression in distinct functional groups, especially in myelin-related genes and genes involved in protein trafficking. Although these results suggest that multiple pathways may be important for neuropathology and altered neuronal function observed in alcoholism, they also exemplify the broad scope of this technology. *The ability to analyze global gene expression from individual brain structures in individual samples from human alcoholics may provide an important vehicle with which to bring much of this disparate information into a coherent, biological narrative.*

C. Summary

Extensive discussion in the literature has been devoted to the fact that although functional genomics (gene expression profiling) has tremendous potential to advance our knowledge about how specific patterns of gene expression relate to disease state, it is unable to provide a complete picture. This is particularly true in the area of protein expression, including post-translational modification of proteins and/or alternative splicing of mRNA species to produce multiple different, but related, protein species. It is entirely possible, for example, that the presence of the alcoholic phenotype will engender unique patterns of protein expression that illuminate important new molecular aspects of the disease process and may contribute to development of effective pharmacotherapies for either direct reduction of alcohol intake or reversal of toxicological effects on end organs (e.g., liver, pancreas).

III. Proteomics Methodologies for Biomarker Discovery

The *proteome* may be defined as the sum of all proteins species (the protein complement, if you will) of a specific cell, tissue, or entire organism (Graves and Haystead, 2002; Rappsilber and Mann, 2002). Data generated from the proteome and the functional genome represent two different, important aspects of understanding disease processes. Given the post-translational complexity of the proteome, there are several important technical aspects to proteomics (Fountoulakis, 2001; Rappsilber and Mann, 2002). In general, to provide for high throughput and high capacity analyses of a proteome, three events must take place: (1) a complex protein mixture is fractionated (via two-dimensional electrophoresis or selective chromatography approaches); (2) proteins are visualized and quantified to illuminate differential expression of selected protein species; and (3) the proteins are identified through sensitive mass spectrometry (MS) technologies or direct protein sequencing.

In considering the central dogma of gene expression, it is widely accepted that the genetic legacy (the genome) is first transcribed to mRNA, and that the message is then translated into functional protein. Clearly, the consequences of a condition such as alcoholism, as manifested in gene expression, will be functionally realized at the level of protein. So why has there been such a recent emphasis on high throughput functional genomics and microarray technologies? The answer is that multiplex analysis of mRNA (so-called functional genomics) is easier than the corresponding analysis of proteins (proteomics). For a number of reasons, DNA microarrays have proven to be more robust and accessible than proteomics—particularly for the academic user (for review, see Freeman *et al.*, 2000; Vrana *et al.*, 2001; Walker *et al.*, 2002). To summarize: (1) a blueprint for the human genome is now known; (2) most microarrays start with known genes; (3) for most molecular biology laboratories, microarrays are only incrementally more difficult than northern blots (although the same cannot be said for the attendant bioinformatics); and (4) once an investigator has a differential result, he or she has an answer (or at least a strong target).

Proteomics, however, has a unique set of problems (Fountoulakis, 2001; Graves and Haystead, 2002; Rappsilber and Mann, 2002), which include (1) there is not a clear and absolute relationship between one gene and one protein; (2) there is a wealth of post-transcriptional (RNA splicing–processing; differential translation start sites) and post-translational (protein phosphorylation, glycosylation, lipid addition, proteolytic processing) activity involved in creating the mature and functional protein; (3) proteins historically had to be physically separated prior to proteomic analysis; and (4) once illuminated, differentially expressed proteins must be identified (no small task). Therefore the biomedical field performs functional genomics because it is technically feasible. However, many labs have recently undertaken broad-based proteomics for the following reasons:

- Functional genomics does not provide all the answers; that is, mRNA does not have to reflect protein (functional disconnect between transcription and translation, as well as the previously described processing issues).
- Proteins are, in fact, the business end of gene expression. Therefore important elements of neurological (and other) disorders will be gleaned from post-translational modification of proteins.
- The proteins in a specific anatomical compartment—for example, serum or cerebrospinal fluid—need not have originated with mRNA in that compartment (e.g., proteins secreted from liver, adrenal, kidney, pituitary).
- Recent advances in several technologies—ProteinChips, immobilized pH gradients (IPGs), enhanced protein staining, more powerful bioinformatics, and more sensitive mass spectrometry platforms—have made large-scale proteomics more accessible to the academic researcher.

There are several options for performing proteomic analysis. We will discuss three approaches, with the emphasis on the SELDI-TOF MS approach.

A. Two-Dimensional Gel Electrophoresis

In two-dimensional gel electrophoresis (2 DE) approach, proteins are resolved into two-dimensional space through a combination of isoelectric focusing (resolution dependent on the inherent charge of a molecule) and its molecular weight [using sodium dodecyl sulfate (SDS)-polyacrylamide gel electrophoresis] (Graves and Haystead, 2002; Rappsilber and Mann, 2002). The resulting protein spots are then visualized and their intensities compared. Those protein species showing a differential expression can then be directly extracted and subjected to protease digestion. The peptide fingerprinting and bioinformatic identification is acheived using matrix-assisted laser desorption ionization (MALDI) mass spectrometry.

Differentially expressed proteins will be revealed by comparison of 2D-PAGE (polyacrylamide gel electrophoresis) gel patterns obtained from experimental and control specimens. This approach has the advantage of increasing the size range of proteins that can be observed. 2D gels can visualize larger proteins (up to approximately 100 kilodattons [kDa]) as well as smaller proteins (down to approximately 8 kDa). It also provides orthogonal separation methods based on isoelectric point, followed by separation on the basis of size (Fountoulakis, 2001; Graves and Haystead, 2002; Rappsilber and Mann, 2002). These parameters can be used to increase confidence in protein identification. Candidate proteins, revealed by 2D gels as being differentially expressed, can be identified using three analytical approaches (in addition to SELDI-TOF MS analysis) (1) direct chemical sequence analysis using Edman degradation; (2) peptide mass finger-printing following digestion of the candidate protein with a protease (e.g., trypsin, endo-Lys C [2] and [3]); MSMS sequencing by techniques such as electrospray-ionization mass spectrometry (ESI MS).

Although initial successes have been realized using old generation gels and ampholytes, new experiments and the future of 2D-PAGE analysis will be in the area of IPGs. The new IPG technologies provide tremendous advantages in the areas of ease of use, reproducibility, and sensitivity. The immobilized pH gradient is created by incorporating a gradient of acidic and basic buffering groups into the polyacrylamide backbone at the time the gel is polymerized. Notably, commercially available IPG strips from Amersham Biosciences, for example, come in a variety of ranges, from pH 3 to pH 10. Because the strips come in quality controlled batches and merely need to be rehydrated before use, they offer flexibility, speed, and consistency that will increase throughput. In addition, where preliminary experiments suggest interesting species at a particular pH, experiments can be reperformed at increasing resolution by using a narrower range IPG strip. For instance, a pH 3- to pH 10-experiment can be followed by a pH 4.5–5.0 or a pH 6–9 range experiment, depending on the species of interest.

B. LIQUID-CHROMATOGRAPHY-MASS SPECTROMETRY

Liquid-chromatograph-mass spectrometry (LC-MS) represents another versatile approach of peptide and protein analysis (see reviews by Clarke *et al.*, 2003; Mann *et al.*, 2001; Mitchell, 2003). It combines the traditional liquid chromatography separation technologies with electrospray MS. The most common configuration of LC-MS uses the reverse-phase LC separation because the proteins and peptides separated through the column are suitable for ionization in the ESI MS analysis. The ability of one-dimensional (LC) or two-dimensional (LC/LC) separation of complex protein and peptide mixtures is one of its advantages for analysis of complex biological samples. The LC separation may be used alone for direct processing of biological samples, or in combination with 1-D or 2-D electrophoresis or other separation technology as a further dimension of separation to enhance its ability of separating proteins and peptides in complex biological samples. The most commonly used MS instrumentation consists of coupling the eluted samples from the LC separation into a nanospray probe capable of nanoliter per minute flow rate for sample delivery (Mann *et al.*, 2001; Srinivas *et al.*, 2002). However, the basic configuration of 1-D LC-MS has its limitation in analyzing proteins in complex samples directly. Proteins tend to denature the buffer conditions used in the reverse phase separation conditions, thus making quantitative elution somewhat difficult. In addition, 1-D reverse-phase separation of proteins and peptides in complex biological samples such as serum of tissue lysis is not sufficient in achieving the necessary sample resolution needed for the MS analysis. Measurement of the molecular mass alone is not sufficient for identification of protein or peptide biomarkers. The LC-MS technology has been improved for analysis of proteins and peptides in complex biological samples with the introduction of LC/LC-tandem MS approach: "shotgun proteomics" method, first by Yates and co-workers (Mitchell, 2003; Wolters *et al.*, 2001), and subsequently commercialized as the MudPIT technology. To increase the separation of complex proteins and to identify the peptides detected, the MudPIT technology requires global digestion of proteins in complex biological samples, prior to separation, first by a reverse-phase capillary column and then by a strong anionic exchange column, followed by delivery of samples into an electrode spray tandem MS instrument, typically with an ion trap setup. LC/LC separation can also be coupled to a tandem TOF-TOF or Fourier-transformed mass spectrometry (FT-MS) instrumentation. The advantage of this improved technology is its ability to separate complex proteins and peptides into two LC columns, and to identify the proteins and peptides directly by sequencing the peptides by tandem MS. However, it has not found widespread use in biomarker discovery in which throughput and quantitative reproducibility are critical. The need for global digest of all proteins generates enormous data of protein and peptide fragments in which peptides from different proteins are scrambled and multiplexed (Wolters *et al.*, 2001). This leads to potential loss of information on protein complexes, *in vivo* truncation, and splicing and post-translation modification of proteins, which are important to the biological relevance of differentially expressed proteins, or potential biomarkers. It may become difficult to pinpoint the intact forms of differentially expressed biomarkers. However, global digest may render it possible to detect high mass proteins in complex biological samples that may otherwise not be detected because of the molecular size and limitation of maximum mass range of most high resolution MS instruments (Bischoff and Luider, 2004). The enormous amount of data of digested protein fragments can post challenges in data flow and high throughput data analysis. Like the 2DE-MS method, the LC-MS is essentially a low throughput technology at its current state in both sample processing and data analysis, though much improvement has been made in instrumentation, sample processing methods, and data analysis tools in recent years. Its use in clinical proteomics research, particularly for high throughput biomarker discovery, is still limited. Its most common use is for identification of proteins.

C. ProteinChip SELDI-TOF-MS Technology

In this relatively new approach proteins are fractionated from complex mixtures on chemically derivatized solid surfaces. The ProteinChip system is actually a collection of several physical surfaces designed to bind proteins of differing biophysical characteristics (Merchant and Weinberger, 2000). For instance, anion exchange, cation exchange, hydrophobic, metal-chelate, and normal phase are all surfaces (Fig. 1). After protein mixtures are bound to the surface, they are washed at increasing stringencies in an effort to reduce the complexity of the proteins on the chip surface. At that point, SELDI mass spectrometry technologies are employed to direct individual ionic species into a time-of-flight (TOF) mass spectrometer that simultaneously measures the molecular weight of the species and determines its relative abundance. The resulting spectra display individual protein species based on mass and allow for comparisons of the protein expression levels between samples. The next task is to use that differential expression information for choosing interesting targets for identification. This can be performed by peptide fingerprinting on the SELDI-TOF platform (following protease digestion) or MALDI-TOF approaches with the higher energy and increased resolution MALDI-TOF approaches. In fact, purified proteins can be subjected to direct protein sequencing in an effort to identify the protein species. This approach has proved quite powerful in advancing our understanding of biological systems (Vehmas *et al.*, 2001).

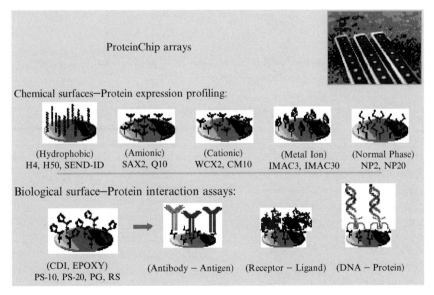

ProteinChip arrays

Chemical surfaces—Protein expression profiling:

| (Hydrophobic) H4, H50, SEND-ID | (Amionic) SAX2, Q10 | (Cationic) WCX2, CM10 | (Metal Ion) IMAC3, IMAC30 | (Normal Phase) NP2, NP20 |

Biological surface—Protein interaction assays:

| (CDI, EPOXY) PS-10, PS-20, PG, RS | (Antibody – Antigen) | (Receptor – Ligand) | (DNA – Protein) |

Fig. 1. Many different surface chemistries are available with SELDI-TOF-MS technology. (See Color Insert.)

IV. Principles of SELDI-TOF-MS

A. PROTEINCHIP SYSTEM

Ciphergen's ProteinChip System is composed of a ProteinChip Reader integrated with ProteinChip Software and a standard personal computer for analysis of protein captured on the arrays. The reader is a laser desorption/ionization TOF mass spectrometer that uses state-of-the-art ion optic and laser optic technology (Fig. 2). The ProteinChip System detects and calculates the mass of compounds ranging from small molecules of less than 1000 Da up to proteins of 500 kDa or more based on measured TOF.

B. EXPERIMENTAL DESIGN

The following example is a description of the preparation of proteins from serum samples, but these protocols can be readily adapted to accomplish protein analysis from any complex mixture (e.g., tissue homogenates, cell lysates). The initial preparation is outlined in Fig. 3.

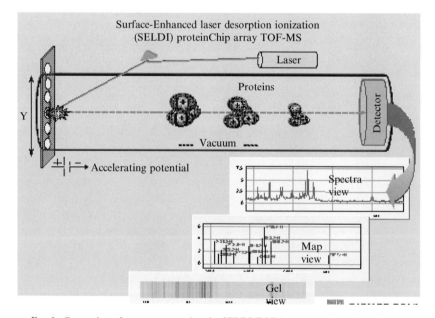

FIG. 2. Generation of mass spectra using the SELDI-TOF instrument. (See Color Insert.)

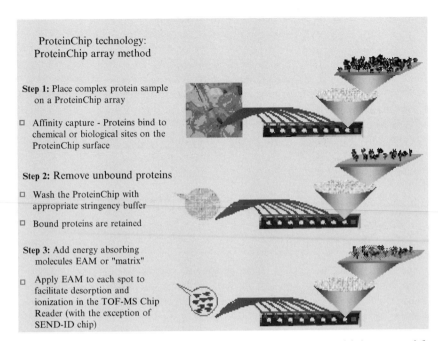

ProteinChip technology:
ProteinChip array method

Step 1: Place complex protein sample
on a ProteinChip array

☐ Affinity capture - Proteins bind to
chemical or biological sites on the
ProteinChip surface

Step 2: Remove unbound proteins

☐ Wash the ProteinChip with
appropriate stringency buffer

☐ Bound proteins are retained

Step 3: Add energy absorbing
molecules EAM or "matrix"

☐ Apply EAM to each spot to
facilitate desorption and
ionization in the TOF-MS Chip
Reader (with the exception of
SEND-ID chip)

FIG. 3. Steps in the process of protein binding to the chip surface and being prepared for detection in the mass spectrometer. (See Color Insert.)

Sample Preparation: Serum samples are received in frozen 50 μl aliquots. This amount is sufficient to perform the SELDI-TOF MS and 2-D gel experiments. Protein concentration is determined for each sample (e.g., using the BCA Protein assay kit from Pierce and following the standard protocols of the manufacturer). In selected applications, to reduce sample complexity and increase detection of mid to low abundant proteins, the crude biological sample (serum) will be prefractionated to separate proteins based on their isoelectric point Fig. 4. This is a solution chemistry analog to the isoelectric focusing gel. Specifically, the samples will be captured (at a high pH of 9) on a disposable Q-Ceramic HyperD anion exchange column. The proteins are then batch-eluted with buffers at increasingly lower pH. The fractions are then analyzed on individual chips.

Analysis of Samples on a ProteinChip: Samples are diluted (typically 1:2 to 1:10) into buffers dictated by the specific type of Ciphergen ProteinChips being tested (e.g., for the H50 or hydrophobic chip, a high salt concentration is recommended). Each ProteinChip has its own chemistry; therefore the protocols are slightly different for each one. Each chip is equilibrated with buffer before sample is added. Depending on the concentration of the samples, they can either be spotted directly onto the chip surface, or a bioprocessor can be used if the volume needed is higher than 3 μl. All samples spotted should be at the same volume in

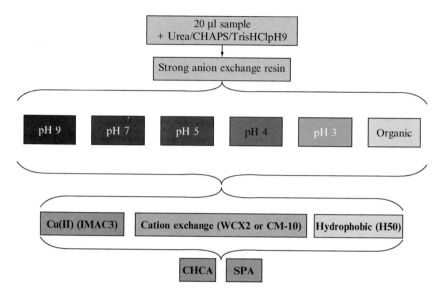

FIG. 4. Fractionation and expression profiling for serum. (See Color Insert.)

the recommended binding buffer for that chip. Each chip has 16 spots, so the two samples can be spotted onto 8 locations each to allow for differential wash conditions to obtain optimal spectra for analysis. Once spotted, the chip is incubated in a humidity chamber for 30–60 minutes. Following incubation, the chip is washed and allowed to air dry and an energy absorbing molecule, sinapinic acid (SPA), is spotted onto the chip and allowed to air dry. The chip can then be analyzed using the Ciphergen PBSII instrument, and the control and treated spectra can then be captured and stored for analysis with the biomarker software.

Based on experience with our Ciphergen PBSII system, we begin with a laser intensity of 220 ($\sim$10 μJ) and a detector setting of 7. The range for the laser is 0–300, and for the detector, the range is 1–10. Single exposures of the laser are taken from each spot on the chip to determine the best settings that will give an optimal spectra. Once these settings are determined, 130 laser illuminations are made from sites on each spot to produce the composite spectra for that spot. There are 100 positions on each spot to which the laser can be directed. Typically, the data collection starts at position 20, 10 laser illuminations are collected, then the laser is indexed up by 5 transients until the final collection is performed at position 80. Data from human serum that had been separated into six fractions and scanned for low (3000–18,000 Da) and high (18,000–200,000 Da) molecular weight proteins can be seen in Fig. 5. The ProteinChips themselves can be stored and, if necessary, reanalyzed at a later time.

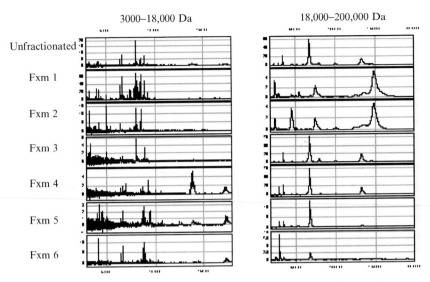

3000–18,000 Da   18,000–200,000 Da

Unfractionated

Fxm 1

Fxm 2

Fxm 3

Fxm 4

Fxm 5

Fxm 6

FIG. 5. Human serum: Whole serum and six fractions profiled on the WCX2 chip.

Data Analysis: Samples are typically analyzed in triplicate, and each ProteinCh-ip (16 spots/chip) is spotted with a pooled serum sample prepared for internal quality control (QC) and instrument normalization. Initial data analysis is per-formed using the Biomarker Patterns Software (termed CART for classification and regression tree) program from Ciphergen, a decision-classification tree algo-rithm. Peak detection is performed using Ciphergen's SELDI software version 2.1 b, with mass ranges from 2000–40,000 Da, as previously described (Adam *et al.*, 2002; Qu *et al.*, 2002). Peak detection involves: (1) baseline subtraction, (2) mass accuracy calibration, (3) automatic peak detection, and (4) peak alignment determination. All labeled peaks are then exported from SELDI to an Excel spreadsheet. A PeakMiner algorithm (Adam *et al.*, 2002) is used to sort all peaks based on mass values from low to high mass. The validity and accuracy of the classification algorithm will then be challenged with a test data set consisting of 25% of the tested samples and blinded to the investigator performing the data analysis. The CART program also possesses an internal cross-validation compo-nent. Specificity and sensitivity is calculated as described (Adam *et al.*, 2002). The software discovers patterns in the (define) training set and presents the results in a tree model (Fig. 6) that can then be updated with additional sample data or used to classify unknowns. The results also include assignment scores of clinical sensitivity (percentage of positive cases) and specificity (percentage of negative cases).

Additional algorithms used for data analysis: SELDI has the potential to measure very large numbers of proteins present in a single sample. Therefore

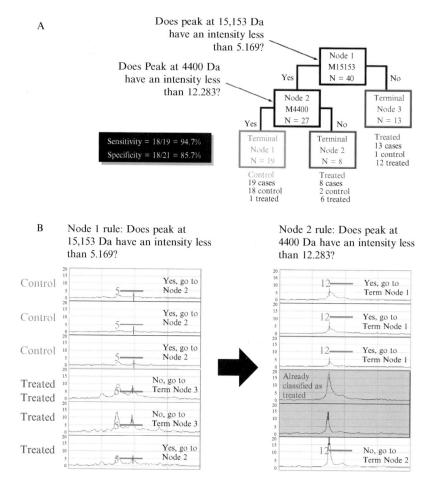

FIG. 6. Classification tree sample. (A) Each node (blue square) is a decision point. Each sample is sifted down the tree based on how it answers the question in each node. For example, the first node asks the question, "Does peak at molecular weight 15,153 Da have a peak intensity less than 5.169?" If the answer is yes, the sample goes to the left node 2; otherwise, it goes to the right terminal node 3. Terminal nodes are stopping points, and the majority of samples determine the classification of each terminal node. In terminal node 3, there is 1 control and 12 treated samples; the control is misclassified and the treated samples are classified correctly. Sensitivity is calculated as the ratio of the number of correctly classified treated samples to the total number of treated samples. Similarly, specificity is calculated as the ratio of the number of control samples to the total number of controls. (B) How the rules in the classification tree manifest themselves in the raw data. In this subset of six spectra from the study used to generate the tree in (A), we can see how the classification tree uses peak intensities to classify each sample. (Reprinted with permission from Fung and Enderwick, 2002.) (See Color Insert.)

the assumption is that with the appropriate choice of sample group, enough phenotype-reflective protein profile differences will be detected. The major challenge to this approach is to develop an adequate computational tool to analyze this information. The Ciphergen Biomarker Patterns Software and SAS (statistical) packages are used routinely to process the SELDI data. Two other computational approaches, wavelet discriminate learning algorithms and binary marker combination approaches, have been used with great success in analyzing serum prostate cancer samples (Adam *et al.*, 2002; Qu *et al.*, 2002).

V. SELDI-TOF-MS in Clinical Proteomics Research

Proteomic analysis involves the separation, identification, and characterization of proteins in a biological sample. By comparing samples from diseased individuals with those from non diseased individuals, it is possible to identify changes in expression of protein that potentially may be related to organ toxicity. Although functional genomics (mRNA expression profiling) has proven very useful is examining *tissue* gene expression, analysis of body fluids (e.g., serum, urine, Cerebrospinal fluid [CSF], synovial fluid) is restricted (largely) to proteomics. Proteomic analysis can therefore yield information on disease processes and potential responses to treatment (Kennedy, 2001).

The ProteinChip platform using SELDI-TOF-MS has been used successfully to discover and analyze biomarkers in areas as diverse as cancer, neuroscience, and pathogenic microorganisms. In particular, differentially expressed protein profiling has proved to be invaluable when discovering proteins with potential application as diagnostic biomarkers for detection of prostate (Adam *et al.*, 2001), bladder (Adam *et al.*, 2001), and ovarian cancers (Petricon *et al.*, 2002). In each case these biomarkers were discovered directly from biological fluids or histological samples. In addition to the early detection of cancer and identification of the stage of cancer progression (Watkins *et al.*, 2001), the ProteinChip Array was used to develop an assay for different amyloid beta peptides, potential diagnostic markers for Alzheimer's disease onset (Davies *et al.*, 1999).

A study by Mittleman *et al.* (1997) examined CSF from patients with three neuropsychiatric diseases (childhood-onset schizophrenia, obsessive-compulsive disorder [OCD], and attention-deficit hyperactivity disorder [ADHD]) of childhood for the presence and level of several cytokines relevant to cell-mediated (type 1) and humoral (type 2) immunity. The cytokines measured included IL-2, IFN-γ, TNF-β/LT, IL-4, IL-5, IL-10, and TNF-α. Their findings suggest CSF cytokine profiles are skewed toward type 1 in patients with OCD, whereas in schizophrenia, the bulk of the mediators are type 2. Profiles for ADHD were intermediate between OCD and schizophrenia.

In another study, proteomic profiling approaches were used with human CSF samples to identify low-abundant proteins. Several neuron-related proteins such as amyloid precursor-like protein, chromogranins A and B, glial fibrillary acid protein, beta-trace, transthyretin, ubiquitin, and cystatin C were identified in CSF. The use of this strategy in proteome studies of CSF/brain tissue is expected to offer new perspectives in studies of the pathology of neurodegenerative diseases and to reveal new potential biomarkers for brain disorders (Davidsson *et al.*, 2001).

Finally, the SELDI-TOF approach was applied to serum from patients chronically infected with hepatitis C virus (HCV; Marrero *et al.*, 2003), monitoring progression from non cirrhotic to cirrhotic disease, and subsequent development of HCV-associated hepatocellular carcinoma (HCC). A subset of clinically defined serum samples (33 patients with HCV-associated HCC, 22 patients with HCV cirrhosis, 27 patients with chronic noncirrhotic HCV, and 39 normal individuals) were applied to IMAC-Cu chips in duplicate. All sample loading, processing, and analysis steps were automated. Clustering and classification analyses of the resulting data were performed using the Ciphergen Biomarker Wizard and Biomarker Patterns software packages, respectively. The cross-validation test is a 1/10 sample removal validation of the classification trees; it has been observed empirically that cross-validation values of greater than 80% indicate a robust analysis. Of note, sera from healthy subjects were readily distinguishable from sera of patients with HCV disease ($\geq$92% specificities/ 100% sensitivities). Sera from patients with chronic liver disease (HCV infected, cirrhotic and noncirrhotic) were also readily distinguishable from sera of patients with HCV-associated HCC. The least sensitive assay was the ability to distinguish HCV-infected sera from subjects without cirrhosis versus subjects with HCV-associated cirrhosis (85% spec/75% sens). Even for this last data set, these numbers could represent a clinical assay far superior to anything currently available for monitoring HCV disease progression.

VI. Biomarkers in Specific Diseases

In the following four subsections, we discuss examples of the search for biomarkers in specific diseases that have a neurological basis. In the discussion of alcoholism, we will present findings from proteomic analysis of serum in a nonhuman primate model of alcoholism.

A. ALCOHOLISM

The diagnosis of chronic ethanol consumption is necessary both for early detection and intervention of potential alcohol abuse and to monitor medical intervention after chronic alcoholism has been diagnosed in the clinic. Classical diagnostic tools and biomarkers, although providing many unique advantages over self-reporting, still suffer from a variety of limitations as to how they may be used. This arises, in part, because of the overall heterogeneity of the human alcoholic population (e.g., gender differences in response to alcohol; consumption pattern differences [e.g., binging/abstinence, versus continuous]; total alcohol consumption history differences; variations in individual co-morbidity with other substances of abuse; differential health status, both related and unrelated to alcohol abuse; and the [un]reliability of self-reporting). As a result of these many sources of individual variation, one of the most serious informational deficits concerns *how various biomarkers characterize alcohol use* (Allen *et al.*, 2001). Although there are several markers of subacute and chronic heavy alcohol use available, there is vast room for improvement given their variability and suboptimal sensitivity levels.

The ability to objectively and reliably diagnose both the risk for and the presence of excessive alcohol consumption is a clinical imperative. Alcoholism research and treatment have been hampered by the lack of reliable markers for alcohol abuse. Historically, the most common method for assessing alcohol use and abuse has relied on standardized questionnaires about alcohol-related behaviors (e.g., CAGE, AUDIT). Given that these self-report tests suffer from considerable under-reporting (Ernhart *et al.*, 1988; Russell *et al.*, 1996), quantifiable biochemical markers have been sought. Common markers currently being used clinically in the United States include gamma-glutamyl transferase (GGT), carbohydrate-deficient transferrin (CDT), and mean corpuscular volume (MCV) (reviewed in Allen *et al.*, 2000; Meerkerk *et al.*, 1999; Salaspuro, 1999). Although each of these is correlated with heavy and/or recent alcohol use, none is absolutely diagnostic and there is considerable evidence that their utility varies with subject demographics (e.g., clinical versus nonclinical samples) and drinking characteristics (Allen *et al.*, 2000; Brathen *et al.*, 2000; Halm *et al.*, 1999; Hermansson *et al.*, 2000; Mundle *et al.*, 1999; Nomura *et al.*, 2000; Szegedi *et al.*, 2000; van Pelt *et al.*, 2000). Both the research scientist and the clinician would be greatly assisted by the availability of a noninvasive and sensitive metric for alcohol use (i.e., a blood test for alcohol abuse). For this reason, we propose to examine the pattern of protein expression in serum from a well-characterized sampling of alcoholics and nonalcoholic controls derived from a clinical setting.

In a study performed in our laboratory, serum from cynomolgus monkeys (*Macaca fasicularis*) in an ethanol self-administration protocol was collected from the ethanol naive state through 9 months of heavy ethanol consumption and then into a period of enforced abstinence. Serum was subjected to SELDI-TOF-MS. Analysis on a hydrophobic (H4) ProteinChip illuminated two prominent serum proteins, one at 27.9 kDa and another at 8.7 kDa, which were observed to be differentially expressed (Fig. 7). Identification of these potential biomarkers was

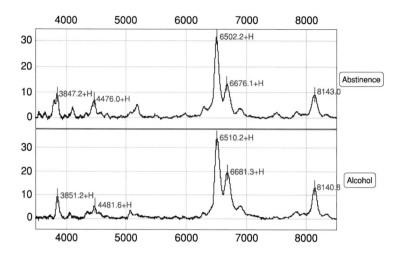

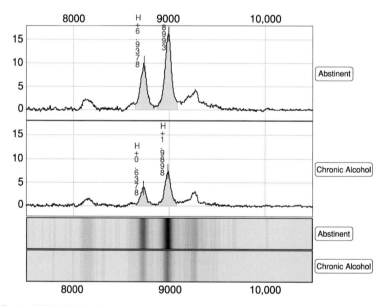

Fɪɢ. 7. SELDI-TOF-MS analysis of serum protein profiles in drinking and nondrinking monkeys. Serum samples from cynomolgus macaques that had been self-administering large amounts of alcohol for nine months were compared to non drinking controls using the Ciphergen ProteinChip system. The majority of the proteins were unchanged, as illustrated by the profile in the upper panel (for a collection of proteins analyzed on a WCX weak cation exchange chip surface). On the other hand, proteins were identified on a number of surfaces that did appear to be dierentially regulated. In this case, hydrophobic proteins (analyzed on an H4 hydrophobic binding surface) were dierentially regulated. Proteins at approximately 9000 daltons appeared to be reduced by ethanol self-administration (lower panel). The bottom of the lower panel shows a "pseudo-gel" representation of the relative expression levels of the various proteins. (See Color Insert.)

then carried out using 1D PAGE with trypsin digestion and mass spectroscopic fingerprint identification of excised bands of interest. These bands were identified as apolipoprotein AI (Apo-AI) and apolipoprotein AII (Apo-AII), respectively. Their correspondence with the SELDI-TOF-MS peak was verified with purified human Apo-AI and Apo-AII proteins. Immunoblot analysis of samples from individual animals confirmed that ethanol consumption significantly elevated Apo-AII. However, because of wide interanimal variability, Apo-AI did not show a significant increase. In agreement with previous studies of human ethanol consumption, the current studies suggest that alcohol self-administration produces elevation of lipoproteins associated with cardiovascular protective effects. These findings contribute evidence that it is the ethanol itself that elicits these potential beneficial effects, because they result from administration of pure ethanol.

B. ALZHEIMER'S DISEASE

Alzheimer's disease (AD) is the most common form of progressive, neurode-generative disease leading to dementia in the elderly population. It accounts for 50–60% of overall cases of progressive dementia in the elderly. At present, clinical diagnosis often requires detailed neurological, neuropsychological, and neuropsychiatric assessment, in addition to a range of pathological tests. Unfortunately, often the most unambiguous diagnosis is made by postmortem examination of the brain. At present, it lacks a good set of molecular markers for both early detection and monitoring of disease progression. A wealth of pathological evidence points to the presence of plagues of aggregated β-amyloid (Aβ) proteins and the formation of neurofibrillary tangles formed by the accumulation of hyperphosphorylated tau protein (Austen et al., 2000; Cai et al., 2001; Carrette et al., 2003; Lewczuk et al., 2003; Netzer et al., 2003; Shi et al., 2003). Aβ is a small peptide of up to 42 amino acids that is derived from the enzymatic cleavage of the amyloid precursor glycoprotein (APP) of 695–770 residues. Cleavage of APP by β-secretase, followed by γ-secretase, releases either the Aβ peptides 1–40 or 1–42 and the C-terminal fragments. Thus the formation of the Aβ peptides depends on the activities of β-secretase and γ-secretase. Understanding the mechanism of the formation of the Aβ peptides, the development of a simple biochemical test, and deriving a strategy to inhibit the production of the Aβ has been much of the focus in Alzheimer's disease research.

The ability of SELDI-ProteinChip technology to detect proteins and peptide selectively, either by the physicochemical or biological affinity of the target proteins with the ProteinChip arrays, and thus resolving the various cleaved forms of the target proteins or peptides by their mass difference, renders this technology uniquely suited for study of the formation of Aβ, and thus in AD. Austen and co-workers (Austen et al., 2000; Davies et al., 1999) first reported the use of SELDI technology in studying Alzheimer's disease, using a ProteinChip array covalently coupled with anti-NTA 4–22 antibody to detect the various forms of Aβ peptides in Aβ-transfected HEK 293 cells. In a single experiment, Aβ fragments ranging from 1–15 to 1–42 were detected and resolved by their mass difference. Similarly, detection of various Aβ fragments in neuronal cells shows the evidence of β-secretase as the key enzyme for the generation of Aβ peptides (Cai et al., 2001). Lewczuk et al. (2003) reported the evidence of the novel carboxyterminally elongated Aβ peptide based on the Aβ peptides detected in human CSF and brain homogenates of AD patients. Accumulation of Aβ peptides 1–40 and 1–42 in human lenses of AD patients was also reported from the detection of the peptides with a ProteinChip, coupled with antibody against Aβ (6E10) (Goldstein et al., 2003). A different approach with the sandwich enzyme-linked immunosorbent assay (ELISA) method would not have resolved the different cleavage fragments because of the common epitope shared among these different fragments. Furthermore, because the interaction between the Aβ peptides with the 6E10 antibody is specific, for this type of experiment the target Aβ peptides may be captured by the antibody directly from the complex samples such as tissue and cell lysis or CSF, thus providing added robustness of the technology. The 6E10 antibody ProteinChip can also be optimized for high throughput format, allowing the simultaneous detection and analysis of up to 192 samples in a single sample cassette. In addition to detecting Aβ peptides on the antibody arrays, the peptides can also be captured on antibody-coupled beads, followed by SELDI analysis (Shi et al., 2003). Taking advantage of the selectivity of the chemical arrays of SELDI ProteinChips, differentially expressed Aβ peptides in CSF may also be detected in AD patients compared to normal controls. Carrette and co-workers (2003) reported a panel of five peptide and protein markers of masses ranging from 4.8–13.4 kDa, as detected by the strong anion exchange ProteinChip. The use of the chemical ProteinChips also yielded the information guiding the scale-up purification of the peptide and proteins markers. These novel CSF markers were identified by peptide mapping to be cystatin C, β2-microglobulin isoforms, an unknown 7.7-kDa polypeptide, and a 4.8-kDa vascular growth factor (VGF) polypeptide. None of these novel markers discovered by the SELDI technology were part of the Aβ family of peptides, making it unique as a potential diagnosis biomarker for AD, and may lead to new areas in the understanding of the mechanism of this disease.

C. AUTISM

Autism (MIM 209850) is a severe neuropsychiatric disorder characterized by social and communication impairments and repetitive, stereotyped behaviors and interests. The condition was first described by one of the founders of child psychiatry, Leo Kanner, in 1943. In a study of 11 children, Kanner noted that in most cases the childs' behavior was abnormal from early infancy, and therefore probably the result of an inborn, presumably genetic, defect (Kanner, 1943). Affected children either fail to reach normal developmental milestones in the first years of life, or they develop normally up to a point and then lose many of their learned behaviors, including the ability to speak (nonverbal regressive autism). Although there are diagnostic criteria to describe autism, no two autistic children share identical clinical characteristics. Moreover, although the basic components of the phenotype of autism are well defined, there is no consensus as to the underlying causes. Currently, there are no biologically based diagnostic markers for autism spectrum conditions—a situation that poses a significant impediment to early intervention—because of the delay in diagnosis.

We have performed a pilot study in conjunction with Ciphergen Biosystems. The main goal of this pilot study was to determine the feasibility of screening serum from autistic patients to uncover unique patterns of protein expression. The protocol was a small, 4×4 design (i.e., four autistic samples and four nonautistic sibling control samples) carried out on a comprehensive number of chromatographic chip surfaces under various wash conditions. Approximately 750 mass spectra were generated in this initial screen.

The general protocol will be outlined here. Briefly, for each of the eight samples, 20 μl serum (performed in duplicate) was diluted into the appropriate sample buffer and then applied to a Q Hyper D column for fractionation. Elution was accomplished by varying the pH of column wash buffer (fraction 1 = flow through; fraction 2 eluted at pH 8; fraction 3 eluted at pH 7; fraction 4 eluted at pH 5; fraction 5 eluted at pH 3; fraction 6 = organic phase). Each of these six fractions from the eight individual serum samples (n = 48) were then assayed on four different ProteinChip surfaces: (1) weak cationic exchange (WCX2) at pH 4; (2) WCX2 at pH 7; (3) metal affinity with copper (IMAC-Cu) at pH 7 and; (4) hydrophobic (H4) at pH 7. Spectral data were generated at both a low and a high laser intensity (to bias toward low molecular weight and high molecular weight proteins, respectively) for each sample. This protocol resulted in more than 750 mass spectra that were then compared for differences between autistic and control samples under the various conditions. Some pattern differences are apparent in serum fraction 4, assayed on the weak cationic exchange surface and eluted at pH 5 (Fig. 8). From these data, it appears the autistic samples are lacking (or have a much reduced amount compared to nonautistic samples) proteins at 6457 and 6650 Da see Fig. 8).

Although the differences found in this pilot study cannot be verified as to their significance with this data by itself, they illustrate the point that differences in protein profiles among sample groups can be seen with this type of approach. In a standard biomarker profiling experiment, one would look at a minimum of 40 samples (20 control and 20 affected), fractionated as described here and assayed

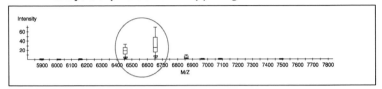

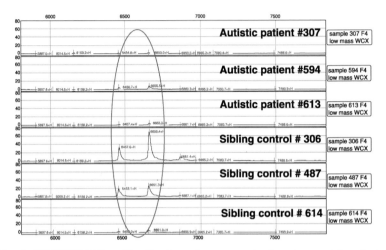

FIG. 8. SEDLI-TOF-MS profiles. Fractionated serum samples from three autistic patients and three non autistic siblings were assayed on a weak cationic exchange surface and eluted at pH 5. Data presented here show that fraction 4 in two of the three control samples contains two proteins, at 6450 and 6650 daltons, that are absent in autistic samples. (See Color Insert.)

under each of the various chip conditions, to create a training set. A sophisticated software package (e.g., the Biomarker Patterns Software from Ciphergen) would be necessary to do this type of pattern recognition from such a large dataset. Once the patterns within the training set have been discovered, this information is used to either add more data to the training set or to assay unknown samples to measure the validity of the biomarker pattern as a diagnostic tool.

D. AMYOTROPHIC LATERAL SCLEROSIS

Amyotrophic lateral sclerosis (ALS; also known as Lou Gehrig disease) is a fatal neurodegenerative disease that attacks nerve cells and pathways in the brain and spinal cord. The average life expectancy of a person diagnosed with ALS is between 2 and 5 years from the time of diagnosis. Obviously, identification of diagnostic biomarkers for this condition would be highly useful for medications development and testing. In a recent presentation by Dr. Robert Bowser from the University of Pittsburgh School of Medicine (at the 11th annual meeting of the International Alliance of ALS/MND Associations and the 14th international symposium on ALS/MND in Milan, Italy), he described a study of biomarker profiling in ALS patients. His group identified protein biomarkers by looking at CSF from 25 ALS patients and 35 control subjects. CSF was used because it is in close contact with motor neurons and glial cells affected by ALS and therefore was thought to harbor high concentrations of diagnostic biomarkers. Using mass spectrometry to characterize protein peaks that showed statistically significant alterations between ALS patients and control samples, the group claims to have identified biomarkers that diagnose ALS with nearly 100% specificity and sensitivity. A CSF-based test may potentially lead to a faster diagnosis, as well as allow physicians to monitor the patient during treatment to determine the efficacy of drugs and drug combinations. Dr. Bowser's group is working to confirm its results in a larger patient population.

VII. Metabolomics

The nontargeted profiling of metabolites (metabolomics–metabonomics) is gaining momentum as an important complementary (to functional genomics and proteomics) strategy for integrative biochemical profiling. The integration of methods based on gas chromatography-mass spectrometry (GC-MS) and liquid chromatography-mass spectrometry (LC-MS; described in Section III.B of this chapter) for the comprehensive identification and, particularly, the accurate quantitation of metabolites has attained a technical robustness that is comparable or even better than conventional mRNA or protein profiling technologies (Weckwerth, 2003). Owing to our incomplete knowledge of quantitative mRNA-protein-metabolite interactions, integrative profiling approaches that combinine metabolomics, proteomics, and transcriptomics will greatly enhance our ability to determine relationships among system components (Weckwerth, 2003; Fig. 9).

Combining functional genomic and metabonomic methods, Coen et al. (2004) demonstrated that together the two technology platforms offer a complementary view into cellular responses to toxic processes. Liver tissue from mice was dosed with various levels of paracetamol (acetaminophen) and then examined by gene expression analysis and metabonomic analysis (by ^{1}H, ^{13}C-NMR spectroscopy) for hepatotoxic response. The metabonomic observations were consistent with the altered levels of gene expression relating to lipid and energy metabolism in

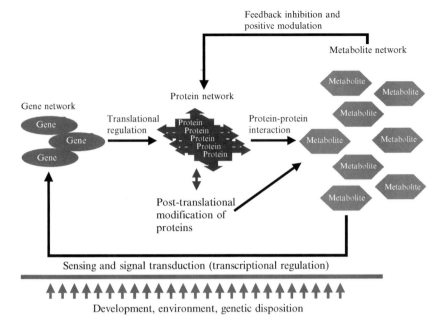

Feedback inhibition and
positive modulation

Metabolite network

Protein network

Gene network

Translational
regulation

Protein-protein
interaction

Post-translational
modification of
proteins

Sensing and signal transduction (transcriptional regulation)

Development, environment, genetic disposition

FIG. 9. Amplification of a metabolic network and feedback regulation in response to developmental and environmental conditions. (Reprinted from Weckwerth, 2003, with kind permission from the author.)

liver, which both preceded and were concurrent with the metabolic perturbations. They conclude that metabonomics has demonstrated profound changes in glucose–glycogen and lipid metabolism that confirm the genomic and proteomic data.

VIII. Conclusions

Clinical medicine is rapidly moving into an era in which individualized diagnosis and treatment of a variety of neurological disease processes will become a reality. Central to this revolution is the continued development and refinement of the necessary clinical tools. Current approaches that integrate findings from mRNA expression, protein expression, and metabolite production to yield a "fingerprint" of distinct responses to therapeutics are of paramount importance. Molecular profiling of relevant tissues such as blood, CSF, and brain continues to provide novel insight into disease processes and moves us ever closer to the goal of individualized treatment.

References

Adam, B. L., Vlahou, A., Semmes, O. J., and Wright, G. L., Jr., (2001). Proteomic approaches to biomarker discovery in prostate and bladder cancers. *Proteomics* **9**, 1264–1270.

Adam, B. L., Qu, Y., Davis, J. W., Ward, M. D., Clements, M. A., Cazares, L. H., Semmes, O. J., Schellhammer, P. F., Yasui, Y., Feng, Z., and Wright, G. L., Jr., (2002). Serum protein fingerprinting coupled with a pattern-matching algorithm distinguishes prostate cancer from benign prostate hyperplasia and healthy men. *Cancer Res.* **62**, 3609–3614.

Allen, J. P., Litten, R. Z., Fertig, J. B., and Sillanaukee, P. (2000). Carbohydrate-deficient transferrin, gamma-glutamyltransferase, and macrocytic volume as biomarker of alcohol problems in women. *Alcohol Clin. Exp. Res.* **24**, 492–496.

Allen, J. P., Litten, R. Z., Strid, N., and Sillanaukee, P. (2001). The role of biomarkers in alcoholism medication trials. *Alcohol Clin. Exp. Res.* **25**, 1119–1125.

Austen, B., Frears, E. R., and Davies, H. (2000). The use of SELDI ProteinChip arrays to monitor the production of Alzheimer's β-amyloid in transfected cells. *J. Pept. Sci.* **6**, 459–469.

Bailey, W. J., and Ulrich, R. (2004). Molecular profiling approaches for identifying novel biomarkers. *Expert Opin. Drug Saf.* **3**, 137–151.

Baker, K. G., Harding, A. J., Halliday, G. M., Kril, J. J., and Harper, C. G. (1999). Neuronal loss in functional zones of the cerebellum of chronic alcoholics with and without Wernicke's encephalopathy. *Neuroscience* **91**, 429–438.

Bischoff, R., and Luider, T. M. (2004). Methodological advances in the discovery of protein and peptide diseases markers. *J. Chromatogr.* **803**, 27–40.

Brathen, G., Bjerve, K. S., Brodtkorb, E., and Bovim, G. (2000). Validity of carbohydrate deficient transferrin and other markers as diagnostic aids in the detection of alcohol related seizures. *J. Neurol. Neurosurg. Psychiatr.* **68**, 342–348.

Cai, H., Wang, Y., McCarthy, D., Wen, H., Borchelt, D. R., Price, D. L., and Wong, P. C. (2001). BACE1 is the major β-secretase for generation of Aβ peptides by neurons. *Nat. Neurosci.* **4**, 233–234.

Carrette, O., Demalte, I., Scherl, A., Yalkinoglu, O., Corthals, G., Burkhard, P., Hochstrasser, D. F., and Sanchez, J.-C. (2003). A panel of cerebrospinal fluid potential biomarkers for the diagnosis of Alzheimer's disease. *Proteomics* **3**, 1486–1494.

Clarke, W., Zhang, Z., and Chan, D. W. (2003). The application of clinical proteomics to cancer and other diseases. *Clin. Chem. Med.* **41**, 1562–1570.

Coen, M., Ruepp, S. U., Lindon, J. C., Nicholson, J. K., Pognan, F., Lenz, E. M., and Wilson, I. D. (2004). Integrated application of transcriptomics and metabonomics yields new insight into the toxicity due to paracetamol in the mouse. *J. Pharm. Biomed. Anal.* **35**, 93–105.

Davidsson, P., Paulson, L., Hesse, C., Blennow, K., and Nilsson, C. L. (2001). Proteome studies of human cerebrospinal fluid and brain tissue using a preparative two-dimensional electrophoresis approach prior to mass spectrometry. *Proteomics* **1**, 444–452.

Davies, H., Lomas, L., and Austen, B. (1999). Profiling of amyloid β peptide variants using SELDI-ProteinChip® arrays. *Biotechniques* **27**, 1258–1261.

Diamond, I., and Gordon, A. S. (1997). Cellular and molecular neuroscience of alcoholism. *Physiol. Rev.* **77**, 1–20.

Ernhart, C. B., Morrow-Tlucack, M., Sokol, R. J., and Martier, S. (1988). Under-reporting of alcohol use in pregnancy. *Alcohol Clin. Exp. Res.* **12**, 506–511.

Fan, L., van der Brug, M., Chen, W.-B., Dodd, P. R., Matsumoto, I., Niwa, S., and Wilce, P. A. (1999). Increased expression of a mitochondrial gene in human alcoholic brain revealed by differential display. *Alcohol Clin. Exp. Res.* **23**, 408–413.

Fountoulakis, M. (2001). Proteomics: Current technologies and applications in neurological disorders and toxicology. *Amino Acids* **21,** 363–381.

Freeman, W. M., Roberston, D. J., and Vrana, K. E. (2000). Fundamentals of DNA hybridization arrays for gene expression analysis. *Biotechniques* **29,** 1042–1055.

Goldstein, L. E., Muffat, J. A., Cherny, R. A., Moir, R. D., Ericsson, M. H., Huang, X., Mavros, C., Coccia, J. A., Faget, K. Y., Fitch, K. A., Masters, C. L., Tanzi, R., Chylack, L. T., Jr., and Bush, A. I. (2003). Cytosolic βamyloid deposition and supranuclear cataracts in lenses from people with Alzheimer's disease. *Lancet* **361,** 1258–1265.

Graves, P. R., and Haystead, T. A. (2002). Molecular biologist's guide to proteomics. *Microbiol. Mol. Biol. Rev.* **66,** 39–63.

Halm, U., Tannapfel, A., Mossner, J., and Berr, F. (1999). Relative versus absolute carbohydrate-deficient transferrin as a marker of alcohol consumption in patients with acute alcoholic hepatitis. *Alcohol Clin. Exp. Res.* **23,** 1614–1618.

Hermansson, U., Helander, A., Huss, A., Brandt, L., and Ronnberg, S. (2000). The Alcohol Use Disorders Identification Test (AUDIT) and carbohydrate-deficient transferrin (CDT) in a routine workplace health examination. *Alcohol Clin. Exp. Res.* **24,** 180–187.

Kanner, L. (1943). Autistic disturbances of affective contact. *Nervous Child* **2,** 217–250.

Kennedy, S. (2001). Proteomic profiling from human samples: The body fluid alternative. *Tox. Lett.* **120,** 379–384.

Lewczuk, P., Esselmann, H., Meyer, M., Wollscheid, V., Neumann, M., Otto, M., Maler, J. M., Ruther, E., Kornhuber, J., and Wiltfang, J. (2003). The amyloid-β (Aβ) peptide pattern in cerebrospinal fluid in Alzheimer's disease: Evidence of a novel carboxyterminally elongated Aβpeptide. *Rapid Commun. Mass Spectrom* **17,** 1291–1296.

Lewohl, J. M., Crane, D. I., and Dodd, P. R. (1997). Expression of the alpha 1, alpha2 and alpha 3 isoforms of the GABAA receptor in alcoholic brain. *Brain Res.* **751,** 102–112.

Mann, M., Hendrickson, R. C., and Pandey, A. (2001). Analysis of proteins and proteomes by mass spectrometry. *Annu. Rev. Biochem.* **70,** 437–473.

Marrero, J. A., Su, G. I., Wei, W., Emick, D., Conjeevaram, H. S., Fontana, R. J., and Lok, A. S. (2003). Des-gamma carboxyprothrobin can differentiate hepatocellular carcinoma from nonmalignant chronic liver disease in American patients. *Hepatology* **37,** 1114–1121.

Mayfield, R. D., Lewohl, J. M., Dodd, P. R., Herlihy, A., Liu, J., and Harris, R. A. (2002). Patterns of gene expression are altered in the frontal and motor cortices of human alcoholics. *J. Neurochem.* **81,** 802–813.

Meerkerk, G. J., Njoo, K. H., Bongers, I. M., Trienekens, P., and van Oers, J. A. (1999). Comparing the diagnostic accuracy of carbohydrate-deficient transferrin, gamma-glutamyltransferase, and mean cell volume in a general practice population. *Alcohol Clin. Exp. Res.* **23,** 1052–1059.

Merchant, M., and Weinberger, S. R. (2000). Recent advancements in surface-enhanced laser desorption/ionization-time of flight-mass spectrometry. *Electrophoresis* **21,** 1164–1177.

Miles, M. F. (1995). Alcohol's effects on gene expression. *Alcohol Health Res. World* **19,** 237–243.

Mitchell, P. (2003). In the pursuit of industrial proteomics. *Nat. Biotech.* **21,** 233–237.

Mittleman, B. B., Castellanos, F. X., Jacobson, L. K., Rapoport, J. L., Swedo, S. E., and Shearer, G. M. (1997). Cerebrospinal fluid cytokines in pediatric neuropsychiatric disease. *J. Immunol.* **159,** 2994–2999.

Mundle, G., Ackermann, K., Munkes, J., Steinle, D., and Mann, K. (1999). Influence of age, alcohol consumption and abstinence on the sensitivity of carbohydrate-deficient transferrin, gamma-glutamyltransferase and mean corpuscular volume. *Alcohol and Alcoholism* **34,** 760–766.

Netzer, W. J., Dou, F., Cai, D., Veach, D., Jean, S., Li, Y., Bornmann, W. G., Clarkson, B., Xu, H., and Greengard, P. (2003). Gleevec inhibits β-amyloid production but not notch cleavage. *Proc. Natl. Acad. Sci.* **100,** 12444–12449.

Nomura, F., Itoga, S., Tamura, M., Harada, S., Iizuka, Y., and Nakai, T. (2000). Biological markers of alcoholism with respect to genotypes of low-Km aldehyde dehydrogenase (ALDH2) in Japanese subjects. *Alcohol Clin. Exp. Res.* **24**(4 Suppl S), 30S–33S.

Petricon, E. F., III, Ardekani, A. M., Hitt, B. A., *et al.* (2002). Use of proteomic patterns in serum to identify ovarian cancer. *Lancet* **359**, 572–577.

Qu, Y., Adam, B. L., Yasui, Y., Ward, M. D., Cazares, L. H., Schellhammer, P. F., Feng, Z., Semmes, O. J., and Wright, G. L., Jr., (2002). Boosted decision tree analysis of surface-enhanced laser desorption/ionization mass spectral serum profiles discriminates prostate cancer from noncancer patients. *Clin. Chem.* **48**, 1835–1843.

Rappsilber, J., and Mann, M. (2002). What does it mean to identify a protein in proteomics? *Trends Biochem. Sci.* **20**, 74–78.

Russell, M., Martier, S. S., Sokol, R. J., Mundar, P., Jacobson, S., and Jacobson, J. (1996). Detecting risk drinking during pregnancy: A comparison of four screening questionnaires. *Am. J. Public Health* **86**, 1435–1439.

Salaspuro, M. (1999). Carbohydrate-deficient transferrin as compared to other markers of alcoholism: A systematic review. *Alcohol* **19**, 261–271.

Schafer, G. L., Crabbe, J., and Wiren, K. M. (2001). Ethanol-regulated gene expression of neuroendocrine specific protein in mice: brain region and genotype specificity. *Brain Res.* **897**, 139–149.

Shi, X.-P., Tugusheva, K., Bruce, J. E., Lucka, A., Wu, G.-X., Chen-Dodson, E., Price, E., Yueming, Li, Xu, M., Huang, Q., Sardana, M. K., and Hazuda, D. J. (2003). β-Secretase cleavage at amino acid residue 34 in the amyloid β peptide is dependent upon β-secretase activity. *J. Biol. Chem.* **278**, 21286–21294.

Srinivas, P. P., Verma, M., Zhao, Y., and Sprivastava, S. (2002). Proteomics for cancer biomarker discovery. *Clin. Chem.* **48**, 1160–1169.

Sullivan, E. V., Deshmukh, A., Desmond, J. E., and Lim, K. O. (2000a). Cerebellar volume decline in normal aging, alcoholism, and Korsakoff's syndrome: Relation to ataxia. *Neuropsychology* **14**, 341–352.

Szegedi, A., Muller, M. J., Himmerich, H., Anghelescu, I., and Wetzel, H. (2000). Carbohydrate-deficient transferrin (CDT) and HDL cholesterol (HDL) are highly correlated in male alcohol dependent patients. *Alcohol Clin. Exp. Res.* **24**, 497–500.

Torvik, A., and Torp, S. (1986). The prevalence of alcoholic cerebellar atrophy: A morphometric and histological study of an autopsy material. *J. Neurol. Sci.* **75**, 43–51.

van Pelt, J., Leusink, G. L., van Nierop, P. W. M., and Keyzer, J. J. (2000). Test characteristics of carbohydrate-deficient transferrin and gamma-glutamyltransferase in alcohol-using perimenopausal women. *Alcohol Clin. Exp. Res.* **24**, 176–179.

Vehmas, A. K., Borchelt, D. R., Price, D. L., McCarthy, D., Wills-Karp, M., Peper, M. J., Rudow, G., Luyinbazi, J., Siew, L. T., and Troncoso, J. C. (2001). Beta-amyloid peptide vaccination results in marked changes in serum and brain Abeta levels in APPswe/PS1DeltaE9 mice, as detected by SELDI-TOF-based ProteinChip technology. *DNA & Cell Biol.* **20**, 713–721.

Victor, M., Adams, R. D., and Mancell, E. L. (1959). A restricted form of cerebellar degeneration occurring in alcoholic patients. *Arch. Neurol.* **1**, 577–688.

Victor, M., Adams, R. D., and Collins, G. H. (1989). "The Wernicke-Korsakoff Syndrome and Related Neurologic Disorders Due to Alcoholism and Malnutrition" ed 2. F. A. Davis, Philadelphia.

Vrana, K. E., Freeman, W. M., Vaccaro, D., and Castrodale, B. (2001). "DNA Microarrays and Related Technologies: Miniaturization and Acceleration of Genomic Research."Cambridge Healthtech Institute's Genomic Pathways Reports Series, Report 8; Cambridge, Mass, 152 pp.

Walker, S. J., Howard, T. D., Hawkins, G. A., Lockwood, D., Branca, M., and Vrana, K. E. (2002). "High Throughput Genomics: Maximizing Efficiency and Productivity for Drug Discovery and Development."Cambridge Healthtech Institute's Genomic Reports; Cambridge, Mass, 182 pp.

Watkins, B., Szo, R., Ball, S., Knubovets, T., Briggman, J., Hlavaty, J. J., Kusinitz, F., and Steig, A. (2001). Detection of early stage cancer – by serum protein analysis. *Amer. Lab.* 26–32.

Weckwerth, W. (2003). Metabolomics in systems biology. *Annu. Rev. Plant Biol.* **54,** 669–689.

Wolters, D. A., Washburn, M. P., and Yates, J. R. (2001). An antomaticed multidimensional protein identification technology for shotgun proteomics. *Anal. Chem.* **73,** 5683–5690.

World Health Organization (1993). *Environmental health information: Air quality guidelines.* www.who.int/environmental_information/Air/Guidelines/ann3.htm; Accessed online 11/23/03.

Worst, T. J., Lack, A. K., Hallak, H., Freeman, W. M., Walker, S. J., and Vrana, K. E. (2004). Ethanol decreases SNARE protein gene expression in cerebellar cultures. *Alcohol Clin. Exp. Res.* In press.

PROTEOMIC ANALYSIS OF MITOCHONDRIAL PROTEINS

Mary F. Lopez,* Simon Melov,[†] Felicity Johnson,[†] Nicole Nagulko,[†]
Eva Golenko,* Scott Kuzdzal,[‡] Suzanne Ackloo,[§] and Alvydas Mikulskis*

*PerkinElmer Life and Analytical Sciences, Boston, Massachusetts 02118
[†]Buck Institute for Age Research, Novato, California 94945
[‡]PerkinElmer Life and Analytical Sciences, Shelton, Connecticut 06484
[§]MDS Sciex, Concord, Ontario, Canada L4K 4V8

I. Introduction

Approximately one billion years ago eukaryotic cells acquired the distant
α-proteobacterial progenitors of modern mitochondria (Burger and Lang, 2003).
Over the course of mitochondrial evolution, many of the bacterial progenitor
genes were lost and many proteins of nonmitochondrial origin were added to the
mitochondrial proteome (Hermann and Neupert, 2003). As a result, the mitochondria in modern organisms are composed of approximately 1000 proteins,
with only a handful of very hydrophobic proteins being contributed directly by
the mitochondrial genome. The rest of the mitochondrial proteins are derived
from genes that reside in the host's nucleus and are translocated into the
organelle.

Eukaryotes exhibit a large diversity of mitochondrial DNA (mtDNA).
Mitochondrial genomes range in size from 15.8 (*Chlamydomonas reinhardtii*) to
366.9 (*Arabidopsis thaliana*) kilobases, with the human circular mitochondrial
genome weighing in at 16.6 kilobases. However, mammalian mitochondria are
extraordinarily well conserved among species, hence their utility in inferring
evolutionary relationships (Boore, 1999).

Mitochondria are a target of intense research because of their central role in multiple cellular processes such as survival, death, signaling pathways, oxidative stress, and multiple anabolic and catabolic pathways (Lopez and Melov, 2002). In addition, mitochondrial dysfunction has been implicated in the cause of numerous diseases and disorders, including defects in energy metabolism, Alzheimer's and Parkinson's diseases, cancer, type 2 diabetes, osteoarthritis, cardiovascular disease, and many drug side effects (Beal *et al.*, 1997; Beckman and Ames, 1998; Behl, 1999; Brown *et al.*, 1992; Dahl, 1998; Delatycki, *et al.*, 2000; Leonard and Schapira, 2000a,b; Plasterer *et al.*, 2001; Schapira, 1999; Scheffler, 1999; Stadtman, 1992).

A comprehensive, detailed map of the mitochondrial proteome, providing information on identity, function, and protein-protein interactions, would be invaluable for the understanding of the complex mechanisms of cellular function and disease. Such a database would be useful to many types of researchers, including academic institutions and hospitals, biopharmaceutical companies, clinical laboratories, and the toxicology industry.

II. Model Systems

Any proteomic study of mitochondria must take into account that mitochondria from different tissues are not necessarily identical and the manifestation of different types of diseases with mitochondrial involvement will be a reflection of this fact. As a result, a study of human mitochondrial proteomics should encompass various tissue sources such as skeletal muscle, heart, brain and liver. In addition, fluids such as blood may contain mitochondrial proteins released during a diseased state, and these proteins may be useful as disease biomarkers.

Because of the difficulty in obtaining human tissues, and because of the highly conserved nature of mammalian mitochondria, mouse models are highly useful for the study of human diseases. Numerous researchers have developed mouse models of human mitochondrial diseases by using homologous recombination (Melov, 2000; Melov *et al.*, 1999a). The mouse models encompass several categories of disease, including reactive oxygen species (ROS) toxicity, adenosine triphosphate (ATP) deficiency and mtDNA depletion–transcription deficiency (Melov, 2000).

Although yeast model systems may have limited applicability to human studies, recently the proteome of mitochondria from *Saccharomyces cerevisiae* has been extensively well documented with the identification of up to 90% of the proteins (Sickmann *et al.*, 2003). This comprehensive database of yeast mitochondrial proteins will undoubtedly be extremely useful for the cross-species characterization of mitochondrial functions and diseases.

III. Technological Approaches

A. Mass Spectrometry-Based Proteomics

The application of mass spectrometry (MS) to protein and peptide mixtures from cells (and subcellular fractions such as mitochondria) has arguably been the major driving force behind the rapidly evolving discipline of proteomics. Mass spectrometry techniques in proteomics studies can be roughly categorized into two main tracks (Aebersold and Mann, 2003).

The first and most common approach combines tryptic digests of proteins separated on 2D-PAGE (two-dimensional polyacrylamide gel electrophonesis) gels (typically) with MALDI-TOF (matrix-assisted laser desorption/ionization time-of-flight) mass spectrometry to derive peptide mass fingerprints. These fingerprints are used to indirectly identify proteins based on the correlation of experimentally derived peptide masses with peptide masses calculated from theoretical tryptic digests of proteins in genomic sequence databases (Henzel et al., 1993; James et al., 1993; Mann et al., 1993; Pappin et al., 1993; Yates et al., 1993). The success of this method depends entirely on both the availability of comprehensive genomic databases and the high sensitivity and mass accuracy of the MALDI-TOF technique. Advantages are that 2-D gels are not only a powerful tool for the parallel purification of thousands of proteins simultaneously, but they are also quantitative and therefore provide a clear basis for the discovery of differentially expressed proteins between diseased and normal samples. In addition, pI and molecular weight information from the 2-D gels can be combined with the peptide masses to increase the confidence of putative protein identifications. Finally, post-translational modifications are easily observed on 2-D gels, and multiple isoforms of proteins can be analyzed to help trace their involvement in disease mechanisms (Lopez and Melov, 2002; Rabilloud, 2002). Although 2D-PAGE/MALDI-TOF peptide mass fingerprinting is a mature technique that has been in use for at least 10 years, 2-D gels have clear limitations with respect to dynamic range, ability to resolve hydrophobic proteins, throughput, and ease of use.

In an effort to circumvent the limitations of 2-D gels, several researchers developed the other major proteomic technology track, peptide LC-MS/MS (Link et al., 1999; Wolters et al., 2001). In this method, protein mixtures (often excised from 1-D gels) are digested with trypsin. The peptides are then separated with multidimensional high-performance liquid chromatography (HPLC), followed by electrospray-ionization (ESI) tandem mass spectrometry. Individual precursor peptide ions are fragmented to produce collision-induced spectra (CID). The CID spectra are not used to produce de novo sequence data, but instead are processed with a variety of algorithms, including cross correlation, peptide sequence tag generation, and probability based matching. Protein identifications are based on pattern matching with genomic or protein sequence databases (Aebersold and Mann, 2003). Advantages of this approach are its throughput, ease of automation, and high confidence protein identifications. Unfortunately, the LC-MS/MS method is not quantitative per se, and must be combined with some type of stable isotope dilution to determine the differential expression of proteins in samples. Proteins may be labeled with heavy and light isotopes, either *in vivo* or *in vitro*, using a variety of methods (Aebersold and Mann, 2003; Gygi *et al.*, 2002; Han *et al.*, 2001). The ratios of heavy to light labeled but otherwise chemically identical analytes may be calculated, thus indicating their relative abundance. Because of the multiple steps involved in LC-MS/MS experiments, larger amounts of sample are needed vis-à-vis 2D-PAGE/MALDI-TOF experiments. In addition, LC-MS/MS with stable isotope dilution also suffers from a limited dynamic range as a result of the large numbers of peptides that will be preferentially generated by tryptic digests versus low abundance proteins (Patton *et al.*, 2002).

Clearly, no single method developed to date has the capability to identify all proteins in an entire proteome. However, the techniques are complementary, and in a recent study combining many of the aforementioned techniques, up to 90% of the yeast mitochondrial proteome were identified (Sickmann, 2003).

B. Descriptive Proteomics

1. *Mitochondrial Protein Maps*

The application of the previously described technologies to mitochondrial fractions has rapidly led to the generation of mitochondrial protein maps of increasing complexity (DaCruz *et al.*, 2003; Lopez *et al.*, 2000; Mootha *et al.*, 2003; Ozawa *et al.*, 2003; Rabilloud *et al.*, 1998; Sickmann *et al.*, 2003; Taylor *et al.*, 2003; Westermann and Neupert, 2003). In 2000, Lopez *et al.* used 2D-PAGE/MALDI-TOF peptide mass fingerprinting in combination with microscale affinity fractionation as part of a high-throughput platform to characterize rat liver mitochondrial proteins. Approximately 70 proteins were identified over the course of 3 days in this study. In that same year Patterson *et al.* (2000) identified 79 proteins from mitochondria undergoing permeability transition with a novel application of LC-MS/MS techniques. Using a combination of sucrose density fractionation and 1D-PAGE/LC-MS/MS, 82 mitochondrial proteins from the human heart (40 of which had not previously been reported) were identified by Taylor *et al.* in 2002, and shortly thereafter the same group (Taylor *et al.*, 2003) identified a total of 615 proteins or approximately 45% of predicted proteins from human heart mitochondria. Mootha *et al.* (2003) recently performed an LC-MS/MS–based proteomic survey from mouse brain, heart, kidney, and liver. Combining the results with existing gene annotations, a list of 591 mitochondrial proteins including 163 not previously associated with the organelle, was produced. Finally, the most recent and comprehensive mitochondrial protein map was recently published (Sickmann *et al.*, 2003), which catalogued 750 different yeast mitochondrial proteins.

C. Functional Proteomics

1. *Protein-Protein Interactions*

Many mitochondrial proteins function as part of large complexes such as the oxidative phosphorylation machinery, proteins involved in RNA, DNA and protein synthesis, ion transport, and lipid metabolism. In general, two main approaches have been applied to analyze protein complexes in proteomic experiments: *i,* bait presentation followed by affinity purification of the complex and analysis of the components; and *ii,* sucrose gradient, or blue native electrophoresis, purification of intact complexes with subsequent analysis by mass spectrometry. Bait-based methods such as immunoprecipitation, tandem affinity purification (TAP) *tagging,* and two-hybrid assays have not been generally applied to mitochondrial proteins and have recently been reviewed elsewhere (Phizicky *et al.*, 2003).

Because of the extraordinarily high complement of very hydrophobic proteins, mitochondrial protein complexes are well suited to analysis by sucrose gradient fractionation or blue native electrophoresis, and several studies have focused on this approach (Brookes *et al.*, 2002, 2004; Lin *et al.*, 2002; Taylor *et al.*, 2002, 2003). Brookes and colleagues coupled blue-native gel electrophoresis with 2D-PAGE and peptide mass fingerprinting with MALDI-TOF to create functional maps of mitochondrial protein complexes. In a variation of this approach, Lin *et al.* (2002) prelabeled thiols in mitochondrial proteins with 4-iodobutyl triphenylphosphonium (IBTP) and then subjected the proteins to blue native gel electrophoresis. Labeling with IBTP allowed the specific analysis of protein thiol redox state following oxidative stress. Sucrose gradient fractionation of mitochondrial protein complexes with subsequent analysis by 1D PAGE and mass specrometry was used by Taylor *et al.* (2002, 2003) to identify more than 90% of the subunits of the oxidative phosphorylation machinery in human heart mitochondria.

Koc *et al.* (2000, 2001) used a proteogenomic approach to study the small, subunit ribosomal proteins in mammalian mitochondria. Ribosomal proteins were subjected to 2D-PAGE, and individual protein spots were digested with trypsin or endoproteinase Lys-C. The resulting peptides were analyzed by electrospray tandem mass spectrometry, and the peptide sequences were used to screen human, mouse, and rat expressed sequence tag databases. Complete consensus cDNA for the different species were deduced *in silico*, and the corresponding protein sequences were then characterized by comparison to known ribosomal proteins in protein databases. Novel homologues to ribosomal proteins from prokaryotes were identified using this technique.

2. Post-Translational Modifications

Many proteins are processed into their mature form by post-translational addition of residues such as carbohydrates, phosphates, lipids, and other molecules. Protein phosphorylation plays a central role in regulatory mechanisms and cell signaling, and therefore mapping of phosphorylation sites has been a goal of many functional proteomic studies (Knight *et al.*, 2003; Schulenberg *et al.*, 2003; Whelan and Hart, 2003; Zhou *et al.*, 2001) Errors in protein glycosylation have been implicated in diseases such as rheumatoid arthritis and others (Castellani *et al.*, 2001; Corthay *et al.*, 2001; Doyle and Mamula, 2002; Meri and Baumann, 2001; Zhou *et al.*, 2002), making glycosylated proteins also a target for proteomic analysis. The analysis of post-translational modifications (PTMs) has been carried out using a variety of methods. Mass spectrometric methods have focused on purified proteins and peptide mapping to determine the site and type of modifications. This process is typically manual, and therefore low throughput, because it requires the determination of as much of the protein sequence as possible, with the protein modifications being deduced by differences between the measured mass and predicted mass of modified peptides (Aebersold and Mann, 2003; Ficarro *et al.*, 2002; Steen *et al.*, 2002). This type of analysis is made even more difficult by the fact that many modifications, especially protein phosphorylation, are present in low amounts.

Two methodological approaches have been developed to try to circumvent this problem. In the first approach, specific types of PTMs are enriched with affinity fractionation techniques. Antibodies specific to phosphotyrosine were used by Pandey *et al.* (2000) and Steen *et al.* (2002) to isolate phosphorylated proteins from epidermal growth factor stimulated cells. Few researchers have used this particular approach with mitochondrial proteins; however, Lopez *et al.* (2000) enriched and identified glycoproteins, calcium binding proteins, and hydrophobic proteins from rat liver mitochondria using microscale affinity columns. In the second approach, a fluorescence-based, multiplexed staining technology is combined with sucrose fractionation, 2-D gels, and mass spectrometry to identify phosphorylated proteins. Schulenberg *et al.* (2003) pioneered this technique and characterized the steady-state levels of human heart mitochondrial proteins.

Finally, a recent report (Knight *et al.*, 2003) describes a novel strategy for specific proteolysis at sites of serine and threonine phosphorylation, facilitating the identification of the phosphorylation site directly from the cleavage pattern without the sequencing of any individual peptide. The authors visualize extensions of this approach to analyze protein glycosylation and possibly other enzyme-based tools for selective interrogation of all PTMs.

3. *Proteomic Expression Profiling*

a. 2-D gel/MALDI-TOF or LC-MS/MS-based Differential Protein Expression Studies. The application of proteomics to disease mechanisms and metabolic dysfunction invariably requires the discovery and identification of differentially expressed proteins. A number of these types of studies have been carried out on mitochondrial proteins.

Mitochondrial antioxidant systems were investigated by Rabilloud *et al.* (2001) in a 2-D gel-based approach, and several mitochondrial proteins were found to be induced by oxidative stress. In a follow-up study the same group (Rabilloud *et al.*, 2002), using similar techniques, demonstrated a quantitative decrease in nuclear encoded subunits of cytochrome c oxidase in mitochondria with single point tRNA mutations. Another group initiated the study of effects of aging in mitochondria. Chang *et al.* (2003) characterized a 2-D gel-based system that resolved *ca* 500 mouse mitochondrial proteins with a gel-to-gel and animal-to-animal coefficient of variation that was less than 50%. Recently, Danial *et al.* (2003) investigated the connection between glycolysis and apoptosis by using a proteogenomic LC-MS/MS approach. This study demonstrated a previously unanticipated role for BAD, a proapoptotic BCL-2 family member that was found to reside in a mitochondrial protein complex with glucokinase. Using a novel, quantitative Western blotting technique, the relative copy numbers of proteins involved in oxidative phosphorylation were determined by Murray *et al.* (2002).

The role of mitochondrial superoxide dismutase (SOD2) deficiency in sideroblastic anemia was investigated by Friedman *et al.* (2004) SOD2 deficient reticulocytes revealed striking mitochondrial proliferation and mitochondrial membrane thickening. Oxidative damage to proteins was increased in SOD2 deficient cells, and proteomic analysis of red cells demonstrated that several proteins involved in folding/chaperone function, redox regulation, ATP synthesis, and red cell metabolism exhibited altered expression in SOD2 deficient cells. Hinerfeld *et al.* (2003) investigated differentially expressed proteins in brain mitochondria isolated from SOD2 nullizygous mice treated with an efficacious antioxidant treatment. The activities of respiratory chain complexes I, II, III, IV, and V and the tricarboxylic acid cycle enzymes α-ketoglutarate dehydrogenase and citrate synthase were monitored. Differential sensitivities of mitochondrial proteins to oxidative stress were observed in this study.

4. *Differential Protein Expression Studies Using Protein Arrays*

The need for a strategy to capture the global differences in protein expression that occur during disease or altered biological states has prompted the development of protein arrays. Although somewhat analogous to genomic arrays and transcriptional profiling, proteins present a number of challenges to this type of approach because of their highly heterogeneous nature, lability, differences in optimum conditions for activity, etc. One of the greatest challenges in the global analysis of protein expression using protein arrays is the lack of comprehensive sets of affinity capture agents such as antibodies (Hanash, 2003). Nevertheless, progress has been made in profiling some types of cancer (Knezevic *et al.*, 2001; Madoz-Gurpide *et al.*, 2001; Paweletz *et al.*, 2001) and autoimmune disorders (Robinson *et al.*, 2002).

A novel strategy for the combination of mass spectrometry and protein capture arrays has recently been developed for the discovery of disease biomarker patterns (Petricoin *et al.*, 2002; Wulfkuhle *et al.*, 2003). In this technique, samples are applied directly to the surface of a plate that has been derivatized with a protein capture reagent such as ion exchange or affinity. The bound proteins are then directly analyzed by MALDI-TOF. The spectral patterns that are obtained are used to distinguish between disease and normal samples. A remarkable level of sensitivity and specificity in distinguishing several types of cancer from normal samples has been achieved with this method (Conrads *et al.*, 2003; Petricoin *et al.*, 2002).

IV. Differential Expression of Proteins in Mouse Brain Mitochondria from Cortex and Synaptosomes

An illustration of a 2-D gel/mass spectrometry-based differential protein expression profiling study is presented in this chapter. As part of an ongoing study on the effects of oxidative stress on neuronal function, mitochondrial proteins, and neurological disease, differential expression of mitochondrial proteins isolated from mouse brain cortex and isolated synaptosomes was investigated using a combination of 2-D gels and a novel orthogonal MALDI-TOF mass spectrometer. Figure 1 is a schematic illustration of the experimental strategy. Mitochondria from cortical tissue and synaptosomes were purified and the solubilized proteins were run on large-format 2-D gels. Five replicate gels each were run from cortex and synaptosomal samples. The digitized gel images were acquired with a CCD (charged-coupled device) camera imaging system

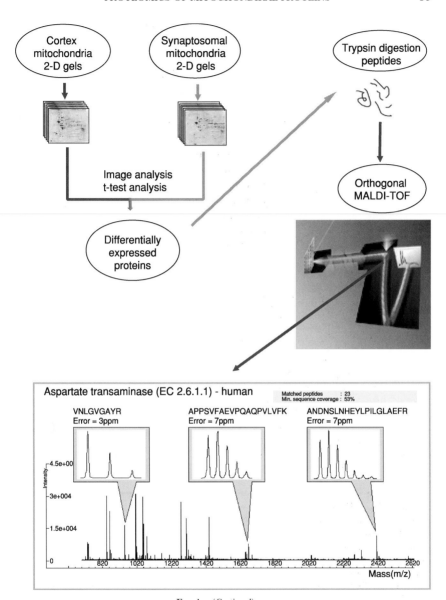

FIG. 1. (*Continued*)

(ProXPRESS, PerkinElmer, Boston) and analyzed (Progenesis Discovery, Non-linear Dynamics Ltd, United Kingdom). The resulting list of corresponding normalized spot volumes was exported into a customized Excel (Microsoft, Redmond, Wash.) template to allow further calculations for downstream analysis. Heteroscedastic t-test calculations were carried out on the normalized spot volumes and subsequently, the ratios of normalized volumes between the synaptosomal and cortex matched spots were calculated. The candidate differentially expressed protein spots identified by this process were validated for accurate matching and quantification by relocating them on the original images in Progenesis. Only the validated protein spots were excised for further analysis by prOTOF (PerkinElmer, Boston) orthogonal MALDI-TOF mass spectrometry. Figure 2 shows a 2-D gel image of cortical mitochondria with the differentially expressed spots indicated. The designated proteins were excised and subjected to trypsin digestion and subsequent peptide mass fingerprinting by orthogonal MALDI-TOF mass spectrometry. Table I is a preliminary list of some identified

---

Fig. 1. 2-D gel/MALDI-TOF-based strategy for the identification of differential protein expression in mitochondria isolated from mouse brain cortex and synaptosomes.Mitochondria and synaptosomes were prepared using a method from Lai and Clark (1976) with the following modifications. All animal procedures were carried out in accordance with approved IACUC (Institutional Animal Care and Use Committees) animal protocols at the Buck Institute in Novato, Calif. Cerebral hemispheres of wild-type mice at 18–21 days of age were harvested, cut into small pieces and homogenized with a Dounce homogenizer in cold H buffer (0.21 M mannitol, 70 mM sucrose, 1 mM EGTA, 0.1 (wt/vol) BSA, and 5 mM HEPES at pH 7.2) before being centrifuged at 1000 Xg for 10 minutes at 4 °C. The supernatant was centrifuged at 8500 Xg, and the pellet was carefully drained. The resuspended pellet was layered onto a step gradient of 15%, 12%, 9%, and 6% ficoll solution (wt/vol). After centrifugation at 75,000 Xg for 45 minutes at 4 °C, the synaptosomes and mitochondrial bands were removed. Mitochondria were washed twice in H buffer (-)BSA and stored at − 20 °C until further use. The two synaptosomal bands were washed and the mitochondria present inside the synaptosomes were isolated via a method modified from those of Lai and Clark (1976) and Asakura *et al.* (1989). Briefly, the synaptosomes were osmotically shocked in water, then resuspended in a 3% ficoll solution and layered onto a 3–6% ficoll cushion. After centrifugation at 11,500 Xg for 30 minutes at 4 °C, the synaptic mitochondria in the pellet were washed before storage at −20 °C. Protein concentrations were estimated using the Bradford assay (Bio-Rad, Hercules, Calif.) according to the manufacturer's protocol. Proteins from the cortical and synaptosomal mitochondria were prepared and run on large-format 2-D gels (Lopez *et al.*, 2000). Five replicate gels were run from each sample. Gel images were acquired with a CCD camera imaging system (ProXPRESS, PerkinElmer, Boston) and analyzed (Progenesis Discovery, Nonlinear Dynamics Ltd, United Kingdom). Normalized spot volumes were exported into a customized Excel (Microsoft, Redmond, Wash.) template and used in heteroscedastic t-test calculations. The ratios of synaptosomal and cortex matched spots were calculated, and the candidate differentially expressed spots were validated for accurate matching and quantification by relocation on the original gel images in Progenesis. Validated protein spots were excised, digested with trypsin, and analyzed with prOTOF (PerkinElmer, Boston) orthogonal MALDI-TOF mass spectrometry. Peptide mass fingerprinting and protein identification was done using TOFWorks software (PerkinElmer). (See Color Insert.)

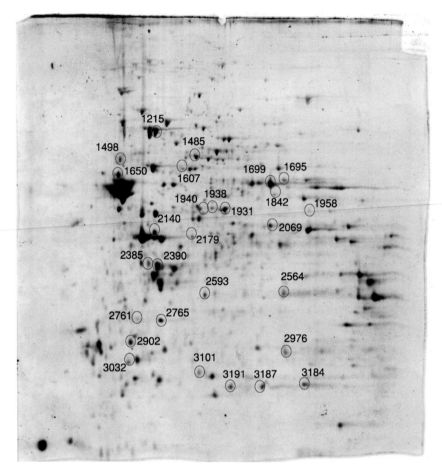

Fig. 2. 2-D gel image of cortical mitochondrial proteins with the differentially expressed spots indicated. Differentially expressed proteins in synaptosomal and cortex mitochondria (see Fig. 1) are indicated. The designated proteins were excised and subjected to trypsin digestion and subsequent peptide mass fingerprinting by orthogonal MALDI-TOF mass spectrometry (see description in Fig. 1 and Table I). (See Color Insert.)

proteins; a complete list of identifications is in progress. The preliminary list of identified proteins in Table I includes mitochondrial proteins pyruvate DH and cytochrome c reductase, and tubulin, which has recently been demonstrated to be an integral part of the mitochondrial membrane associated with the voltage-dependent anion channel (Carre *et al.*, 2002). Other identified proteins are Rabphilin, a member of a family of proteins involved in protein transport in synaptic vesicles, and a cell cycle dependent kinase.

TABLE I

DIFFERENTIALLY EXPRESSED PROTEINS IN MITOCHONDRIA ISOLATED FROM MOUSE BRAIN CORTEX AND SYNAPTOSOMES

Spot ID	Accession #	Protein name	kDa	pI	# Matched peptides	Coverage	ppm error	Expression in synaptosomal mitochondria versus cortex mitochondria	P-value
3101	gi 28515714	Rabphilin 3A like	33.03	5.8	2	13	1	1.49	0.089179
2976	gi 136708	Ubiquinol-cytochrome C reductase	27.96	9.2	4	20	11	3.16	0.04639
2385	gi 7710104	Mixture of tropomodulin	39.50	4.8	4	13	3	0.04	0.054662
	gi 6755901	Tubulin, alpha 1	50.80	4.9	4	13	3		
2390	gi 7710104	Mixture of tropomodulin	39.50	4.8	4	13	3	0.58	0.067203
	gi 6755901	Tubulin, alpha 1	50.80	4.9	4	13	3		
2052	gi 5453257	Cyclin-dependent kinase 6	32.98	6.2	4	17	10	2.62	0.009472
2069	gi 6679261	Pyruvate DH E1 alpha subunit	43.9	9.0	7	29	9	1.40	0.053963

gi; pI, isoelectric point; ppm, parts per million.

V. Conclusions

Mitochondria generate the energy that drives the maintenance, repair, and turnover of cellular machinery and are therefore central to survival. The dysfunction of mitochondria is linked to various diseases, aging, and tumorigenicity (Beal et al., 1997; Beckman and Ames, 1998; Behl, 1999; Brown et al., 1992; Dahl, 1998; Delatycki et al., 2000; Leonard et al., 2000a,b; Lopez and Melov, 2002; Plasterer et al., 2001; Schapira, 1999; Scheffler, 1999; Stadtman et al., 1992). The in-depth study of the proteomics associated with these disease mechanisms has been facilitated by the availability of appropriate animal models and the development of powerful technical approaches. The rapid evolution of mass spectrometry–based tools in conjunction with protein purification methods such as 1-D gels, 2-D gels, fractionation techniques, and liquid chromatography has allowed the development of increasingly more comprehensive mitochondrial protein maps. These descriptive studies are now being complemented with functional proteomics studies that explore protein-protein interactions in mitochondrial complexes, differential protein expression, and the search for biomarkers of disease states.

Impairment of brain energy metabolism can lead to neuronal damage or facilitate the deleterious effects of some neurotoxic agents. Specifically, the buildup of damage caused by ROS (produced by the mitochondrion itself during oxidative phosphorylation) (Dahl, 1998; Delatycki et al., 2000; Hinerfeld et al., 2003; Melov et al., 1999a,b, 2001) is thought to play a major role in aging and neurological diseases. The investigation of specific changes in protein expression in neuronal mitochondria will undoubtedly aid in understanding the mechanisms of neurological diseases such as Alzheimer's, Huntington's or amyotrophic lateral sclerosis (ALS). Arias et al. (2002) presented evidence suggesting that synapses may be particularly sensitive to metabolic perturbation and providing experimental support to the hypothesis that certain risk factors such as metabolic dysfunction and amyloid accumulation may interact to exacerbate Alzheimer's disease. LaFontaine et al. (2002) demonstrated that administration of a mitochondrial inhibitor, 3-nitropropionic acid (3-NP), in an animal model led to pathology similar to that of Huntington's disease, including massive loss of striatal neurons associated with oxidative stress. Oxidative stress induced by 3-NP also extended to the cortex; however, in that case a minimum of neuron loss occurred. A lipid bilayer-specific probe demonstrated that in cortical synaptosomes, membrane fluidity increased in animals treated with 3-NP, whereas in striatal synaptosomes, membrane fluidity decreased in animals treated with 3-NP. These results suggested that oxidatively induced changes in membrane fluidity may be involved in mechanisms by which selective striatal neuronal loss occurs in this animal model of Huntington's disease. The involvement of oxidative stress and p53 in neuronal apoptosis was recently investigated by Gilman *et al.* (2003). Levels of active p53 increased in isolated cortical synaptosomes exposed to oxidative and excitotoxic insults. Synaptosomes from p53-deficient mice exhibited increased resistance to oxidative and excitotoxic insults, as indicated by stabilization of mitochondrial membrane potential and decreased production of reactive oxygen species. These findings provided evidence for the mechanism of action of p53 in synapses and suggest that p53 may contribute to the dysfunction and degeneration of synapses that occurs in various neurodegenerative disorders. In a study on the effects of aging on synaptosomal mitochondria from rat brain, Joyce *et al.* (2003) showed that the flux through the substrate oxidation system in synaptosomes from old rats was impaired as compared to synaptosomes from young animals. These results support the hypothesis that age-dependent impairment of mitochondrial energy production may result in increased susceptibility to neurodegeneration. A preliminary list of differentially expressed mitochondrial and associated proteins in mouse brain cortex tissue and synaptosomes identified by 2-D gel/orthogonal MALDI-TOF peptide mass fingerprinting was documented in this report. One of the identified proteins, Rabphilin, is involved in synaptic vesicle protein transport and has been shown to contact Rab3A, a small G protein important in neurotransmitter release.

The clear trend emerging from these and other studies is the increasing importance of integrating proteomic information within a global "systems biology" approach. Future studies will undoubtedly correlate genomic, proteomic, and array data in an effort to more clearly elucidate the molecular mechanisms of mitochondria and ultimately, whole cells.

References

Aebersold, R., and Mann, M. (2003). Mass spectrometry-based proteomics. *Nature* **422,** 198–207.

Arias, C., Montiel, T., Quiroz-Baez, R., and Massieu, L. (2002). Beta-amyloid neurotoxicity is exacerbated during glycolysis inhibition and mitochondrial impairment in the rat hippocampus in vivo and in isolated nerve terminals: Implications for Alzheimer's disease. *Exp. Neurol.* **176,** 163–174.

Asakura, T., Ikeda, Y., and Matsuda, M. (1989). Distribution of activity converting 4-aminobutyraldehyde to γ-aminobutyric acid in subcellular fractions of mouse brain. *J. Neurochem.* **52,** 448–452.

Beal, M. F., Howell, N., and Bodis Wallner, I. (Eds.) (1997). *"Mitochondria and Free Radicals in Neurodegenerative Diseases."* Wiley-Liss, New York.

Beckman, K. B., and Ames, B. N. (1998). The free radical theory of aging matures. *Physiol. Rev.* **78,** 547–581.

Behl, C. (1999). Alzheimer's disease and oxidative stress: Implications for novel therapeutic approaches. *Prog. Neurobiol.* **57,** 301–323.

Boore, J. L. (1999). Animal mitochondrial genomes. *Nucleic Acids Res.* **27,** 1767–1780.

Brookes, P. S., and Darley-Usmar, V. M. (2004). Role of calcium and superoxide dismutase in sensitizing mitochondria to peroxynitrite-induced permeability transition. *Am. J. Physiol. Heart Circ. Physiol.* **286,** 39–46.

Brookes, P. S., Pinner, A., Ramachandran, A., Coward, L., Barnes, S., Kim, H., and Darley-Usmar, V. M. (2002). High throughput two-dimensional blue-native electrophoresis: A tool for functional proteomics of mitochondria and signaling complexes. *Proteomics* **2,** 969–977.

Brown, M. D., Voljavec, A. S., Lott, M. T., Macdonald, I., and Wallace, D. C. (1992). Leber's hereditary optic neuropathy: A model for mitochondrial neurodegenerative diseases. *FASEB J.* **6,** 2791–2799.

Burger, G., and Lang, B. F. (2003). Parallels in genome evolution in mitochondria and bacterial symbionts. *Life* **55,** 205–212.

Carre, M., Andre, N., Carles, G., Borghi, H., Brichese, L., Briand, C., and Braguer, D. J. (2002). Tubulin is an inherent component of mitochondrial membranes that interacts with the voltage-dependent anion channel. *J. Biol. Chem.* **277,** 33664–33669. Epub. 2002 Jun. 26.

Castellani, R. J., Harris, P. L., Sayre, L. M., Fujii, J., Taniguchi, N., Vitek, M. P., Founds, H., Atwood, C. S., Perry, G., and Smith, M. A. (2001). Active glycation in neurofibrillary pathology of Alzheimer disease: N(epsilon)-(carboxymethyl) lysine and hexitol-lysine. *Free Radic. Biol. Med.* **31,** 175–180.

Chang, J., Van Remmen, H., Cornell, J., Richardson, A., and Ward, W. F. (2003). Comparative proteomics: Characterization of a two-dimensional gel electrophoresis system to study the effect of aging on mitochondrial proteins. *Mech. Ageing Dev.* **124,** 33–41.

Conrads, T. P., Zhou, M., Petricoin, E. F., III, Liotta, L., and Veenstra, T. D. (2003). Cancer diagnosis using proteomic patterns. *Expert Rev. Mol. Diagn.* **3,** 411–420.

Corthay, A., Backlund, J., and Holmdahl, R. (2001). Role of glycopeptide-specific T cells in collagen-induced arthritis: An example how post-translational modification of proteins may be involved in autoimmune disease. *Ann. Med.* **33,** 456–465.

Da Cruz, S., Xenarios, I., Langridge, J., Vilbois, F., Parone, P. A., and Martinou, J. C. (2003). Proteomic analysis of the mouse liver mitochondrial inner membrane. *J. Biol. Chem.* **278,** 41566–41571. Epub. 2003 Jul. 15.

Dahl, H-HM. (1998). Getting to the nucleus of mitochondrial disorders: Identification of respiratory chain-enzyme genes causing Leigh syndrome. *Am. J. Hum. Genet.* **63,** 1594–1597.

Danial, N. N., Gramm, C. F., Scorrano, L., Zhang, C. Y., Krauss, S., Ranger, A. M., Datta, S. R., Greenberg, M. E., Licklider, L. J., Lowell, B. B., Gygi, S. P., and Korsmeyer, S. J. (2003). BAD and glucokinase reside in a mitochondrial complex that integrates glycolysis and apoptosis. *Nature* **424,** 952–956.

Delatycki, M. B., Williamson, R., and Forrest, S. M. (2000). Freidreich ataxia: An overview. *J. Med. Genet.* **37,** 1–8.

Doyle, H. A., and Mamula, M. J. (2002). Posttranslational protein modifications: New flavors in the menu of autoantigens. *Curr. Opin. Rheumatol.* **14,** 244–249.

Ficarro, S. B., McCleland, M. L., Stukenberg, P. T., Burke, D. J., Ross, M. M., Shabanowitz, J., Hunt, D. F., and White, F. M. (2002). Phosphoproteome analysis by mass spectrometry and its application to Saccharomyces cerevisiae. *Nat. Biotechnol.* **20,** 301–305.

Friedman, J. S., Lopez, M. F., Fleming, M. D., Rivera, A., and Doctorow, S. R. (2004). SOD2 deficiency anemia: Protein oxidation and altered protein expression reveal targets of damage, stress response and anti-oxidant responsiveness. *Blood* Epub ahead of print.

Gilman, C. P., Chan, S. L., Guo, Z., Zhu, X., Greig, N., and Mattson, M. P. (2003). p53 is present in synapses where it mediates mitochondrial dysfunction and synaptic degeneration in response to DNA damage, and oxidative and excitotoxic insults. *Neuromolecular Med.* **3,** 159–172.

Gygi, S. P., Rist, B., Griffin, T. J., Eng, J., and Aebersold, R. (2002). Proteome analysis of low-abundance proteins using multidimensional chromatography and isotope-coded affinity tags. *J. Proteome Res.* **1,** 47–54.

Han, D. K., Eng, J., Zhou, H., and Aebersold, R. (2001). Quantitative profiling of differentiation-induced microsomal proteins using isotope-coded affinity tags and mass spectrometry. *Nat. Biotechnol.* **19,** 946–951.

Hanash, S. (2003). Disease proteomics. *Nature* **422,** 226–231.

Henzel, W. J., Billeci, T. M., Stults, J. T., Wong, S. C., Grimley, C., and Watanabe, C. (1993). Identifying proteins from two-dimensional gels by molecular mass searching of peptide fragments in protein sequence databases. *Proc. Natl. Acad. Sci. USA* **90,** 5011–5015.

Hermann, J. M., and Neupert, W. (2003). Protein insertion into the inner membrane of mitochondria. *Life* **55,** 219–225.

Hinerfeld, H., Traini, M. D., Weinberger, R. P., Cochran, B., Doctrow, S. R., Harry, J., and Melov, S. (2004). Endogenous mitochondrial oxidative stress: Neurodegeneration, proteomic analysis, specific respiratory chain defects, and efficacious antioxidant therapy in superoxide dismutase 2 null mice. *J. Neurochem.* **88,** 657–667.

James, P., Quadroni, M., Carafoli, E., and Gonnet, G. (1993). Protein identification by mass profile finger printing. *Biochem. Biophys. Res. Commun.* **195,** 58–64.

Joyce, O. J., Farmer, M. K., Tipton, K. F., and Porter, R. K. (2003). Oxidative phosphorylation by in situ synaptosomal mitochondria from whole brain of young and old rats. *J. Neurochem.* **86,** 1032–1041.

Knezevic, V., Leethanakul, C., Bichsel, V. E., Worth, J. M., Prabhu, V. V., Gutkind, J. S., Liotta, L. A., Munson, P. J., Petricoin, E. F., III, and Krizman, D. B. (2001). Proteomic profiling of the cancer microenvironment by antibody arrays. *Proteomics* **1,** 1271–1278.

Knight, Z. A., Schilling, B., Row, R. H., Kenski, D. M., and Gibson, B. W. (2003). Phosphospecific proteolysis for mapping sites of protein phosphorylation. *Nat. Biotechnol.* **21,** 1047–1054.

Koc, E. C., Burkhart, W., Blackburn, K., Koc, H., Moseley, A., and Spremulli, L. L. (2001). Identification of four proteins from the small subunit of the mammalian mitochondrial ribosome using a proteomics approach. *Protein Sci.* **10,** 471–481.

Koc, E. C., Burkhart, W., Blackburn, K., Moseley, A., Koc, H., and Spremulli, L. L. (2000). A proteomics approach to the identification of mammalian mitochondrial small subunit ribosomal proteins. *J. Biol. Chem.* **275,** 32585–32591.

LaFontaine, M. A., Geddes, J. W., and Butterfield, D. A. (2002). 3-Nitropropionic acid-induced changes in bilayer fluidity in synaptosomal membranes: Implications for Huntington's disease. *Neurochem. Res.* **27,** 507–511.

Lai, J. C. K., and Clark, J. B. (1976). Preparation and properties of mitochondria derived from synaptosomes. *Biochem. J.* **154,** 423–432.

Leonard, J. V., and Schapira, A. H. (2000a). Mitochondrial respiratory chain disorders I: Mitochondrial DNA defects. *Lancet* **355,** 299–304.

Leonard, J. V., and Schapira, A. H. (2000b). Mitochondrial respiratory chain disorders II: Neurodegenerative disorders and nuclear gene defects. *Lancet* **355,** 389–394.

Lin, T. K., Hughes, G., Muratovska, A., Blaikie, F. H., Brookes, P. S., Darley-Usmar, V., Smith, R. A., and Murphy, M. P. (2002). Specific modification of mitochondrial protein thiols in response to oxidative stress: A proteomics approach. *J. Biol. Chem.* **277,** 17048–17056.

Link, A. J., Eng, J., Schieltz, D. M., Carmack, E., Mize, G. J., Morriss, D. R., Garvik, B. M., and Yates, J. R., III. (1999). Direct analysis of protein complexes using mass spectrometry. *Nat. Biotechnol.* **17,** 696–682.

Lopez, M. F., and Melov, S. (2002). Applied proteomics: Mitochondrial proteins and effect on function. *Circ. Res.* **90,** 380–389.

Lopez, M. F., Kristal, B. S., Chernokalskaya, E., Lazarev, A., Shestopalov, A. I., Bogdanova, A., and Robinson, M. (2000). High-throughput profiling of the mitochondrial proteome using affinity fractionation and automation. *Electrophoresis* **21,** 3427–3440.

Madoz-Gurpide, J., Wang, H., Misek, D. E., Brichory, F., and Hanash, S. M. (2001). Protein based microarrays: A tool for probing the proteome of cancer cells and tissues. *Proteomics* **1,** 1279–1287.

Mann, M., Hojrup, P., and Roepstorff, P. (1993). Use of mass spectrometric molecular weight information to identify proteins in sequence databases. *Biol. Mass. Spectrom.* **22,** 338–345.

Melov, S., Coskun, P. E., and Wallace, D. C. (1999a). Mouse models of mitochondrial disease, oxidative stress and senescence. *Mutation. Res.* **434,** 233–242.

Melov, S., Coskun, P., Patel, M., Tuinistra, R., Cottrell, B., Jun, A. S., Zastawny, T. H., Dizdaroglu, M., Goodman, S. I., Huang, T., Miziorko, H., Epstein, C. J., and Wallace, D. C. (1999b). Mitochondrial disease in superoxide dismutase 2 mutant mice. *Proc. Natl. Acad. Sci. USA* **96,** 846–851.

Melov, S. (2000). Mitochondrial oxidative stress. Physiologic consequences and potential for a role in aging. *Ann. NY Acad. Sci.* **908,** 219–225.

Melov, S., Doctrow, S. R., Schneider, J. A., Haberson, J., Patel, M., Coskun, P. E., Huffman, K., Wallace, D. C., and Malfroy, B. (2001). Lifespan extension and rescue of spongiform encephalopathy in superoxide dismutase 2 nullizygous mice treated with superoxide dismutase catalase mimetics. *J. Neurosci.* **21,** 8348–8353.

Meri, S., and Baumann, M. (2001). Proteomics: Posttranslational modifications, immune responses and current analytical tools. *Biomol. Eng.* **18,** 213–220.

Michalewski, M. P., Kaczmarski, W., Golabek, A. A., Kida, E., Kaczmarski, A., and Wisniewski, K. E. (1999). Posttranslational modification of CLN3 protein and its possible functional implication. *Mol. Genet. Metab.* **66,** 272–276.

Mootha, V. K., Lepage, P., Miller, K., Bunkenborg, J., Reich, M., Hjerrild, M., Delmonte, T., Villeneuve, A., Sladek, R., Xu, F., Mitchell, G. A., Morin, C., Mann, M., Hudson, T. J., Robinson, B., Rioux, J. D., and Lander, E. S. (2003). Identification of a gene causing human cytochrome c oxidase deficiency by integrative genomics. *Proc. Natl. Acad. Sci. USA* **100,** 605–610. Epub. 2003 Jan. 14.

Murray, J., Gilkerson, R., and Capaldi, R. A. (2002). Quantitative proteomics: The copy number of pyruvate dehydrogenase is more than 10(2)-fold lower than that of complex III in human mitochondria. *FEBS Lett.* **529,** 173–178.

Ozawa, T., Sako, Y., Sato, M., Kitamura, T., and Umezawa, Y. (2003). A genetic approach to identifying mitochondrial proteins. *Nat. Biotechnol.* **23,** 287–293. Epub. 2003 Feb. 10.

Pandey, A., Podtelejnikov, A. V., Blagoev, B., Bustelo, X. R., Mann, M., and Lodish, H. F. (2000). Analysis of receptor signaling pathways by mass spectrometry: Identification of vav-2 as a substrate of the epidermal and platelet-derived growth factor receptors. *Proc. Natl. Acad. Sci. USA* **97,** 179–184.

Pappin, D. J. C., Hojrup, P., and Bleasby, A. J. (1993). Rapid identification of proteins by peptide-mass fingerprinting. *Curr. Biol.* **3,** 327–332.

Patterson, S. D., Spahr, C. S., Daugas, E., Susin, S. A., Irinopoulou, T., Koehler, C., and Kroemer, G. (2000). Mass spectrometric identification of proteins released from mitochondria undergoing permeability transition. *Cell Death Differ.* **7,** 137–144.

Patton, W. F., Schulenberg, B., and Steinberg, T. H. (2002). Two-dimensional gel electrophoresis; Better than a poke in the ICAT? *Curr. Opin. Biotechnol.* **13,** 321–328.

Paweletz, C. P., Charboneau, L., Bichsel, V. E., Simone, N. L., Chen, T., Gillespie, J. W., Emmert-Buck, M. R., Roth, M. J., Petricoin, E. F., and Liotta, L. A. (2001). Reverse phase protein microarrays which capture disease progression. *Oncogene* **20,** 1981–1989.

Petricoin, E. F., Zoon, K. C., Kohn, E. C., Barrett, J. C., and Liotta, L. A. (2002). Clinical proteomics: Translating benchside promise into bedside reality. *Nat. Rev. Drug Discov.* **1,** 683–695.

Phizicky, E., Bastiaens, P. H., Zhu, H., Snyder, M., and Fields, S. (2003). Protein analysis on a proteomic scale. *Nature* **422,** 208–215.

Plasterer, T. N., Smith, T. F., and Mohr, S. C. (2001). Survey of human mitochondrial diseases using new genomic/proteomic tools. *Genome Biol.* **2,** RESEARCH0021. Epub. 2001 Jun. 01.

Rabilloud, T. (2002). Two-dimensional electrophoresis in proteomics: old, old fashioned, but it still climbs up the mountains. *Proteomics* **2,** 3–10.

Rabilloud, T., Heller, M., Rigobello, M. P., Bindoli, A., Aebersold, R., and Lunardi, J. (2001). The mitochondrial antioxidant defense system and its response to oxidative stress. *Proteomics* **1,** 1105–1110.

Rabilloud, T., Kieffer, S., Procaccio, V., Louwagie, M., Courchesne, P. L., Patterson, S. D., Martinez, P., Garin, J., and Lunardi, J. (1998). Two-dimensional electrophoresis of human placental mitochondria: Toward a human mitochondrial proteome. *Electrophoresis* **19,** 1006–1014.

Rabilloud, T., Strub, J. M., Carte, N., Luche, S., Van Dorsselaer, A., Lunardi, J., Giege, R., and Florentz, C. (2002). Comparative proteomics as a new tool for exploring human mitochondrial tRNA disorders. *Biochemistry* **4,** 144–150.

Robinson, W. H., DiGennaro, C., Hueber, W., Haab, B. B., Kamachi, M., Dean, E. J., Fournel, S., Fong, D., Genovese, M. C., de Vegvar, H. E., Skriner, K., Hirschberg, D. L., Morris, R. I., Muller, S., Pruijn, G. J., van Venrooij, W. J., Smolen, J. S., Brown, P. O., Steinman, L., and Utz, P. J. (2002). Autoantigen microarrays for multiplex characterization of autoantibody responses. *Nat. Med.* **8,** 295–301.

Schapira, A. H. (1999). Mitochondrial disorders. *Biochim. Biophys. Acta* **1410,** 99–102.

Scheffler, I. E. (1999). "Mitochondria." Wiley-Liss, New York.

Schulenberg, B., Aggeler, R., Beecham, J. M., Capaldi, R. A., and Patton, W. F. (2003). Analysis of steady-state protein phosphorylation in mitochondria using a novel fluorescent phosphosensor dye. *J. Biol. Chem.* **278,** 27251–27255.

Sickmann, A., Reinders, J., Wagner, Y., Joppich, C., Zahedi, R., Meyer, H., Schonfisch, B., Perchill, I., Chacinska, A., Guinard, B., Rehling, P., Pfanner, N., and Meisinger, C. (2003). *Proc. Natl. Acad. Sci. USA* **100,** 13207–13212. Epub. 2003 Oct. 23.

Stadtman, E. R. (1992). Protein oxidation and aging. *Science.* **257,** 1220–1224.

Steen, H., Kuster, B., Fernandez, M., Pandey, A., and Mann, M. (2002). Tyrosine phosphorylation mapping of the epidermal growth factor receptor signaling pathway. *J. Biol. Chem.* **277,** 1031–1039.

Taylor, S. W., Fahy, E., Zhang, B., Glenn, G. M., Warnock, D. E., Wiley, S., Murphy, A. N., Gaucher, S. P., Capaldi, R. A., Gibson, B. W., and Ghosh, S. S. (2003). Characterization of the human heart mitochondrial proteome. *Nat. Biotechnol.* **21,** 281–286. Epub. 2003 Feb. 18.

Taylor, S. W., Warnock, D. E., Glenn, G. M., Zhang, B., Fahy, E., Gaucher, S. P., Capaldi, R. A., Gibson, B. W., and Ghosh, S. S. (2002). An alternative strategy to determine the mitochondrial proteome using sucrose gradient fractionation and 1D PAGE on highly purified human heart mitochondria. *J. Proteome Res.* **1,** 451–458.

Westermann, B., and Neupert, W. (2003). 'Omics' of the mitochondrion. *Nat. Biotechnol.* **21,** 239–240.

Whelan, S. A., and Hart, G. W. (2003). Proteomic approaches to analyze the dynamic relationships between nucleocytoplasmic protein glycosylation and phosphorylation. *Circ. Res.* **93,** 1047–10458.

Wolters, D. A., Washburn, M. P., and Yates, J. R., III. (2001). An automated multidimensional protein identification technology for shotgun proteomics. *Anal. Chem.* **73,** 5683–5690.

Wulfkuhle, J. D., Liotta, L. L., and Petricoin, E. F. (2003). Proteomic applications for the early detection of cancer. *Nature Reviews* **3,** 267–276.

Yates, J. R., III, Speicher, S., Griffin, P. R., and Hunkapiller, T. (1993). Peptide mass maps: A highly informative approach to protein identification. *Anal. Biochem.* **214,** 397–408.

Zhou, Z., and Menard, H. A. (2002). Autoantigenic posttranslational modifications of proteins: Does it apply to rheumatoid arthritis? *Curr. Opin. Rheumatol.* **14,** 250–253.

Zhou, Z., Watts, J. D., and Aebersold, R. (2001). A systematic approach to the analysis of protein phosphorylation. *Nat. Biotechnol.* **19,** 375–378.

SECTION II

PROTEOMIC APPLICATIONS

NMDA RECEPTORS, NEURAL PATHWAYS, AND PROTEIN INTERACTION DATABASES

Holger Husi

Division of Neuroscience
University of Edinburgh
Edinburgh EH8 9JZ, United Kingdom

I. Introduction

Proteomics in general aims to provide a comprehensive view and analysis of the characteristics and function of every protein within a given biological system at a given point of time and throughout the life span of the protein, and how the integration of all the protein components are orchestrating the cellular dynamics and cell-cell cross talk. On the other hand, the genome, which encodes the entire complement of genes in an organism, has been seen as the fundamentally complex component of cells underpinning the proteome. However, it has emerged in recent years that the genome's complexity is overshadowed by that of the transcriptome, which describes the full complement of mRNA transcripts transcribed from the genome of the cell. This in turn gives rise to yet another level of complexity in the form of the cellular proteome. This proteome is derived from the variety of alternative splicing events that occur at the level of transcription and translation, including the use of alternative start and stop sites and frame-shifting, which occurs at the level of translation. This complexity is raised even more by the approximately 300 different protein modifications that have been reported (Aebersold and Goodlett, 2001), of which phosphorylation and glycosylation are the most common. Comprehensive proteome analysis also seeks to elucidate protein subcellular distribution, protein quantification, and protein–protein interactions, which are crucial in determining the integration of large numbers of proteins into interaction networks, and functional molecular complexes that ultimately perform a myriad of cellular functions. Furthermore, the proteome is highly dynamic and temporal and undergoes constant perturbations, and thus describes the complement of proteins expressed in a cell at a single time.

Synaptic proteomics falls into the field of organellar proteomics, in which subcellular organelles and structures rather than whole cells are investigated (Taylor *et al.*, 2003). These subcellular organelles represent attractive targets for global proteome analysis because they represent discrete functional units, their complexity in protein composition is reduced relative to whole cells and, when abundant cytoskeletal proteins are removed, lower abundance proteins specific to the organelle are revealed (Fig. 1).

The postsynaptic density (PSD), which is an important dense structure located directly beneath the postsynaptic side, contains receptors with associated signaling and scaffolding proteins that organize signal-transduction pathways near the postsynaptic membrane. The PSD plays an important role in synaptic plasticity, and protein phosphorylation is critical to the regulation of PSD function, including learning and memory. Recent studies have investigated the protein constituents of the PSD and substrate proteins for various protein kinases by proteomic analysis, showing the importance of the molecular properties of PSD proteins, substrates of protein kinases, and their regulation by phosphorylation in synaptic plasticity (Grant and Husi, 2001; Husi and Grant, 2001a; Li *et al.*, 2003; Yamauchi, 2002). Functional grouping of the identified proteins indicated that the PSD in itself is a structurally and functionally complex organelle that may be involved in a broad range of synaptic activities. These activities include the receptors and ion channels for glutamate neurotransmission, proteins for maintenance and modulation of synaptic architecture, sorting and trafficking of membrane proteins, generation of anaerobic energy, scaffolding and signaling, local protein synthesis, and correct protein folding and breakdown of synaptic proteins. Together these results imply that the postsynaptic density may have the ability to function (semi-) autonomously and may direct various cellular functions in order to integrate synaptic physiology.

II. NMDA Receptor

The N-methyl-D-aspartate (NMDA) receptor (NMDAR) is an ion-channel receptor found at most excitatory synapses, where it responds to the neurotransmitter glutamate, and therefore belongs to the family of glutamate receptors. The glutamate receptors mediate excitatory neurotransmission in the brain and are important in memory acquisition, learning, and neurodegenerative disorders. The excitatory amino acid receptors can be grouped into ionotropic receptors

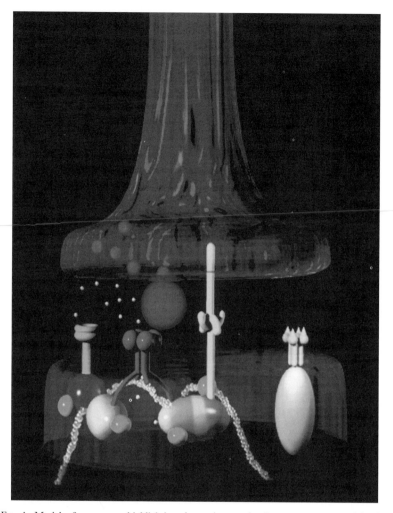

Fig. 1. Model of a synapse highlighting the various molecular components participating in synaptic function. Neurotransmitters (purple) are released from the presynaptic terminal and target postsynaptic receptors (turquoise and red), which are either channels for other small molecules such as calcium (gray), or are transmitting signals through other means such as G-proteins (blue). Other signaling machineries (green) then convey signals through specific pathways to downstream targets. Linkage between these molecules is by and large provided by cytoskeletal molecules (brown and white), and the presynaptic and postsynaptic side is tethered together by cadherins and other cell-adhesion–related molecules (yellow). (See Color Insert.)

(i.e., those in which receptor activation is directly coupled to a membrane ion channel) and metabotropic receptors (i.e., those in which receptor activation is coupled to an intracellular biochemical cascade; this may eventually lead to opening or closing of membrane ion channels, among other effects). The ionotropic receptors were the first to be classified pharmacologically (Watkins and Evans, 1981), and the broad scheme of NMDA receptors and non-NMDA (alpha-amino-3-hydroxy-5-methyl-4-isoxazolepropionate/kainate [AMPA/kainate]) ionotropic receptors, based on responses evoked by the selective agonists NMDA, AMPA, and kainate, is still in use (Watkins, 1991). Subsequently, metabolic responses to excitatory amino acid agonists were discovered (Foster and Roberts, 1981; Manzoni *et al.*, 1991; Nicoletti *et al.*, 1986), and this ultimately led to the characterization of the metabotropic glutamate receptors (mGluRs) (Pin and Duvoisin, 1995; Watkins and Collingridge, 1994) (Fig. 2). Molecular biological techniques have so far revealed the existence of four glutamate receptor subunits (GluR1–GluR4), which can be regarded as AMPA receptor subunits, and five receptor subunits, which can be regarded as kainate receptor subunits (GluR5–GluR7 and KA1, KA2). Both of these subunit groups can form homomeric and heteromeric channel assemblies with other members of their groups (Gasic and Hollmann, 1992; Hollmann and Heinemann, 1994). The NMDA-receptor-channel complex has been studied extensively, and it is known that it has a relatively higher Ca^{2+} permeability than the non-NMDA ionotropic receptors, it is blocked by Mg^{2+} in a voltage-dependent manner, it has

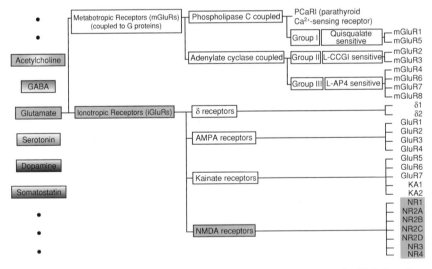

FIG. 2. The glutamate receptor family. Glutamate receptors are classified based on pharmacological properties and whether they contain seven transmembrane spanning regions and are coupled to G-proteins (metabotropic glutamate receptors), or whether they form Na^+/K^+- and/or Ca^{2+}-permeable channels (ionotropic glutamate receptors). The molecules belonging to the NMDA receptor family are highlighted in blue. (See Color Insert.)

a requirement for glycine as a coagonist, and it has modulatory sites for poly-amines, reducing agents, Zn^{2+}, and protons (McBain and Mayer, 1994). Molec-ular biological techniques have revealed that the NMDA-channel complex comprises two subunits (NR1 and NR2–NR4). There are eight splice variants of NR1, and it is thought that NR1 is a component of all native NMDA receptors, although NR1 subunits can be assembled into homomeric NR1 channels. There are four NR2 subunit types (NR2A–NR2D), which when coex-pressed with NR1, are thought to form native NMDA-receptor-channel com-plexes (Gasic and Hollmann, 1992; Hollmann and Heinemann, 1994; McBain and Mayer, 1994). Recently, two new subtypes were identified (NR3 and NR4), which are thought to be similar to the NR2 subtype; however, little is known about their actual functions in the context of glutamate-based signaling.

The NMDAR is mainly found in the postsynaptic density; however, its presynaptic localization has also been described (Froemke et al., 2003). Altera-tions in the glutamatergic system have been proposed to play a key role in the neurochemical disruptions underlying diseases such as Alzheimer's (Doraiswamy, 2003), schizophrenia (Coyle et al., 2002; McGuffin et al., 2003), Parkinson's (Blandini et al., 1996), and nociception (Petrenko et al., 2003). In particular, the similarities between the symptoms of schizophrenia and the hallucinogenic effects of some noncompetitive NMDAR antagonists such as phencyclidine indicate that a hypofunctional state of the NMDAR might underlie schizophrenia.

Largely through the use of pharmacological antagonists, the NMDAR was shown to be involved in synaptic plasticity (long-term potentiation [LTP], long-term depression [LTD]) and activation of cytoskeletal, translational, tran-scriptional, and dendritic structural changes (Sanes and Lichtman, 1999). This multitude of cellular events must be driven by a signal-transduction machinery coupled to the receptor and must be highly organized to allow a specific signal induced at the receptor to reach its predestined target.

III. Molecular Clustering

The contribution of glutamate to synaptic transmission, plasticity, and develop-ment is well established, and current evidence is based on diverse approaches to decipher function and malfunction of this principal transmitter. With respect to learning and memory, it is possible to identify more specifically the role played by the three main glutamate receptor classes in learning and memory. The key component appears to be the NMDAR, with overwhelming evidence proving its involvement in the actual learning process (encoding). Evidence for the contribution of the AMPA receptors (AMPARs) is less clear-cut due to the general problem of specifi-city, whereby a block of AMPARs will shut down neuronal communication, and this will affect various components essential for learning. Therefore the role of AMPARs cannot be established in isolation. Metabotropic glutamate receptors may contribute very little to the actual acquisition of new information. However, memory formation appears to require mGluRs, through the modulation of consolidation and/or recall (Riedel *et al.*, 2003). The studies of isolated receptors can sometimes be problematic to reveal even the potential role they have in a larger signal-transduction network, and hence large-scale analysis on interconnected protein networks might shed light on molecular modulatory roles.

Protein–protein interactions are the basis on which the cellular structure and function are built, and interaction partners are an immediate lead into biological function that can be exploited for therapeutic purposes. Proteomics has been shown to make a crucial contribution to the study of protein–protein interactions (Neubauer *et al.*, 1997). Proteomic approaches to tackle multiprotein complexes usually involve purification of the entire complex by a variety of affinity methods and protein identification by western blotting or mass-spectrometry based approaches. The first proteomic analysis of multiprotein complexes relevant to the brain was the purification and identification of the molecular constituents of the NMDA receptor complexes (NRC) (Husi and Grant, 2001b; Husi *et al.*, 2000), and this will be described as a prototypic approach to multiprotein complex proteomics.

A. NMDA Receptor Complex

Like most neurotransmitter receptors, the NMDAR has a very low abundance in neurons in comparison to the overall protein content. Therefore it is very important to generate highly enriched samples containing the target molecule(s). This can be achieved by a variety of methods, generally involving affinity chromatography steps. These steps can range from ligand affinity (e.g., drugs, substrates, cofactors, peptide ligands) to the more widely used approach of immunoprecipitation, involving specific antibodies to the molecule of interest (Husi and Grant, 2001b). A major drawback in using antibody-based approaches for proteomic analysis is the introduction of the antibody itself, which will interfere with the analysis by overshadowing proteins of interest that comigrate during the gel separation. This very same problem arises with protein-affinity–based methods, in which a recombinant protein carries one or several affinity tags (e.g., polyhistidines) or is expressed as a Glutathione-S-Transferase (GST)-fusion protein. This problem can be eliminated using either the Tandem Affinity Purification (TAP) method (Rigaut *et al.*, 1999) or non-protein based methods that exploit substrate or ligand affinities, such as peptide-based isolation procedures (Husi and Grant, 2001b). All of these ligands, groups, or proteins are then coupled to a resin, either irreversibly (usually in the case of small molecules) or through a secondary affinity linkage specific for the bait-molecule. Protein extracts are then incubated with the resins bearing the bait and bound molecules separated from each other, as well as from the matrix, by conventional gel analysis.

Identification of isolated proteins can be readily achieved using western blotting or mass spectrometry. Western blotting (also known as immunoblotting) uses specific antibodies to detect a protein that has been transferred from a gel onto a membrane. A major advantage of western blotting is its sensitivity and ability to detect amounts of protein beyond the range of current sequencing-based or mass spectrometry methodologies. It is obvious that this approach is biased by the assumption that a given molecule might be present, and therefore the approach cannot be used to identify unknown or unsuspected proteins. However, there is a large amount of neurobiological evidence concerning the putative involvement of molecules that influence many target proteins, and such proteins pose ideal targets for western blotting approaches. Additionally, changes in protein levels as a result of modulation or modification in the receptor's environment can easily be visualized using specific antibodies against the proteins under investigation. A disadvantage of this method is its labor-intensive nature and thus difficulty in performing on a large scale.

The main approaches to protein identification are peptide-mass fingerprinting using matrix-assisted laser desorption ionization (MALDI) (Henzel et al., 1993; Shevchenko et al., 1996) and electrospray ionization using a tandem mass spectrometer, (Shevchenko et al., 1997) or a combination of both (Shevchenko et al., 2000a). Recent developments led to new methodologies that use direct liquid chromatography/tandem mass spectrometry (LC-MS/MS) techniques, which allow fast and reliable mapping of very low amounts of peptides in an almost completely automated fashion (Shevchenko et al., 2000b). Furthermore, using this method, it is also possible to determine if a protein or peptide carries any post-translational modifications such as glycosylation or phosphorylation (Pandey et al., 2000b).

The sample is usually separated on a gel and the bands of interest excised and treated with trypsin to generate fragments of proteins that can subsequently be extracted from the gel slice. There are several reasons for analyzing peptides rather than proteins. The peptide's mass can be measured with much greater precision than the mass of intact proteins. Peptides give rise to a library of molecular masses that are directly derived from the proteins, which can be identified using computational techniques (Berndt et al., 1999).

Using such proteomic approaches, it was recently shown that the NMDAR is part of a network composed of more than 77 molecules, of which 30 are implicated from binding studies and another 19 participate in NMDAR signaling (Fig. 3) (Husi et al., 2000). The NRC consists of: (1) glutamate receptors—both NMDAR and metabotropic mGluRs are found within the same complexes; however, another important-glutamate receptor, the AMPA receptor, could not be detected; (2) adaptor proteins, which include PSD-95; (3) second messenger

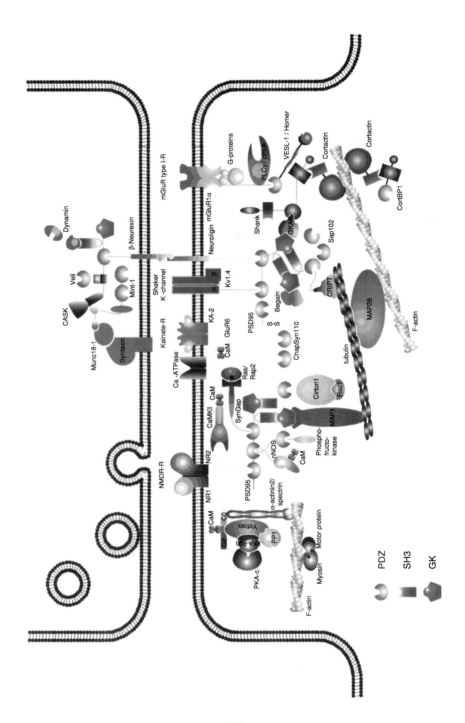

enzymes, including protein kinases and phosphatases; (4) cytoskeletal proteins and (5) cell-adhesion proteins. A striking feature of the composition is that there appear to be "modules" or sets of signaling proteins known to comprise key components of signal-transduction pathways that can be distinctly regulated. For example, all of the molecules necessary to induce the phosphorylation of mito-gen-activated protein kinase (MAPK) following NMDAR stimulation are present in the NRC (including *Ca^{2+} calmodulin-dependent protein kinase II* [CaMKII], *synaptic GTPase-activating protein* [SynGAP], Ras, c-Raf1, *MAPK/ERK kinase* [MEK] and *extracellular signal-regulated kinase* [ERK] (see Fig. 3). These modules may allow the NMDAR and mGluR to integrate signals within the complex and then couple to downstream cellular effector mechanisms, such as trafficking of AMPA receptors and cytoskeletal changes that mediate structural and physiological plasticity. Furthermore, at least 18 NRC constituents are regulated by synaptic activity, indicating that the composition of the complex is dynamic. In hippocampus, these activity-dependent genes are known to undergo specific temporal changes following the induction of plasticity.

Genetic or pharmacological interference with 15 NRC proteins impairs learning, and with 22 proteins alters synaptic plasticity in rodents. Mutations in three human genes (*neurofibromatosis type 1* [NF1], *ribosomal subunit kinase 2* [Rsk-2], L1) are associated with learning impairments, indicating the NRC also participates in human cognition.

This NRC dataset was further expanded using a combination of peptide affinity chromatography and mass spectrometry identification of new components of the complex (Husi *et al.*, 2003). Purification of MASCs (*membrane-associated guanylate kinases* [MAGUK]-associated signaling complexes) was achieved by peptide affinity chromatography, using a hexapeptide corresponding to the C-terminus of the NMDA-R2B subunit. This approach extended the NRC dataset to comprise 184 proteins, which constitute the MASC (Husi *et al.*, 2003). Also, AMPA complexes were purified using immunoaffinity chromatography, resulting in the identification of 10 unique proteins. These two receptor complex datasets, togeth-er with the PSD, provide for the first time a general composition of the postsynaptic proteome, which totaled 698 distinct proteins. The main overlap was seen between MASC and the PSD, with 108 common proteins (Husi *et al.*, 2003).

FIG. 3. Schematic diagram of synaptic multiprotein complexes. Postsynaptic complexes of proteins associated with the NMDA receptor and PSD-95, found at excitatory mammalian synapses, are shown. Individual proteins are illustrated with arbitrary shapes, and known interactions are indicated. Proteins shown in color are those found in a proteomic screen, whereas those shown in gray are inferred from bioinformatic studies. The specific protein–protein interactions are predicted, based on published reports from yeast two-hybrid studies. Membrane proteins (e.g., receptors, channels, and adhesion molecules) are attached to a network of intracellular scaffold, signaling, and cytoskeletal proteins, as indicated. (See Color Insert.)

B. Other Receptor Complexes

Since the *characterization* of the NRC, other receptor complexes have been reported. P2X receptors are adenosine triphosphate (ATP)-gated ion channels in the plasma membrane, and activation of the P2X7 receptor also leads to rapid cytoskeletal rearrangements such as membrane distortions. *Eleven* proteins in human embryonic kidney cells that interact with the rat P2X7 receptor were identified by affinity purification followed by mass spectroscopy and immuno-blotting (Kim *et al.*, 2001). Using a proteomic approach based on peptide affinity chromatography and mass spectrometric and immunoblotting analysis, another study identified 15 proteins that interact with the C-terminal tail of the 5-hydroxytryptamine 2C (5-HT$_{2C}$) receptor (Becamel *et al.*, 2002). These proteins include several synaptic multidomain proteins that contain one or several PDZ domains (PSD-95 and the proteins of the tripartite complex Veli3-CASK-Mint1), proteins of the actin/spectrin cytoskeleton, and signaling proteins. Coimmuno-precipitation experiments showed that 5-HT$_{2C}$ receptors interact with PSD-95 and the Veli3-CASK-Mint1 complex *in vivo*. Electron microscopy also indicated a synaptic enrichment of Veli3 and 5-HT$_{2C}$ receptors and their co-localization in microvilli of choroidal cells. These results indicate that the 5-HT$_{2C}$ receptor is associated with protein networks that are important for its synaptic localization and its coupling to the signaling machinery (Becamel *et al.*, 2002). Additionally, in neurons and glia, plasma membrane microdomains containing NCX1 (*Na$^+$/Ca^{2+} exchanger subtype 1*) and Na$^+$ pumps form Ca^{2+}-signaling complexes with underlying endoplasmic reticulum containing the sarcoplasmic reticulum Ca^{2+} ATPase SERCA2 (*sarco [endo] plasmic reticulum Ca^{2+} ATPase-2*) and the inositol *triphosphate* receptor IP(3)R-1, and these components appear to be linked through the cytoskeletal spectrin network (Lencesova *et al.*, 2003).

It is now emerging that multiprotein signaling complexes or "signaling machines," of which the NRC is prototypic, are responsible for orchestrating the complex signaling events at ionotrophic glutamate receptors (Husi *et al.*, 2000), ATP receptors (Kim *et al.*, 2001), and G-protein coupled receptors (Becamel *et al.*, 2002; *GPCR*). They seem to share a common *organization* of receptor, protein scaffold (in which the signaling molecules are *localized*), and membrane to cytoskeletal interactions. Therefore study of individual receptor multiprotein complexes such as the NRC will most likely provide a mechanistic basis that will be very useful and applicable for the systematic identification and study of membrane receptor complexes associated with the estimated 100 other receptor types believed to exist in the brain. This paradigm of "fate or guilt by association" (i.e., pathways lined by physical interactions) has several key aspects: the bypassing of random events, unilateral downstream processing, and high efficiency. This tethering of signaling components also introduces time-delay signaling via branched signal transduction (i.e., direct tagging found in phosphorylation cascades) and diffusional signaling through Ca^{2+} release, for example.

IV. Signal Transduction Pathways

Interactions of neurotransmitters with their cognate receptors led to the generation of second messengers such as cyclic AMP and Ca^{2+}, which regulate the activity of intracellular protein kinases and protein phosphatases, which in turn alters the binding properties of other molecules. Such post-translational modifications are important tagging mechanisms within a living cell and serve to indicate specific properties of a protein, such as stability, turnover, localization, activity, and specificity. Proteomic approaches are ideal analytical tools to study these modifications. Activation of several receptors, including the NMDAR, results in tyrosine-phosphorylation of a large set of substrates. These events can be observed by antibody-based techniques (e.g., phosphorylation-state specific antibodies) and mass spectrometry. Several studies used proteomic tools to characterize tyrosine-phosphorylated proteins on epidermal growth factor (EGF) (Steen *et al.*, 2002) or platelet-derived growth factor (PDGF) (Pandey *et al.*, 2000a) stimulation of fibroblasts. In analogy to such effects, it is also possible to induce physiological changes such as ischaemia in living animals (Horsburgh *et al.*, 2000), followed by analysis of the protein changes. It could be shown that ischaemia induction leads to an elevated level of a specific phosphorylation event of the NMDAR subunit NR1 on Ser890, whereas another known phosphorylation site on Ser897 is apparently not, or only very marginally, affected. Activation of the NRC also leads to a down-regulation of proteolytic events of the NMDAR channel components NR1 and NR2B, and lateral molecules of the NMDAR, like PSD-95, are not affected by breakdown processes. A conclusion could be that activation of the NMDA-sensitive network of proteins leads to an increase of phosphorylation events, thereby protecting the molecules from degradation (Bao *et al.*, 2001). Based on results obtained by analyzing the NRC, one potential protease, Calpain, could be the mediator of the integrity of the molecular NRC cluster (Fig. 4).

The facilitation of hippocampus-based, long-lasting synaptic plasticity, which is frequently investigated in model systems such as long-term potentiation and in learning paradigms such as the Morris water maze, is associated with several cellular key events: Ca^{2+} influx through the NMDAR; generation of cyclic AMP (cAMP); and activation of protein kinase A (PKA); phosphorylation of (MAPK) and cAMP-response element-binding protein (CREB); and subsequent transcription of plasticity-associated genes (Figs. 4 and 5). Recently, a signal-transduction cascade from cAMP/PKA to MAPK was discovered, which seems to be neuron-specific and comprises the critical events of hippocampus-based, long-term plasticity into one single cascade. A major alternative to cAMP/PKA-MAPK signaling is the cascades from Ca^{2+} to MAPK via Ras. However, Ras is inhibited by PKA (Waltereit and Weller, 2003).

NMDA and AMPA/kainate receptors act as glutamate-gated cation channels, whereas mGluRs modulate the production of second messengers via G-proteins. Metabotropic glutamate receptors have been shown to stimulate phosphatidylinositol metabolism, and subsequently, liberate Ca^{2+} from intracellular stores. Glutamate can stimulate phosphatidylinositol metabolism, generating inositol-1,4,5-trisphosphate (IP3), and ultimately liberate Ca^{2+} from intracellular

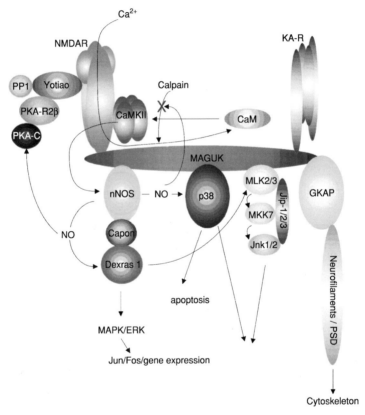

Fig. 4. Schematic representation of a potential signal-transduction pathway following NMDAR activation and Ca^{2+} influx by NRC tethered components. Ca^{2+} leads to activation of Calmodulin (CaM), which in turn activates CaMKII. Nitric oxide (NO) is produced by *neuronal nitric oxide synthase* (nNOS) after activation by CaMKII, and this potent messenger leads to activation of *protein kinase A* (PKA), *dexamethasone-induced RAS protein 1* (Dexras1), p38) *protein kinase*, and *mixed lineage kinase 2/3* (MLK2/3), as well as inhibition of Calpain and ultimately to downstream events, including gene expression. (See Color Insert.)

stores of neurons (Fig. 5) (Nakanishi *et al.*, 1998; Zirpel *et al.*, 1995). This in turn leads to activation of calmodulin (CaM) and ultimately triggers downstream pathways, including the MAPK cascade and gene expression. This exemplifies how the underlying molecular signaling machinery of the NRC is coupled to several receptors and used in a variety of ways; therefore it is not surprising that all of the components of the aforementioned pathways can be found in close vicinity tethered to the NMDAR.

Information contained within signal pathway databases (Table I) can also be used to extend the knowledge of potential additional pathways embedded in the NRC. The expansion of known signaling pathways within a variety of species and integration with other pathways, such as metabolic ones (see Table I), will undoubtedly lead to a better understanding of the molecular interplay within protein networks. The main obstacle is the sheer volume of information to handle, and as technology advances, even more data will be available, which in turn requires automation of data processing and handling.

V. Bioinformatic Analysis

The description of physical protein (and gene) interaction networks will likely provide new insights into cellular regulation and the machinery of signal-transduction networks. Large protein networks are ideal candidates for computational analysis and prediction of protein-protein interactions, as was shown for protein networks in *Saccharomyces cerevisiae* in publications during the last several years (Gavin *et al.*, 2002; Ho *et al.*, 2002; Verma *et al.*, 2000). A similar analysis at a less complex level, using proteins present in the NMDA receptor complex in which all published interactions were taken into consideration, suggests a molecular network such as that shown in Fig. 6, consisting of approximately 250 molecules. Because no real proof exists that such an orchestration of events does occur, it is still a working hypothesis that needs to be tested by various strategies. However, this demonstrates that searching for known interaction partners described in databases can elucidate interactions of novel proteins within networks. The development of computational methods to detect functional linkages among predicted proteins has also helped to accelerate the functional analysis of novel proteins.

The number of comparative *two-dimensional/mass spectrometry* (2D/MS) studies of disease and disease models has increased over the last number of years. This has led to the accumulation of lists of proteins whose expression levels have been shown to be altered in the particular system, but with little integration of these lists to provide a global view. This is an emerging problem in the study of complex diseases, not only at the level of proteomics, but also at the level of study of individual protein function in relation to disease. Complex diseases are

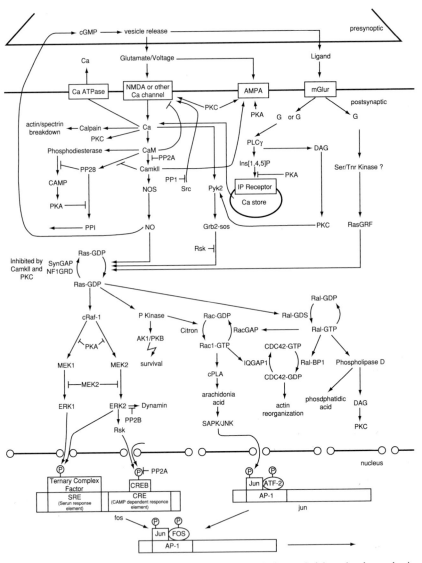

Fig. 5. Potential interplay of glutamate receptors and the underlying signal-transduction machinery. Molecular pathways, which were described in this chapter to play a crucial role in glutamate-triggered molecular events, were assembled and extended where possible based on the presence of proteins found in the NRC. Glutamate receptors (white boxes) are located in the membrane of the post-synaptic side, and once activated trigger the underlying signaling cascades, and eventually lead to gene expression.

TABLE I

Website Addresses of Signaling, Metabolic and Enzymatic Pathway Databases

Signaling pathways	
AfCS	http://www.signaling-gateway.org
aMAZE	http://www.ebi.ac.uk/research/amaze/
BioCarta	http://www.biocarta.com/genes/index.asp
CSNDB	http://geo.nihs.go.jp/csndb/
SPAD	http://www.grt.kyushu-u.ac.jp/eny-doc/spad.html
Metabolic and enzymatic pathways	
BioCyc	http://biocyc.org/
EMP	http://ergo.integratedgenomics.com/EMP/
KLOTHO	http://www.biocheminfo.org/klotho/
MMP	http://home.wxs.nl/~pvsanten/mmp/mmp.html
UM-BBD	http://umbbd.ahc.umn.edu/
Roche pathway map	http://www.expasy.org/cgi-bin/search-biochem-index

ideal candidates to be studied by proteomic approaches. The very nature of the complexity involved, and the underlying molecular anomalities, requires a global approach. An example of one such study relates to the work on the NRC, described earlier in the Chapter.

The identification of NRC and its network properties provides a unique opportunity to explore human cognition and its disorders. Although it is generally accepted that cognitive mechanisms are conserved between mice and humans, it is unclear how much the rodent molecular studies map onto human psychiatric conditions. The possibility that NRC proteins may be involved with human psychiatric and neurological disorders was investigated, and it was found that 46 NRC proteins are implicated in mental illness in the literature (Fig. 7). Although all mental disorders were searched, 26 NRC proteins were found in schizophrenia, 18 in mental retardation, 7 in bipolar disorder, and 6 in depressive illness. This apparent bias toward schizophrenia and mental retardation could be biologically relevant because both illnesses have a major cognitive component to their primary symptoms, unlike the affective disorders.

A number of studies have focused on Alzheimer's disease (AD) and molecules relating to this illness (Schonberger *et al.*, 2001; Tilleman *et al.*, 2002). Analysis of a protein-protein interaction network (Fig. 8) of molecules implicated in AD pathology in relation to functional complexes at the synapse revealed that 54 out of the identified 97 proteins associated with AD are components of the *PSD* proteome, 32 are found in the NRC, and 3 are present in the AMPA receptor complex. This also showed a large overlap of 30 proteins common to the PSD and NRC that are implicated in AD. It is probable that there are subsets of proteins within the large number of proteins associated with AD that represent distinct mechanisms, leading to the formation of amyloid plaques and neurofibrillary tangles characteristic of AD.

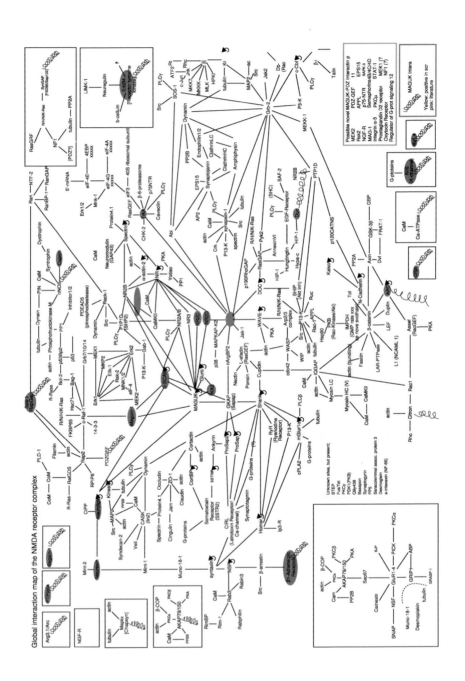

Global interaction map of the NMDA receptor complex

The large numbers of implicated proteins present in the NRC and AMPAR indicate that altered signaling from these membrane receptors may be responsible for the loss of synaptic function and cognitive decline associated with several diseases. Elucidating the involvement of particular pathways in a systematic way should begin to uncover these various molecular routes to the diseased state. This approach of network integration of components of a complex disease should provide a coherent view of the disease process at the molecualr level. Network analysis of many other complex diseases might indicate new leads into the mechanisms of pathology and areas of therapeutic intervention.

VI. Proteomic Databases

The paradigm that molecules within living cells are not only compartmentalized but also associate into modules or complexes, and these modules are then assembled to become part of even larger complexes, is a new concept of biological function. To study these clusters of proteins requires the handling of large datasets, regardless whether they were acquired by mass-spectrometric, antibody-based, or yeast two-hybrid screens. Furthermore, proteomic analysis in any system encompasses many areas, and integration of this data into biologically meaningful knowledge is the ultimate goal. Current efforts in deciphering complete genomes have opened the floodgates of sequence information. However, little is known on a comparative level among species. One major drawback is that currently there is no "unifying" database available that combines all the knowledge gathered so far, which in turn means that any large-scale screen needs to be analyzed manually in one way or another. Such analyses usually involve retrieving sequence information from the databases listed in Table II. Many of these databases contain a high redundancy ratio, and it can therefore be difficult to retrieve large amounts of data with a minimum of repetition.

Another set of databases deals explicitly with protein-interaction data gathered from literature-mining and large-scale analysis from yeast, for example. Several of such proteomic databases describing protein-protein interactions exist today (Table III). Many of these databases are not based on unified sequence databases and hold loosely gathered information for a minority of all proteins found in any proteome. However, even at the current state of many of these data resources, they

---

Fig. 6. Global interaction map of the NRC. Yellow-colored molecules were found in a screen of the NRC, and pink denotes proteins that were shown by individual publications to interact with adjacent molecules. Small boxes denote molecules that tether to PSD-95 and other members of the MAGUK family. The black box contains the AMPA receptor complex, which does not link into the NRC. (See Color Insert.)

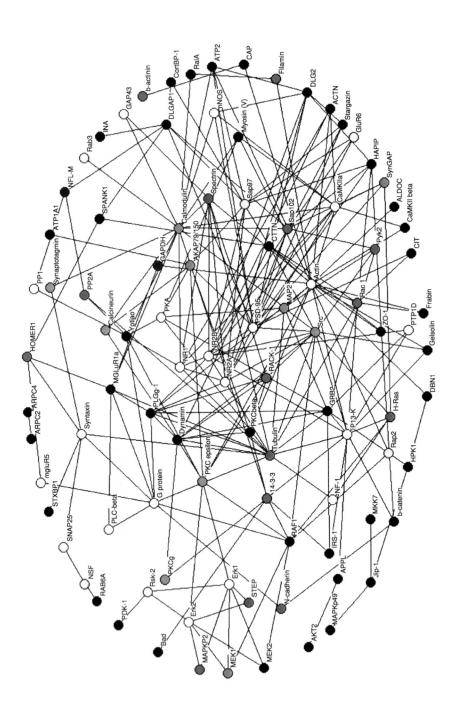

68

are good enough for initial network analysis, but are problematic when trying to use a semi, automated or completely automated attempt. This raises the need for a novel type of database that not only deals with the vast amount of sequence data (and its redundancies), but also contains information about expression, modification, abundance, similarity, homology, and interaction data, preferably across more than one proteome. Additionally, there is also a need to interpret any data obtained from large-scale screens to be analyzed visually e.g., by network drawing and clustering, domain analysis, functional assignments.

Currently, there are a few attempts emerging to integrate this vast amount of information, combining sources from molecular biology, physiology, and other areas. One such combinatorial database can be exemplified by the proteomic analysis database (PADB) (Fig. 9).

This database is filling the gap by unifying molecular entries across several species by using homology and ortholog maps. It is footed on sequence databases such as SwissProt, EMBL, TrEMBL (translated EMBL sequences), RefSeq, and UniGene (see Table II) and the literature database PubMed (www.ncbi.nlm.nih. gov/PubMed/). There is a sub database called SESwiss (Something Else Swiss), which is a sequence and protein feature database. Primary data in SESwiss is acquired by batch processes for whole proteomes from the databases listed in Table II, merged, and made nonredundant by manual database mining using BLAST searches and ClustalW alignments to identify novel splice variants. SESwiss includes the phosphoproteomic database PPO4, which lists phosphorylation sites identified by experimentation and/or publication. A typical entry in PADB holds all protein and gene accession numbers associated with them, protein and gene sequences, post-translational protein modifications, and the OMIM (*Online Mendelian Inheritance in Man*) entry as maintained by Johns Hopkins University in Baltimore (www.ncbi.nlm.nih.gov/entrez/query.fcgi?db=OMIM). Entry points also include protein-binding information together with the literature reference (see Fig. 9). These physical protein-protein interaction maps, complexes, and genetic interactions are held in the subdatabase PPID (protein–protein interaction database). Entries in PPID are retrieved by manual literature searches using protein name entries, including synonyms, analysis of large proteomic

---

FIG. 7. Network representation of NRC proteins with phenotypic annotation. Ninety-seven NRC proteins with known direct protein interactions to other NRC proteins are plotted. The NMDA receptor subunits (NR1, NR2A, NR2B) are located in the center. The association of each protein with plasticity, rodent behavior, or human psychiatric disorders is shown in the color of the node. Key: black-no known association; red-psychiatric disorder; green-plasticity; blue-rodent behavior; yellow-psychiatric disorders and plasticity; cyan-plasticity and rodent behavior; white-all three phenotypes; and orange-psychiatric disorders and rodent behavior. The network provides a common connection or association among these disease molecules. Network simulations also show that disruption of combinations of proteins produce more severe effects on the network. This suggests that combinations of proteins (or mutant alleles) underpin the polygenic nature of a variety of disorders. (See Color Insert.)

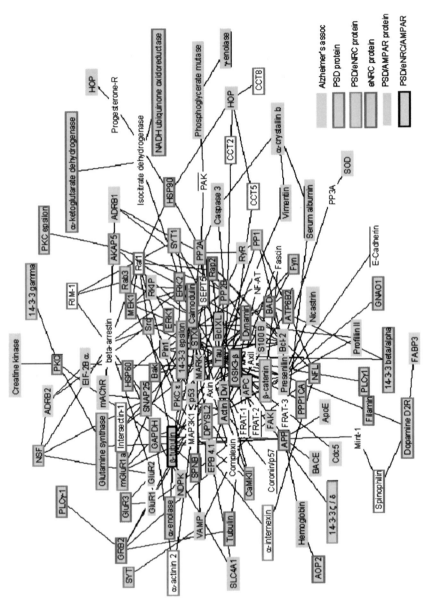

Fig. 8. Network cluster of proteins associated with Alzheimer's disease within the NRC and AMPAR complexes. (See Color Insert.)

TABLE II
WEBSITE ADDRESSES OF PROTEIN AND DNA SEQUENCE DATABASES

Swiss-Prot/TrEMBL	http://www.expasy.org
ENTREZ	http://www.ncbi.nlm.nih.gov/Entrez/index.html
UniGene	http://www.ncbi.nlm.nih.gov/entrez/query.fcgi?db=unigene
EMBL/TIGR	http://www.ebi.ac.uk/embl/index.html
Ensembl	http://www.ebi.ac.uk/ensembl/index.html
RefSeq/RefGen	http://www.ncbi.nlm.nih.gov/RefSeq/
IPI	http://www.ebi.ac.uk/IPI/IPIhelp.html

TABLE III
WEBSITE ADDRESSES OF PROTEIN–PROTEIN INTERACTION DATABASES

BIND	http://www.blueprint.org/bind/bind.php
BRITE	http://www.genome.ad.jp/brite/
Cellzome	http://yeast.cellzome.com/
DIP	http://dip.doe-mbi.ucla.edu/
GRID	http://biodata.mshri.on.ca/grid/index.html
HPRD	http://www.hprd.org/
InterPreTS	http://www.russell.embl.de/interprets/
MINT	http://cbm.bio.uniroma2.it/mint/
MIPS	http://mips.gsf.de/genre/proj/yeast/index.jsp
PathCalling–CuraGen	http://portal.curagen.com/extpc/com.curagen.portal.servlet.Yeast
PIM-Hybrigenics	http://www.hybrigenics.fr/
Riken-PPI	http://fantom21.gsc.riken.go.jp/PPI/
PPID	http://www.ppid.org

studies based on original data only, and inclusion of large datasets from yeast two hybrid studies. Currently, PPID holds approximately 8000 mammalian protein-interaction points and more than 14,000 interactions for yeast proteins. Another aspect of PADB deals with expression maps of proteins in various tissues. This information is stored in the subdatabase EMAP (Expression MAP). Further-more, PADB also holds data relating to orthologs and homologs in the OMAP database. This database was constructed by manual sequence alignments using ClustalW and BLAST searches and the results compared to other ortholog databases such as COG (*clusters of orthologous genes*), MBGD (*microbial genome database*), InParanoid, and HomoloGene. The whole database is manually curated as far as possible to ensure accuracy and quality. Data analysis will be made available offering BLAST and ClustalW searches, and whole datasets can be investigated by batch submission using accession numbers from various databases. These accession numbers are then made nonredundant by conver-sion to PADB internal accession numbers and are submitted via PPID and

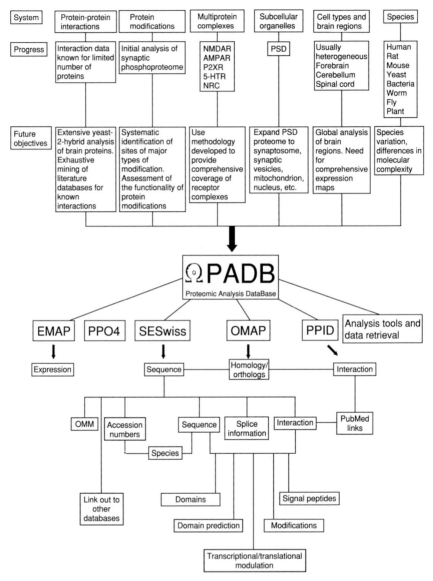

Fig. 9. Overview of the progress and objectives of proteomics and the structure of PADB, a proteomic analysis database.

other parts of the database for network analysis, features, orthologs, diseases, etc., offering a comprehensive system from data retrieval to cluster analysis and beyond.

VII. Future Directions

In general terms the function of the brain could be defined by the number, type, and location of multiprotein complexes. Given that multiprotein complexes act as molecular machines, where the sum of their components is required to perform specific functions, a broad and comprehensive catalogue of complexes would provide a platform for the study of brain function. For example, the NRC contains receptors other than the NMDAR. These complexes are not likely to be unique in this general function, and it is expected that other complexes will also convert activity into cellular changes but with different properties. A list of complexes can provide a basis for maps of interactions or functional connection between complexes. Assessing the function of the complexes in the brain will require a combination of integrated approaches. As a result, it is apparent that there is a growing need for bioinformatic tools and databases to deal with the amount of data being acquired by proteomic methodologies. Integrative proteomic databases such as PADB will be essential for the analysis of such data. The ability to submit whole datasets to such databases and retrieve comprehensive protein information, including protein-protein interactions, will greatly reduce the current bottleneck of manual analysis of large numbers of proteins. Such assembly of proteins into networks has been facilitated by this tailored proteomic

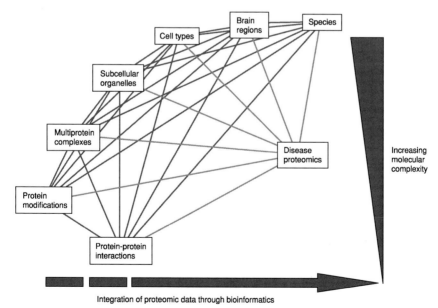

Fig. 10. Overview of levels of proteomic complexity.

database, and such insights into global basic biology would not be possible in its absence. Bioinformatic analysis of proteomes is in its infancy, and future objectives of the comprehensive analysis of many proteomes that exist are ambitious but necessary (Fig. 10). Basic information on protein interactions, protein modifications, and multiprotein complexes has to be obtained for relevant subcellular structures in various cell types and brain regions and integrated with previously published functional information. Within such a framework of biological knowledge, complex biological problems and pathologies can be addressed in a less biased and comprehensive way than ever thought possible. Integration of diverse proteomic data to provide a global view is an ambitious but achievable long-term task, which will only be accomplished by *standardization* of data, very powerful bioinformatic tools, and comprehensive databases.

References

Aebersold, R., and Goodlett, D. R. (2001). Mass spectrometry in proteomics. *Chem. Rev.* **101,** 269–295.

Bao, W. L., Williams, A. J., Faden, A. I., and Tortella, F. C. (2001). Selective mGluR5 receptor antagonist or agonist provides neuroprotection in a rat model of focal cerebral ischemia. *Brain Res.* **922,** 173–179.

Becamel, C., Alonso, G., Galeotti, N., Demey, E., Jouin, P., Ullmer, C., Dumuis, A., Bockaert, J., and Marin, P. (2002). Synaptic multiprotein complexes associated with 5-HT(2C) receptors: A proteomic approach. *EMBO J.* **21,** 2332–2342.

Berndt, P., Hobohm, U., and Langen, H. (1999). Reliable automatic protein identification from matrix-assisted laser desorption/ionization mass spectrometric peptide fingerprints. *Electrophoresis* **20,** 3521–3526.

Blandini, F., Porter, R. H., and Greenamyre, J. T. (1996). Glutamate and Parkinson's disease. *Mol. Neurobiol.* **12,** 73–94.

Coyle, J. T., Tsai, G., and Goff, D. C. (2002). Ionotropic glutamate receptors as therapeutic targets in schizophrenia. *Curr. Drug Target CNS Neurol. Disord.* **1,** 183–189.

Doraiswamy, P. M. (2003). Alzheimer's disease and the glutamate NMDA receptor. *Psychopharmacol. Bull.* **37,** 41–49.

Foster, G. A., and Roberts, P. J. (1981). Kainic acid stimulation of cerebellar cyclic GMP levels: Potentiation by glutamate and related amino acids. *Neurosci. Lett.* **23,** 67–70.

Froemke, R. C., Li, C. Y., and Dan, Y. (2003). A form of presynaptic coincidence detection. *Neuron* **39,** 579–581.

Gasic, G. P., and Hollmann, M. (1992). Molecular neurobiology of glutamate receptors. *Annu. Rev. Physiol.* **54,** 507–536.

Gavin, A. C., Bosche, M., Krause, R., Grandi, P., Marzioch, M., Bauer, A., Schultz, J., Rick, J. M., Michon, A. M., Cruciat, C. M., Remor, M., Hofert, C., Schelder, M., Brajenovic, M., Ruffner, H., Merino, A., Klein, K., Hudak, M., Dickson, D., Rudi, T., Gnau, V., Bauch, A., Bastuck, S., Huhse, B., Leutwein, C., Heurtier, M. A., Copley, R. R., Edelmann, A., Querfurth, E., Rybin, V., Drewes, G., Raida, M., Bouwmeester, T., Bork, P., Seraphin, B., Kuster, B., Neubauer, G., and Superti-Furga, G. (2002). Functional organization of the yeast proteome by systematic analysis of protein complexes. *Nature* **415**, 141–147.

Grant, S. G., and Husi, H. (2001). Proteomics of multiprotein complexes: Answering fundamental questions in neuroscience. *Trends Biotechnol.* **19**, S49–S54.

Henzel, W. J., Billeci, T. M., Stults, J. T., Wong, S. C., Grimley, C., and Watanabe, C. (1993). Identifying proteins from two-dimensional gels by molecular mass searching of peptide fragments in protein sequence databases. *Proc. Natl. Acad. Sci. USA* **90**, 5011–5015.

Ho, Y., Gruhler, A., Heilbut, A., Bader, G. D., Moore, L., Adams, S. L., Millar, A., Taylor, P., Bennett, K., Boutilier, K., Yang, L., Wolting, C., Donaldson, I., Schandorff, S., Shewnarane, J., Vo, M., Taggart, J., Goudreault, M., Muskat, B., Alfarano, C., Dewar, D., Lin, Z., Michalickova, K., Willems, A. R., Sassi, H., Nielsen, P. A., Rasmussen, K. J., Andersen, J. R., Johansen, L. E., Hansen, L. H., Jespersen, H., Podtelejnikov, A., Nielsen, E., Crawford, J., Poulsen, V., Sorensen, B. D., Matthiesen, J., Hendrickson, R. C., Gleeson, F., Pawson, T., Moran, M. F., Durocher, D., Mann, M., Hogue, C. W., Figeys, D., and Tyers, M. (2002). Systematic identification of protein complexes in Saccharomyces cerevisiae by mass spectrometry. *Nature* **415**, 180–183.

Hollmann, M., and Heinemann, S. (1994). Cloned glutamate receptors. *Annu. Rev. Neurosci.* **17**, 31–108.

Horsburgh, K., McCulloch, J., Nilsen, M., McCracken, E., Large, C., Roses, A. D., and Nicoll, J. A. (2000). Intraventricular infusion of apolipoprotein E ameliorates acute neuronal damage after global cerebral ischemia in mice. *J. Cereb. Blood Flow Metab.* **20**, 458–462.

Husi, H., Ward, M. A., Choudhary, J. S., Blackstock, W. P., and Grant, S. G. (2000). Proteomic analysis of NMDA receptor-adhesion protein signaling complexes. *Nat. Neurosci.* **3**, 661–669.

Husi, H., and Grant, S. G. (2001a). Proteomics of the nervous system. *Trends Neurosci.* **24**, 259–266.

Husi, H., and Grant, S. G. (2001b). Isolation of 2000-kDa complexes of N-methyl-D-aspartate receptor and postsynaptic density 95 from mouse brain. *J. Neurochem.* **77**, 281–291.

Husi, H., Choudhary, J., Yu, L., Collins, M. O., Blackstock, W., and Grant, S. G. N. (2004). Composition of the post-synaptic proteome: Analysis of the post-synaptic density, glutamate receptor and scaffolding complexes by mass spectrometry. Submitted.

Kim, M., Jiang, L. H., Wilson, H. L., North, R. A., and Surprenant, A. (2001). Proteomic and functional evidence for a P2X7 receptor signalling complex. *EMBO J.* **20**, 6347–6358.

Lencesova, L., O'Neill, A., Resneck, W. G., Bloch, R. J., and Blaustein, M. P. (2004). Plasma membrane-cytoskeleton-endoplasmic reticulum complexes in neurons and astrocytes. *J. Biol. Chem.* **279**, 2885–2893.

Li, K. W., Hornshaw, M. P., Van Der Schors, R. C., Watson, R., Tate, S., Casetta, B., Jimenez, C. R., Gouwenberg, Y., Gundelfinger, E. D., Smalla, K. H., and Smit, A. B. (2004). Proteomics analysis of rat brain postsynaptic density: Implications of the diverse protein functional groups for the integration of synaptic physiology. *J. Biol. Chem.* **279**, 987–1002.

Manzoni, O. J., Prezeau, L., and Bockaert, J. (1991). beta-N-methylamino-L-alanine is a low-affinity agonist of metabotropic glutamate receptors. *Neuroreport* **2**, 609–611.

McBain, C. J., and Mayer, M. L. (1994). N-methyl-D-aspartic acid receptor structure and function. *Physiol. Rev.* **74**, 723–760.

McGuffin, P., Tandon, K., and Corsico, A. (2003). Linkage and association studies of schizophrenia. *Curr. Psychiatry Rep.* **5**, 121–127.

Nakanishi, S., Nakajima, Y., Masu, M., Ueda, Y., Nakahara, K., Watanabe, D., Yamaguchi, S., Kawabata, S., and Okada, M. (1998). Glutamate receptors: Brain function and signal transduction. *Brain Res. Brain Res. Rev.* **26**, 230–235.

Neubauer, G., Gottschalk, A., Fabrizio, P., Seraphin, B., Luhrmann, R., and Mann, M. (1997). Identification of the proteins of the yeast U1 small nuclear ribonucleoprotein complex by mass spectrometry. *Proc. Natl. Acad. Sci. USA* **94**, 385–390.

Nicoletti, F., Wroblewski, J. T., Novelli, A., Guidotti, A., and Costa, E. (1986). Excitatory amino acid signal transduction in cerebellar cell cultures. *Funct. Neurol.* **1**, 345–349.

Pin, J. P., and Duvoisin, R. (1995). The metabotropic glutamate receptors: Structure and functions. *Neuropharmacology* **34**, 1–26.

Pandey, A., Fernandez, M. M., Steen, H., Blagoev, B., Nielsen, M. M., Roche, S., Mann, M., and Lodish, H. F. (2000a). Identification of a novel immunoreceptor tyrosine-based activation motif-containing molecule, STAM2, by mass spectrometry and its involvement in growth factor and cytokine receptor signaling pathways. *J. Biol. Chem.* **275**, 38633–38639.

Pandey, A., Podtelejnikov, A. V., Blagoev, B., Bustelo, X. R., Mann, M., and Lodish, H. F. (2000b). Analysis of receptor signaling pathways by mass spectrometry: Identification of vav-2 as a substrate of the epidermal and platelet-derived growth factor receptors. *Proc. Natl. Acad. Sci. USA* **97**, 179–184.

Petrenko, A. B., Yamakura, T., Baba, H., and Shimoji, K. (2003). The role of N-methyl-D-aspartate (NMDA) receptors in pain: A review. *Anesth. Analg.* **97**, 1108–1116.

Riedel, G., Platt, B., and Micheau, J. (2003). Glutamate receptor function in learning and memory. *Behav. Brain Res.* **140**, 1–47.

Rigaut, G., Shevchenko, A., Rutz, B., Wilm, M., Mann, M., and Seraphin, B. (1999). A generic protein purification method for protein complex characterization and proteome exploration. *Nat. Biotechnol.* **17**, 1030–1032.

Sanes, J. R., and Lichtman, J. W. (1999). Can molecules explain long-term potentiation? *Nat. Neurosci.* **2**, 597–604.

Schonberger, S. J., Edgar, P. F., Kydd, R., Faull, R. L., and Cooper, G. J. (2001). Proteomic analysis of the brain in Alzheimer's disease: Molecular phenotype of a complex disease process. *Proteomics* **1**, 1519–1528.

Shevchenko, A., Wilm, M., Vorm, O., Jensen, O. N., Podtelejnikov, A. V., Neubauer, G., Shevchenko, A., Mortensen, P., and Mann, M. (1996). A strategy for identifying gel-separated proteins in sequence databases by MS alone. *Biochem. Soc. Trans.* **24**, 893–896.

Shevchenko, A., Chernushevich, I., Ens, W., Standing, K. G., Thomson, B., Wilm, M., and Mann, M. (1997). Rapid '*de novo*' peptide sequencing by a combination of nanoelectrospray, isotopic labeling and a quadrupole/time-of-flight mass spectrometer. *Rapid Commun. Mass Spectrom.* **11**, 1015–1024.

Shevchenko, A., Chernushevich, I., Wilm, M., and Mann, M. (2000a). De novo peptide sequencing by nanoelectrospray tandem mass spectrometry using triple quadrupole and quadrupole/time-of-flight instruments. *Methods Mol. Biol.* **146**, 1–16.

Shevchenko, A., Loboda, A., Shevchenko, A., Ens, W., and Standing, K. G. (2000b). MALDI quadrupole time-of-flight mass spectrometry: A powerful tool for proteomic research. *Anal. Chem.* **72**, 2132–2141.

Steen, H., Kuster, B., Fernandez, M., Pandey, A., and Mann, M. (2002). Tyrosine phosphorylation mapping of the epidermal growth factor receptor signaling pathway. *J. Biol. Chem.* **277**, 1031–1039.

Taylor, S. W., Fahy, E., and Ghosh, S. S. (2003). Global organellar proteomics. *Trends Biotechnol.* **21**, 82–88.

Tilleman, K., Stevens, I., Spittaels, K., Haute, C. V., Clerens, S., Van Den Bergh, G., Geerts, H., Van Leuven, F., Vandesande, F., and Moens, L. (2002). Differential expression of brain proteins in glycogen synthase kinase-3 transgenic mice: A proteomics point of view. *Proteomics* **2**, 94–104.

Verma, R., Chen, S., Feldman, R., Schieltz, D., Yates, J., Dohmen, J., and Deshaies, R. J. (2000). Proteasomal proteomics: Identification of nucleotide-sensitive proteasome-interacting proteins by mass spectrometric analysis of affinity-purified proteasomes. *Mol. Biol. Cell.* **11**, 3425–3439.

Waltereit, R., and Weller, M. (2003). Signaling from cAMP/PKA to MAPK and synaptic plasticity. *Mol. Neurobiol.* **27**, 99–106.

Watkins, J. C., and Evans, R. H. (1981). Excitatory amino acid transmitters. *Annu. Rev. Pharmacol. Toxicol.* **21,** 165–204.

Watkins, J. C. (1991). Some chemical highlights in the development of excitatory amino acid pharmacology. *Can. J. Physiol. Pharmacol.* **69,** 1064–1075.

Watkins, J., and Collingridge, G. (1994). Phenylglycine derivatives as antagonists of metabotropic glutamate receptors. *Trends Pharmacol. Sci.* **15,** 333–342.

Yamauchi, T. (2002). Molecular constituents and phosphorylation-dependent regulation of the post-synaptic density. *Mass Spectrom Rev.* **21,** 266–286.

Zirpel, L., Lachica, E. A., and Rubel, E. W. (1995). Activation of a metabotropic glutamate receptor increases intracellular calcium concentrations in neurons of the avian cochlear nucleus. *J. Neurosci.* **15,** 214–222.

DOPAMINE TRANSPORTER NETWORK AND PATHWAYS

Rajani Maiya* and R. Dayne Mayfield[†]

*Institute for Cellular and Molecular Biology
University of Texas at Austin, Austin, Texas 78712
[†]Waggoner Center for Alcohol and Addiction Research
University of Texas at Austin
Austin, Texas 78712

I. Introduction

An emerging theme in neuronal cell signaling is the assembly of receptors and channels into large macromolecular complexes via protein-protein interactions. Currently, 77 proteins involved in mediating a variety of cellular functions have been found to associate with the N-methyl-D-aspartate (NMDA) receptor (Husi *et al.*, 2000). 5-Hydroxytryptamine 2C (5-HT$_{2C}$) receptors have also been shown to exist as a multi protein complex with several PDZ domain-containing proteins like postsynaptic density (PSD)-95 (Becamel *et al.*, 2000). The search for interacting proteins has been greatly aided by recent advances in mass spectrometry (MS)-based proteomics.

The family of Na$^+$ and Cl$^-$ dependent transporters, which includes the dopamine (DA), and norepinephrine (NE) transporters (DAT and NET, respectively), functions to clear released neurotransmitters from the synaptic cleft (Nelson, 1998). DAT regulates the spatial and temporal aspects of dopaminergic synaptic transmission and is an integral part of the mesostriatal DA system. This system plays a central role in mediating the rewarding and reinforcing effects of various drugs of abuse, such as ethanol (Brodie *et al.*, 1990, 1998; Weiss *et al.*, 1993). DAT is also the site of action for various psychostimulants such as cocaine and amphetamine (Nelson, 1998).

II. Structure and Function of DAT

Monoamine transporters including DAT are 12 transmembrane domain (TMD) containing proteins with intracellular N- and C-termini (Giros *et al.*, 1993). Chimeric constructs between DAT and NET were generated to identify regions on the transporter important for substrate binding, translocation, cocaine, and tricyclic antidepressant affinity (Buck and Amara, 1994; Giros *et al.*, 1994). These studies suggest that a region of the transporter encompassing TMD6–TMD8 is important for cocaine affinity and binding of tricyclic antidepressants. Amino acid residues spanning TMD9 through the carboxyl-terminal tail are important for high affinity substrate binding. The regions of the transporter important for substrate translocation are somewhat controversial, with one study implicating a region spanning TMD4–TMD8 (Giros *et al.*, 1994) and another study suggesting that the first five transmembrane domains are important for this function (Buck and Amara, 1994). The large extracellular loop between TMD3 and TMD4 has several potential glycosylation sites (Giros *et al.*, 1994). DAT is a heavily glycosylated protein *in vivo*, and several studies have shown that DAT glycosylation is necessary for the cell surface expression but not important for substrate affinity (Torres *et al.*, 2003a). Recent studies indicate that DAT at the cell membrane can exist as multimers (Hastrup *et al.*, 2001). Several regions of the transporter have been implicated in oligomerization of DAT. A glycophorin-like motif in TMD6 has been implicated in the formation of DAT dimers. This was demonstrated by symmetrical cross-linking of cysteine residues in the extracellular face of TMD6 (Hastrup *et al.*, 2001). It has been shown that mutations in the leucine repeat region of TMD2 can abolish plasma membrane delivery of DAT, and these mutants also display a dominant negative phenotype when coexpressed with wild-type DAT (Torres *et al.*, 2003a). Fluorescence resonance energy transfer (FRET) studies of tagged human DAT molecules have shown that DAT can exist as an oligomer in the endoplasmic reticulum (ER) and that DAT is internalized as an oligomer upon treatment with drugs such as amphetamines, cocaine, and phorbol esters (Sorkina *et al.*, 2003). Cysteine cross-linking experiments have shown that DAT may exist at the cell surface as a tetramer composed of two symmetrical homodimers (Hastrup *et al.*, 2003). These results suggest that discrete regions on the transporter are involved in transporter oligomerization and reiterate the importance of DAT oligomerization for steady state trafficking of DAT to the cell surface.

DA uptake by DAT is electrogenic and is accompanied by the cotransport of two Na^+ and one Cl^- ion, resulting in the net movement of two positive charges per DA molecule. Studies of transporter-associated currents in heterologous systems suggest at least three different conductances: (1) a substrate coupled conductance, (2) a constitutive leak conductance that is blocked by both substrates and inhibitors of the transporter, and (3) an uncoupled transport-associated conductance (Ingram *et al.*, 2002). A physiological role for these DAT-associated conductances was recently highlighted by two studies. The first study suggests that synaptic activation of somatodendritic DA release in the substantia nigra is DAT dependent. However, the mechanism by which DAT function is reversed to cause DA efflux is still not clear (Falkenburger *et al.*, 2001). A second study describes an endogenous DAT-mediated anion conductance in rat midbrain DA neurons in culture. The anion conductance promotes excitability of DA neurons in culture and suggests an alternative mechanism for DAT-mediated release of DA (Ingram *et al.*, 2002). It is possible that uncoupled substrate-dependent anion conductance could be mediated by proteins (particularly ion channels) associated with DAT. Proteomics-based approaches to investigate DAT-associated proteins could help test this hypothesis.

III. Cellular Localization of DAT

DAT is exclusively expressed in the cell bodies, dendrites, and axonal membranes of dopaminergic neurons. DAT is localized to the plasma membranes and smooth endoplasmic reticulum of dendrites and dendritic spines in the substantia nigra (Nirenberg *et al.*, 1996). Axonal terminals in the striatum demonstrated a perisynaptic labeling of DAT. DAT labeling was also associated with vesicular structures in the dendrites of dopaminergic cell bodies in the ventral tegmental area (VTA) (Nirenberg *et al.*, 1997), suggesting that targeting mechanisms exist to transport DAT to specific perisynaptic sites.

IV. Regulation of DAT

A recurring theme in monoamine transporter regulation is the altered cell surface distribution of DAT. For example, activation of protein kinase C (PKC) by phorbol esters has been shown to induce a rapid down-regulation of DAT in several cell types and striatal synaptosomal preparations (Daniels *et al.*, 1999; Melikian *et al.*, 1999; Zhu *et al.*, 1997). This has been shown to be a dynamin- and clathrin-dependent process (Daniels *et al.*, 1999). The fate of the internalized transporters is somewhat controversial with one group reporting that the internalized transporters are targeted to lysosomes for degradation (Daniels *et al.*, 1999) and another group reporting that transporters are internalized into endosomes and recycled to the cell surface (Melikian *et al.*, 1999). The DAT sequence has several consensus sites for phosphorylation by PKC and protein kinase

A (PKA; Giros *et al.*, 1993). Mutagenesis studies have shown that these consensus sites are not essential for PKC-mediated internalization of DAT, suggesting a role for accessory proteins in PKC regulation of DAT function (Zhu *et al.*, 1997). Drugs of abuse, such as amphetamines, inhibit DAT function by causing internalization of cell surface transporters in a dynamin- and clathrin-dependent manner (Saunders *et al.*, 2000). Experiments carried out in human embryonic kidney (HEK) cells demonstrated that acute exposure to cocaine enhances DAT activity in a time-dependent manner by increasing the number of functional transporters at the cell surface (Daws *et al.*, 2002). Cocaine also increases the number of DAT binding sites in neuro2A cells (derived from mouse neuroblastoma) by altering the intracellular trafficking of DAT (Little *et al.*, 2002).

Ethanol has been shown to affect the function of several members of the Na^+ and Cl^- dependent family of transporters. Experiments in HEK-293 cells stably transfected with glycine transporters (GLYT1 and GLYT2) have shown that relatively high concentrations of ethanol (100–200 millimolar [mM]) inhibit uptake of [^{3}H]glycine by GLYT2 and potentiate [^{3}H]glycine uptake by GLYT1 (Nunez *et al.*, 2000). Also, acute exposure to ethanol has been shown to enhance serotonin transporter (SERT) activity in rat cortical, hippocampal, and brainstem synaptosomes (Alexi *et al.*, 1991). Acute ethanol (10–100 mM) enhances DAT-mediated [^{3}H]DA uptake and transporter-associated currents in a time- and concentration-dependent manner (Mayfield *et al.*, 2001). This potentiation of transporter function was accompanied by an increase in the number of functional cell surface transporters, suggesting that ethanol affects transporter function by altering DAT trafficking. In contrast, electrochemical experiments suggest that NET function is inhibited by ethanol (Lin *et al.*, 1993). The contrasting effects of ethanol on DAT and NET function were exploited to identify sites on DAT that are critical for ethanol regulation of DAT. Chimeric DAT-NET transporters revealed that a region spanning the first three TMDs are important for etha-nol-regulation of DAT function. Site directed mutagenesis experiments suggested that discrete amino acid residues in the second intracellular loop of DAT are important for ethanol sensitivity of DAT (Maiya *et al.*, 2002).

Thus there is substantial evidence that DAT undergoes regulated trafficking both *in vitro* and *in vivo*, and this may be important for the functional and pharmacological sensitivity of the transporter. It is likely that transporter-interacting proteins play a key role in these modes of regulation. The DAT sequence contains numerous motifs for protein-protein interactions, including a PDZ binding domain at the C-terminus, an N-terminal leucine repeat, and two di-leucine motifs (Torres *et al.*, 2003b). Currently, three proteins have been identified that alter DAT function by interacting directly with the transporter. These proteins were identified by the yeast two-hybrid approach using the C-terminal tail of DAT as bait. These proteins are: α-synuclein, the PDZ domain containing protein PICK1 (protein interacting with C kinase 1), and Hic-5 (hydrogen peroxide-inducible protein 5). PICK1 potentiates DAT function by enhancing cell surface distribution of the transporters (Torres *et al.*, 2001). PICK1 was originally identified as a protein that interacts with the catalytic domain of PKC-α (Staudinger *et al.*, 1995). Hence it is tempting to speculate that PICK1 is important for PKC-mediated regulation of DAT function. The interaction of DAT with Hic-5 results in inhibition of DAT function by down-regulating the number of cell surface transporters. Hic-5 is a multiple Lin-11, Isl-1, and Mec-3 (LIM)-domain–containing adaptor protein that has been shown to interact with several kinases, such as focal adhesion kinase and fyn kinase, suggesting that Hic-5 could play a role in linking DAT to diverse cell-signaling pathways (Carniero *et al.*, 2002). α-Synuclein was the first protein shown to interact with the C-terminal tail of DAT (Lee *et al.*, 2001). The functional consequence of DAT-α-synuclein interaction remains controversial, with one group suggesting that DAT interaction with α-synuclein enhances clustering of DAT and cellular uptake of DA (Lee *et al.*, 2001); however, one study suggests that α-synuclein inhibits DAT function (Wersinger and Sidhu, 2003).

V. Mass Spectrometry-Based Proteomics

The term *proteome* refers to the set of all proteins expressed in a cell at a given time under a given set of conditions (Mann and Aebersold, 2003). Mass spectrometry is an analytical technique that identifies proteins by accurately determining the mass of fragments obtained by proteolytic digestion of the proteins and comparing the mass obtained to theoretical digests of known and predicted proteins in databases. Proteomics can be classified into two types: expression and interaction proteomics. Expression proteomics refers to large-scale studies of variations in protein expression. Interaction proteomics refers to the identification of protein-protein interactions within a cell (Mann and Aebersold, 2003). Protein-protein interactions can be enriched by antibody-based or affinity-purification techniques. The classical method for identifying protein-protein interactions is the yeast two-hybrid method, in which the bait proteins are expressed as a fusion to the DNA-binding domain of a yeast transcription factor and the cDNA library insert is expressed as a fusion protein to the activation domain of the transcription factor. Interaction between the bait and library proteins results in the activation of the transcription factor and a reporter gene. The yeast two-hybrid technique has been used successfully in biology to identify protein-protein interactions and is amenable for high throughput applications. MS-based approaches have advantages over the classical yeast two-hybrid approaches in that the interactions are identified in authentic cellular contexts, and hence do not require extensive validations (Mann and Aebersold, 2003). Mass spectrometry methods are very sensitive and highly accurate and can identify proteins whose abundance is in the low femtomole levels.

The two most commonly used MS approaches are MALDI (matrix-assisted laser desorption ionization) and ESI (electrospray ionization) mass spectrometry. The techniques differ in the methods used for ionization of peptides. MALDI analysis requires the digested sample to be mixed in a UV-absorbing matrix and the peptides are ionized with a UV laser beam. In the case of ESI the peptide solution is ionized by high voltages to form multiple protonated species (Rappsilber and Mann, 2002). Thus ESI has higher mass accuracy than MALDI. The first step in identifying a protein by MS is to digest the protein with a specific protease such as trypsin. The resulting peptides are then introduced into a mass spectrometer, where they are ionized and their masses are measured. Sequence information is generated by tandem mass spectrometry in which ions of interest are selected, fragmented, and the masses of the fragmented ions are used to generate an MS/MS or daughter spectrum. Complete sequence information of the entire protein is not determined by MS, but sequence information obtained from a few peptides is used to query a database and identify the protein (Perkins et al., 1999).

VI. Isolation and Validation of the DAT Proteome

We used an interaction proteomics based approach to identify proteins that exist in a complex with DAT. There is growing evidence that protein-protein interactions play a vital role in regulating transporter function. For example, the function of the γ-aminobutyric acid (GABA) transporter, a member of the sodium- and chloride-dependent family of neurotransmitter transporters, is regulated by syntaxin 1A, a protein that is involved in neurotransmitter release, via direct protein-protein interactions (Deken et al., 2000). Furthermore, the function of the SERT is also regulated by protein phosphatase 2A, a protein that has been shown to exist in a complex with SERT (Bauman et al., 2000). However, this approach has not been used to study monoamine transporter function.

DAT-associated proteins were isolated from the striatum by immunoprecipitation techniques using a monoclonal antibody directed to the N-terminus of DAT (Figs. 1A and B; Luo et al., 1997). The immunoprecipitation procedure was validated by examining the association between DAT and α-synuclein, a protein previously shown to exist in a complex with DAT (Lee et al., 2001). α-Synuclein was readily detected in the DAT complex, isolated from the striatum but not the cerebellum, a region devoid of DAT.

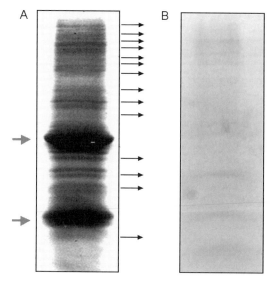

Fig. 1. Coimmunoprecipitation of DAT-associated proteins. (A) DAT-associated proteins were immunoprecipitated from the striata of male DBA/2J mice, and the proteins were separated on a 10% polyacrylamide gel electrophoresis (SDS)-PAGE and visualized with Coomassie staining. (B) Proteins pulled down nonspecifically with the protein A/protein G agarose beads.

VII. Mass Spectrometry

Approximately 20–25 bands ranging from 35–300 kilodaltons (kDa) were excised from the Coomassie-stained gel, and the proteins were identified by liquid chromatography (LC)-ESI-MS. A nonredundant mouse database was queried using the MASCOT (www.matrixscience.com) search engine. Twenty candidate proteins (Table I) were identified and classified as high- and medium-probability hits based on the number of peptides detected and the number of times the protein was pulled down. The presence of five of these proteins in the DAT complex was confirmed by coimmunoprecipitation experiments.

VIII. Confirmation of Members of the DAT Proteome

Eight peptides corresponding to synapsin 1b were detected by MS (see Table I). Reciprocal coimmunoprecipitation experiments using both DAT and synapsin I (both a and b) antibodies were carried out to confirm the presence of

TABLE I

CLASSIFICATION OF HIGH- AND MEDIUM-PROBABILITY PROTEINS

Proteins/accession numbers	Number of peptides detected
Signaling proteins	
Rho GEF (T30867)	6
Ras-GRF2 (P70392)	*3*
Trafficking proteins	
Synapsin I (AAD08933)	8
Dynamin I (Q61358)	5
Synaptojanin 2 (AAC40153)	*3*
Adapter protein 1 beta (Q922E2)	*3*
Cell-adhesion molecules	
Neurocan (S52781)	11
Brevican precursor (S57653)	4
Ion channels	
Kv4.3M (AAD16974)	*3*
Kv2.1 (I56529)	*4*
Cystic Fibrosis transmembrane conductance regulator (A39901)	*14*
Cytoskeletal/motor proteins	
Tubulin (I77426)	4
Actin (CAA27396)	17
Kinesin-related protein (KIF3B) (A57107)	*3*
Aczonin (PDZ) (T42215)	*4*
Metabolic enzymes	
Similar to mitochondrial aconitase (Q99KI0)	4
Fructose bis phosphate aldolase (ADMSA)	10
Triose phosphate isomerase (ISMST)	2
Miscellaneous	
Par-3 (PDZ) (Q99NH2)	2
Brca 2 (Q9BTL1)	*10*

Proteins were grouped according to known cellular function. Proteins were classified into high- and medium-probability (*italics*) hits, as described. A minimum of three peptides was required to identify a protein. Fragmentation patterns and sequence information were analyzed for medium-probability hits.

synapsin I in the DAT complex (Figs. 2A and B). Immunoprecipitations under denaturing conditions were performed to rule out nonspecific association of synapsin with agarose beads. Synapsin 1b belongs to a family of phosphoproteins that are involved in regulating neurotransmitter release (Greengard *et al.*, 1993). Syntaxin 1a, a protein involved in regulating neurotransmitter release, interacts directly with the GABA transporter and regulates its function (Deken *et al.*, 2000), providing a mechanism to couple neurotransmitter release to reuptake. Thus it is tempting to speculate that synapsin 1b may play a similar role in coupling

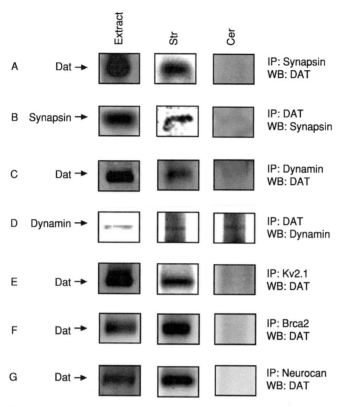

FIG. 2. Immunoprecipitation under nondenaturing conditions was followed by western blotting to confirm the presence of candidate proteins in the DAT complex. (A) Immunoprecipitation with synapsin and western blot using DAT antibody. (B) Immunoprecipitation with DAT antibody and western blot using synapsin antibody. (C) Immunoprecipitation with dynamin antibody and western blot with DAT antibody. (D) Immunoprecipitation with DAT antibody and western blot using dynamin antibody. (E) Immunoprecipitation with Kv2.1 antibody and western blot with DAT antibody. (F) Immunoprecipitation with Brca2 antibody and western blot with anti-DAT antibody. (G) Immunoprecipitation using antineurocan antibody and western blot using anti-DAT antibody. Str = striatum immunoprecipitation, Cer = cerebellum immunoprecipitation; negative control, Str Lysate = striatal lysate; positive control.

transmitter release to DAT function. It is possible that interaction of DAT with synapsin 1b could be indirectly mediated through actin, which is also detected in the DAT complex (see Fig. 3).

Five peptides corresponding to dynamin were detected in the DAT complex by MS. Reciprocal coimmunoprecipitation experiments (nondenaturing and denaturing) confirmed the association of DAT with dynamin (Figs. 2C and D). Dynamin I is a GTPase-involved in mediating endocytosis (Danino *et al.*, 2001). There is evidence that endocytosis of DAT is a dynamin-dependent process.

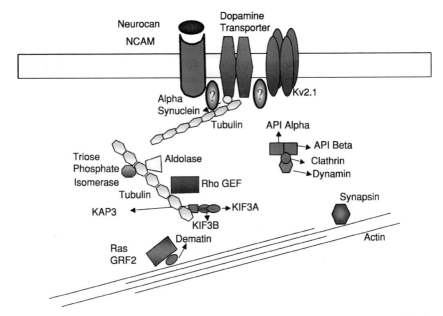

Fɪɢ. 3. Schematic representation of the dopamine transporter proteome. Proteins found in the dopamine transporter complex are shown. Proteins shown in gray were not found in our studies but are known to exist in a complex with one or more proteins that were identified in our screen. (See Color Insert.)

Coexpression of a dominant negative isoform of dynamin resulted in attenuation of PMA's and amphetamine's effects on DAT function (Daniels *et al.*, 1999; Melikian and Buckley, 1999; Saunders *et al.*, 2000). Hence the association of dynamin I with DAT could also have a functional role in regulating DAT trafficking *in vivo*.

Four peptides corresponding to Kv2.1, a delayed rectifier potassium channel, were detected in the DAT complex (Fig. 2E). Association of DAT with Kv2.1 was confirmed by immunoprecipitation (denaturing and nondenaturing conditions) experiments. Kv2.1 alpha subunit is widely expressed in the brain, and its expression is restricted to the soma and proximal dendrites in cortical and hippocampal neurons (Murakhoshi and Trimmer, 1999). In rat cerebellar basket cells there is evidence for expression of Kv2.1 in axons and neuronal terminals (Tan and Llano, 1999). The subcellular localization of Kv2.1 in the striatum has not been examined. Kv2.1 is a major component of the delayed rectifier current in hippocampal neurons (Baranauskas *et al.*, 1999). Recent studies suggest that DAT-associated currents can modulate neuronal excitability (Falkenburger *et al.*, 2001; Ingram *et al.*, 2002) and association of DAT with Kv2.1 could provide a novel mechanism by which DAT could control neuronal excitability and modulate neurotransmitter release. Although functional association of neuro-transmitter receptors with ion channels has been established (Law et al., 2000), this is the first report of association between a neurotransmitter transporter and an ion channel. It still remains to be tested whether this interaction is of any functional consequence.

Ten peptides corresponding to Brca2 were detected in the DAT complex. The presence of Brca2 in the DAT complex was also confirmed by immunoprecipitation experiments (Fig. 2F). Brca2 is a nuclear protein involved in the maintenance of chromosome structure and DNA repair. Mutations in the gene encoding Brca2 render susceptibility to breast and ovarian cancers (Venkitaraman, 2002), but our results point to an additional role for this protein in the brain, perhaps by regulating DAT function.

Eleven peptides corresponding to neurocan were detected in the DAT complex (Fig. 2G). Immunoprecipitations (denaturing and nondenaturing conditions) were performed to confirm neurocan's interaction with DAT. Neurocan is a chondroitin sulphate proteolycan whose expression is developmentally regulated. In adults, neurocan is proteolytically cleaved to a 130 kDa core protein with an average molecular mass of $\sim$200 kDa (Rauch et al., 2001). Neurocan is an extracellular matrix-associated protein that is a ligand for tenascin-R and neural cell adhesion molecule (NCAM) (Dityatev and Schachner, 2003). Neurocan has been implicated in the organization of striatal compartments, although the mechanism by which this occurs is unknown (Charvet et al., 1998).

The cytoskeletal proteins actin and tubulin were detected as high probability hits in our analysis. We also detected kinesin-related protein 3B (KIF3B), a motor protein involved in vesicular transport and highly enriched in the brain (Yamazaki et al., 1995). KIF3B is part of the kinesin II complex, which plays an important role in insulin-stimulated glucose transporter 4 (GLUT4) trafficking (Imamura et al., 2003). Hence it is possible that KIF3B is involved in the transport of vesicles containing DAT to the cell surface. The metabolic enzymes aldolase and triose phosphate isomerase, similar to mitochondrial aconitase, were also detected in the DAT complex. These enzymes are highly expressed in the brain, and it is possible that the association of these enzymes with DAT could be indirect, mediated by their interactions with tubulin (Walsh et al., 1989; see Fig. 3).

Two proteins with scaffolding function were detected in our analysis: aczonin and partitioning defective-3 (PAR-3). Scaffolding proteins are important because of their ability to nucleate multiprotein complexes. Aczonin is a presynaptic cytomatrix protein that is involved in synapse assembly. Aczonin possesses numerous protein interaction motifs, including a C-terminal PDZ domain, and is thought to play a role in localizing exocytic and endocytic machinery (Garner et al., 2000). PAR-3 is a 180-kDa adaptor protein containing 3 PDZ domains. It is highly expressed in embryonic and adult striatum and is known to play a role in the development of neuronal polarity (Lin et al., 2000).

The C-terminal tail of DAT has been shown to interact with PICK1 (a protein that interacts with C-kinase alpha via its PDZ domain), α-synuclein, and Hic-5. α-Synuclein was readily detected in our screen by western blotting, but we were unable to detect PICK1 or Hic-5 in our screen. A possible reason for this could be the comigration of PICK1 and Hic-5 with the immunoglobulin G (IgG) heavy chain. It is also possible that the monoclonal DAT antibody used in this study does not immunoprecipitate PICK1 and Hic-5.

IX. In Silico Analysis of DAT Proteome

To evaluate the functional significance of proteins in the DAT proteome, we used the WebQTL database (http://webqtl.org), a web-based resource for complex trait analysis (Chesler et al., 2003; Wang et al., 2003). This database contains data on more than 600 published phenotypes, more than 500 genetic markers, and 12,000 RNA expression traits tested in a panel of BXD recombinant inbred (RI) mouse strains. BXD RI strains derived through inbreeding of progeny from a cross of C57BL/6 and DBA/2 inbred strains are a powerful tool for quantitative trait loci (QTL) mapping and investigating relationship among complex traits. The relationship among traits can be evaluated by means of genetic correlations, which, if significant, imply a common genetic etiology. Genetic correlation among the traits is assessed using Pearson's product moment correlation, with each strain's mean representing a single data point (Crabbe et al., 1990; Markel et al., 1997).

The WebQTL database was used to answer two questions: (1) Does the expression of 21 DAT-associated proteins (listed in Table I, excluding actin, including DAT, and α-synuclein) co-vary? Co-variation would imply a common pattern of gene expression; (2) Do the common patterns of gene expression (if they exist) correlate with phenotypes functionally related to the transporter? To investigate the first question, we carried out principal component analysis (PCA) based on a correlation matrix of variables of interest. It reduces dimensionality of the data matrix while capturing the underlying variation and relationship among the variables. The proportion of variance explained by PC1 (Principal component 1) generally reflects how well variables correlate with each other. PC1 of the set of 21 DAT proteome genes, accounted for approximately 37% of data variation (data not shown). By comparison, the mean value of PC1 (100 different sets of 21 randomly selected genes) selected from forebrain expression dataset (total of 12,422 expression traits) was 23.6% ± 4.2% standard deviation (SD). Thus the 37% value of DAT proteome PC1 deviates more than 3 SD from the estimated population mean, indicating a nonrandom inter-correlation pattern among the 21 DAT proteome genes, which suggests a common regulatory

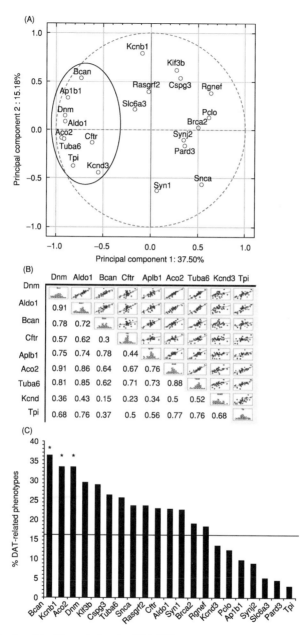

Fig. 4. Results of *in silico* analysis using WebQTL database. Results of PCA on the 21 DAT-related genes are plotted on a two-dimensional diagram (A), with PC1, PC2, and PC3 loadings for each gene being shown. Nine genes with similar loading patterns are encircled. (B) Correlations

mechanism for the expression of these genes. PCA of 21 DAT proteome genes also distinguished a group of 9 genes. These genes had high loading scores (loading score is a measure of the contribution of the variables to the principal component) for PC1 and were colocated in a three-dimensional (PC1 versus PC2) space (Fig. 4A). Most correlations among members of this subset were highly significant (Fig. 4B), implying that this set of genes is a primary target of coregulation.

The second question of functional relevance was addressed by calculating genetic correlations between expression values of 21 DAT proteome genes and 626 published phenotypes. Ninety-nine of these phenotypes could be classified as functionally related to DAT, such as cocaine-induced behaviors (locomotion, stereotypy, and sensitization) dopamine transporter density, and dopamine receptor 1 and 2 densities. We calculated the proportion of these phenotypes among all phenotypes that show significant correlations ($p < 0.05$) with DAT proteome gene expression (Fig. 4C). DAT-related phenotypes represent 16% of the total number of phenotypes in the WebQTL database (represented by a solid line; see Fig. 4C). We then compared this proportion to the proportion of DAT-related phenotypes with significant correlations using χ^2 statistic. Two thirds of DAT proteome genes (14 of 21) showed significant correlations greater than baseline (solid line represented in Fig. 4C). Three of the 14 DAT proteome genes (Brevican, Kv2.1, and similar to mitochondrial aconitase) reached statistical significance (χ^2 values ranging from 4.712 to 5.814; $p < 0.05$).

In summary, the MS approach identified a network of proteins that exist in a complex with DAT. This network is schematically represented in Fig. 3. Proteins that are shaded in gray are missing links; that is, they are not detected in our screen but have been shown in other studies to interact with proteins that are found in the DAT complex in our analysis. This approach will allow comparisons among the DAT, NET, and SERT proteomes to determine if common mechanisms exist for the regulation of monoamine transporter function. Future studies

---

among the nine genes are shown numerically (below major diagonal) and graphically (above major diagonal). Numbers in bold represent significant correlations ($r \geq 0.33$, $p < 0.05$; $r \geq 0.42$, $p < 0.01$). Diagrams located on the major diagonal represent BXD RI strain mean distributions. (C) Proportion of significant genetic correlations ($p < 0.05$) between gene expression and DAT-related phenotypes are shown in columns for each gene. A solid line across columns shows a proportion of DAT-related phenotypes of the total number of phenotypes in the WebQTL database (global proportion). Asterisks indicate significant deviation of the proportion of significantly correlated DAT-related phenotypes from the global proportion (by a χ^2 test). Bcan = brevican, Kcnb1 = Kv2.1, Aco2 = similar to mitochondrial aconitase, Dnm = dynamin, Kif3b = kinesin-related protein 3B, Cspg3 = neurocan, Tuba6 = tubulin, Snca = α-synuclein, Rasgrf2 = Ras GRF2, Cftr = cystic fibrosis transmembrane conductance regulator, Aldo1 = fructose bis phosphate aldolase, Syn1 = synapsin 1, Rgnef = Rho GEF, Kcnd3 = Kv4.3M, Pclo = piccolo, Ap1b1 = adaptor protein 1 beta, Synj2 = synaptojanin2, Slc6a3 = dopamine transporter, Pard3 = Par3, Tpi = triose phosphate isomerase. (See Color Insert.)

will investigate the functional consequences of these interactions and examine how this network is perturbed by psychiatric conditions, drug treatments, and drug addiction.

References

Alexi, T., and Azmitia, E. C. (1991). Ethanol stimulates [3H]5-HT high-affinity uptake by rat forebrain synaptosomes: Role of 5-HT receptors and voltage channel blockers. *Brain Res.* **544,** 243–247.

Baranauskas, G., Tkatch, T., and Surmeir, J. D. (1999). Delayed rectifier currents in rat globus pallidus neurons are attributable to Kv2.1 and Kv3.1/3.2 K^+ channels. *J. Neurosci.* **19,** 6394–6404.

Bauman, A. L., *et al.* (2000). Cocaine and antidepressant-sensitive biogenic amine transporters exist in regulated complexes with protein phosphatase 2A. *J. Neurosci.* **20,** 7571–7578.

Becamel, C., Alonso, G., Galeotti, N., Demey, E., Jouin, P., Ullmer, C., Dumuis, A., Bockaert, J., and Marin, P. (2000). Synaptic multiprotein complexes associated with 5-HT(2C) receptors: A proteomic approach. *EMBO J.* **21,** 2332–2342.

Brodie, M. S., Shefner, S. A., and Dunwiddie, T. V. (1990). Ethanol increases the firing rate of dopamine neurons of the rat ventral tegmental area *in vitro*. *Brain Res.* **508,** 65–69.

Brodie, M. S., and Appel, S. B. (1998). The effects of ethanol on dopaminergic neurons of the ventral tegmental area studied with intracellular recording in brain slices. *Alcohol Clin. Exp. Res.* **22,** 236–244.

Buck, K. J., and Amara, S. G. (1994). Chimeric dopamine-norepinephrine transporters delineate structural domains influencing selectivity for catecholamines and 1-methyl-4-phenylpyridinium. *Proc. Natl. Acad. Sci. USA* **91,** 12584–12588.

Carneiro, A. M., *et al.* (2002). The multiple LIM domain-containing adaptor protein Hic-5 synaptically colocalizes and interacts with the dopamine transporter. *J. Neurosci.* **22,** 7045–7054.

Charvet, I., Hemming, F. J., Feurstein, C., and Saxod, R. (1998). Transient compartment specific expression of neurocan in the developing rat striatum. *J. Neurosci. Research* **51,** 612–618.

Chesler, E. J., *et al.* (2003). Genetic correlates of gene expression in recombinant inbred strains: A relational model system to explore neurobehavioral phenotypes. *Neuroinformatics* **1,** 343–357.

Crabbe, J. C., Phillips, T. J., Kosobud, A., and Belknap, J. K. (1990). Estimation of genetic correlation: Interpretation of experiments using selectively bred and inbred animals. *Alcohol Clin. Exp. Res.* **14,** 141–151.

Daniels, G. M., and Amara, S. G. (1999). Regulated trafficking of the human dopamine transporter. Clathrin-mediated internalization and lysosomal degradation in response to phorbol esters. *J. Biol. Chem.* **274,** 35794–35801.

Daws, L. C., *et al.* (2002). Cocaine increases dopamine uptake and cell surface expression of dopamine transporters. *Biochem. Biophys. Res. Comm.* **290,** 1545–1550.

Deken, S. L., Beckman, M. L., Boos, L., and Quick, M. W. (2000). Transport rates of GABA transporters: Regulation by the N-terminal domain and syntaxin 1A. *Nat. Neurosci.* **3,** 998–1003.

Dityatev, A., and Schachner, A. (2003). Extracellular matrix molecules and synaptic plasticity. *Nat. Rev. Neurosci.* **4,** 456–468.

Falkenburger, B. H., Barstow, K. L., and Mintz, I. M. (2001). Dendrodendritic inhibition through reversal of dopamine transport. *Science* **293,** 2465–2470.

Danino, D., and Hinshaw, J. E. (2001). Dynamin family of mechanoenzymes. *Curr. Opin. Cell. Biol.* **13,** 454–460.

Garner, C. C., Kindler, S., and Gundelfinger, E. D. (2000). Molecular determinants of presynaptic active zones. *Curr. Opin. Neurobiol.* **10,** 321–327.

Giros, B., and Caron, M. G. (1993). Molecular characterization of the dopamine the transporter. *Trends Pharmacol. Sci.* **14,** 43–49.

Giros, B., Wang, Y. M., Suter, S., McLeskey, S. B., Pifl, C., and Caron, M. G. (1994). Delineation of discrete domains for substrate, cocaine, and tricyclic antidepressant interactions using chimeric dopamine-norepinephrine transporters. *J. Biol. Chem.* **269,** 15985–15988.

Greengard, P., Valtorta, F., Czernik, A. J., and Benfenati, F. (1993). Synaptic vesicle phosphoproteins and regulation of synaptic function. *Science* **259,** 780–785.

Hastrup, H., Karlin, A., and Javitch, J. A. (2001). Symmetrical dimer of the human dopamine transporter revealed by cross-linking Cys-306 at the extracellular end of the sixth transmembrane segment. *Proc. Natl. Acad. Sci. USA* **98,** 10055–10060.

Hastrup, H., Sen, N., and Javitch, J. A. (2003). The human dopamine transporter forms a tetramer in the plasma membrane: Cross-linking of a cysteine in the fourth transmembrane segment is sensitive to cocaine analogs. *J. Biol. Chem.* **278,** 45045–45048.

Husi, H., Ward, M. A., Choudhary, J. S., Blackstock, W. P., and Grant, S. G. (2000). Proteomic analysis of the NMDA receptor-adhesion protein signaling complexes. *Nat. Neurosci.* **3,** 661–669.

Imamura, T., Huang, J., Usui, I., Satoh, H., Bever, J., and Olefsky, J. M. (2003). Insulin-induced GLUT4 translocation involves protein kinase C-lambda-mediated functional coupling between Rab4 and the motor protein kinesin. *Mol. Cell. Biol.* **23,** 4892–4900.

Ingram, S. L., Prasad, B. M., and Amara, S. G. (2002). Dopamine transporter-mediated conductances increase excitability of midbrain dopamine neurons. *Nat. Neurosci.* **5,** 971–978.

Law, P. Y., Wong, Y. H., and Loh, H. H. (2000). Molecular mechanisms and regulation of opioid receptor signaling. *Annu. Rev. Pharmacol. Toxicol.* **40,** 389–430.

Lee, F. J., Liu, F., Pristupa, Z. B., and Nixnik, H. B. (2001). Direct binding and functional coupling of alpha-synuclein to the dopamine transporters accelerate dopamine-induced apoptosis. *FASEB J.* **15,** 916–926.

Lin, A. M., Bickford, P. C., Palmer, M. R., and Gerhardt, G. A. (1993). Ethanol inhibits the uptake of exogenous norepinephrine from the extracellular space of the rat cerebellum. *Neurosci. Lett.* **164,** 71–75.

Lin, D., Edwards, A. S., Fawcett, J. P., Mbamalu, G., Scott, J. D., and Pawson, T. (2000). A mammalian PAR-3-PAR-6 complex implicated in Cdc42/Rac1 and aPKC signalling and cell polarity. *Nat. Cell. Biol.* **2,** 540–547.

Little, K. Y., Elmer, L. W., Zhong, H., Scheys, J. O., and Zhang, L. (2002). Cocaine induction of dopamine transporter trafficking to the plasma membrane. *Mol. Pharmacol.* **61,** 436–445.

Luo, J., Wang, Y., Yasuda, R. P., Dunah, A. W., and Wolfe, B. B. (1997). The majority of N-methyl-D-aspartate receptor complexes in adult rat cerebral cortex contain at least three different subunits (NR1/NR2A/NR2B). *Mol. Pharmacol.* **51,** 79–86.

Maiya, R., Buck, K. J., Harris, R. A., and Mayfield, R. D. (2002). Ethanol-sensitive sites on the human dopamine transporter. *J. Biol. Chem.* **277,** 30724–30729.

Mann, M., and Aebersold, R. (2003). Mass spectrometry-based proteomics. *Nature* **422,** 198–207.

Markel, P. D., Bennett, B., Beeson, M., Gordon, L., and Johnson, T. E. (1997). Confirmation of quantitative trait loci for ethanol sensitivity in long-sleep and short-sleep mice. *Genome Res.* **7,** 92–99.

Mayfield, R. D., Maiya, R., Keller, D., and Zahnizer, N. R. (2001). Ethanol potentiates the function of the human dopamine transporter expressed in Xenopus oocytes. *J. Neurochem.* **79,** 1070–1079.

Melikian, H. E., and Buckley, K. M. (1999). Membrane trafficking regulates the activity of the human dopamine transporter. *J. Neurosci.* **19,** 7699–7710.

Murakhoshi, H., and Trimmer, J. S. (1999). Identification of the Kv2.1 K+ channel as a major component of the delayed rectifier K+ current in rat hippocampal neurons. *J. Neurosci.* **19,** 1728–1735.

Nelson, N. (1998). The family of Na+/Cl− neurotransmitter transporters. *J. Neurochem.* **71,** 1785–1803.

Nirenberg, M. J., Vaughan, R. A., Uhl, G. R., Kuhar, M. J., and Pickel, V. M. (1996). The dopamine transporter is localized to dendritic and axonal plasma membranes of nigrostriatal dopaminergic neurons. *J. Neurosci.* **16,** 436–447.

Nirenberg, M. J., Chan, J., Vaughan, R. A., Uhl, G. R., Kuhar, M. J., and Pickel, V. M. (1997). Immunogold localization of the dopamine transporter: An ultrastructural study of the rat ventral tegmental area. *J. Neurosci.* **17,** 4037–4044.

Nunez, E., Lopez-Corcurea, B., Martinez-Maza, R., and Aragon, C. (2000). Differential effects of ethanol on glycine uptake mediated by the recombinant GLYT1 and GLYT2 glycine transporters. *Br. J. Pharmacol.* **129,** 802–810.

Perkins, D. N., Pappin, D. J., Creasy, D. M., and Cottrell, J. S. (1999). Probability-based protein identification by searching sequence databases using mass spectrometry data. *Electrophoresis* **20,** 3551–3567.

Rappsilber, J., and Mann, M. (2002). What does it mean to identify a protein in proteomics? *Trends. Biochem. Sci.* **27,** 74–78.

Rauch, U., Feng, K., and Zhou, X.-H. (2001). Neurocan: A brain chondroitin sulfate proteoglycan. *Cell. Mol. Life Sci.* **58,** 1842–1856.

Saunders, C., Ferrer, J. V., Shi, L., Chen, J., Merrill, G., Lamb, M. E., Leeb-Lundberg, L. M., Carvelli, L., Javitch, J. A., and Galli, A. (2000). Amphetamine-induced loss of human dopamine transporter activity: An internalization-dependent and cocaine-sensitive mechanism. *Proc. Natl. Acad. Sci.* **97,** 6850–6855.

Sorkina, T., Doolen, S., Galperin, E., Zahniser, N. R., and Sorkin, A. (2003). Oligomerization of dopamine transporters visualized in living cells by fluorescence resonance energy transfer microscopy. *J. Biol. Chem.* **278,** 28274–28283.

Staudinger, J., Zhou, J., Burgess, R., Elledge, S. J., and Olson, E. N. (1995). PICK1: A perinuclear binding protein and substrate for protein kinase C isolated by the yeast two-hybrid system. *J. Cell. Biol.* **128,** 263–271.

Tan, Y. P., and Llano, I. (1999). Modulation of K$^+$ channels of action potential-evoked intracellular Ca^{2+} concentration rises in rat cerebellar basket cell axons. *J. Physiol.* **520,** 65–78.

Torres, G. E., *et al.* (2001). Functional interaction between monoamine plasma membrane transporters and the synaptic PDZ domain-containing protein PICK1. *Neuron* **30,** 121–134.

Torres, G. E., Carneiro, A., Seamans, K., Fiorentini, C., Sweeney, A., Yao, W. D., and Caron, M. G. (2003a). Oligomerization and trafficking of the human dopamine transporter. Mutational analysis identifies critical domains important for the functional expression of the transporter. *J. Biol. Chem.* **278,** 2731–2739.

Torres, G. E., Gainetdinov, R. R., and Caron, M. G. (2003b). Plasma membrane membrane monoamine transporters: Structure, regulation and function. *Nat. Rev. Neurosci.* **4,** 13–25.

Venkitaraman, A. R. (2002). Cancer susceptibility and the functions of BRCA1 and BRCA2. *Cell* **108,** 171–182.

Wang, J., Williams, R. W., and Manly, K. F. (2003). WebQTL: Web-based complex trait analysis. *Neuroinformatics* **1,** 299–308.

Walsh, J. L., Keith, T. J., and Knull, H. R. (1989). Glycolytic enzyme interactions with tubulin and microtubules. *Biochem. Biophys. Acta* **999,** 64–70.

Weiss, F., Lorang, M. T., Bloom, F. E., and Koob, G. F. (1993). Oral alcohol self-administration stimulates dopamine release in the rat nucleus accumbens: Genetic and motivational determinants. *J. Pharmacol. Exp. Ther.* **267,** 250–258.

Wersinger, C., and Sidhu, A. (2003). Attenuation of dopamine transporter activity by alpha-synuclein. *Neurosci. Lett.* **340,** 189–192.

Yamazaki, H., Nakata, T., Okada, Y., and Hirokawa, N. (1995). KIF3A/B: A heterodimeric kinesin superfamily protein that works as a microtubule plus end-directed motor for membrane organelle transport. *J. Cell. Biol.* **130,** 1387–1399.

Zhu, S. J., Kavanaugh, M. P., Sonders, M. S., Amara, S. G., and Zahniser, N. R. (1997). Activation of protein kinase C inhibits uptake, currents and binding associated with the human dopamine transporter expressed in Xenopus oocytes. *J. Pharmacol. Exp. Ther.* **282,** 1358–1365.

PROTEOMIC APPROACHES IN DRUG DISCOVERY AND DEVELOPMENT

Holly D. Soares,* Stephen A. Williams,* Peter J. Snyder,* Feng Gao,*
Tom Stiger,* Christian Rohlff,[†] Athula Herath,[†] Trey Sunderland,[‡]
Karen Putnam,[‡] and W. Frost White*

*Pfizer Global Research and Development, Groton, Connecticut 06340
[†]Oxford Glycosciences, Abingdon, United Kingdom OX1 3QX
[‡]National Institute of Mental Health, Bethesda, Maryland 20892

I. Proteomics in Drug Discovery and Development

A. CHALLENGES FACING DRUG DISCOVERY AND DEVELOPMENT

Proteomics, a word coined from protein and genomics, has many definitions in the literature. The most encompassing definition was provided by the National Academy of Science working group to define proteomic mandates in the post-genomic era. Based on a panel consensus, "proteomics represents the effort to establish the identities, quantities, structures, and biochemical and cellular functions of all proteins in an organism, organ or organelle, and how these properties vary in space, time or physiological state" (Kenyon *et al.*, 2002). Although a subset of functional proteomic technologies has been driven by advances in genomics, the study of proteins actually predates the genomic era. Indeed, efforts to develop "protein maps" were well underway before the explosion of genomics (Clark, 1981). Today, improvements in separation techniques (Gygi *et al.*, 1999, 2000), mass spectrometry instrumentation (Chaurand *et al.*, 2002; Gygi and Aebersold, 2000; Le Blanc *et al.*, 2003; Lill, 2003; Lin *et al.*, 2003; Link *et al.*, 1999; Ong *et al.*, 2003; Smith, 2002; Stoeckli *et al.*, 2001; Todd *et al.*, 2001), protein microarrays (Espina *et al.*, 2003; Haab, 2003; Hanash, 2003; Tang *et al.*, 2004; Templin *et al.*, 2003), protein tagging (Adam *et al.*, 2002a; Sekar and Periasamy, 2003), functional strategies (Adam *et al.*, 2002a,b; Gerlt, 2002; Hagenstein *et al.*, 2003; Hanash, 2003; Jarvik *et al.*, 2002; Kozarich, 2003; Templin *et al.*, 2003), and the development of robust informatics software (Boguski and McIntosh, 2003; Chakravarti *et al.*, 2002; Fenyo and Beavis, 2002; Stupka, 2002; Taylor *et al.*, 2003) have yielded sensitive, high-throughput technologies for large-scale identification and quantitation of protein expression, protein modification, subcellular localization, protein function, and protein-protein interactions. Proteomic strategies can yield powerful tools for drug discovery and development by providing insight into target-drug interactions, predicting compound safety, explaining disease heterogeneity, characterizing risk and progression, and identifying targets that may be more directly involved in pathophysiological processes. The challenge remains to apply the technology in a manner focused on overcoming existent discovery and developmental hurdles.

One of the primary hurdles to innovation has been the significant cost associated with bringing drugs to the market. In a study examining data obtained from 12 pharmaceutical companies and encompassing the progress of 93 randomly selected new drugs developed between 1970 and 1982, it was estimated that the capitalized cost to bring a drug to market was approximately $231 million (DiMasi *et al.*, 1991). Updates of the analysis covering development costs of 68 new drugs developed between 1980 and 1999 from 10 pharmaceutical firms showed that the capitalized cost to bring a new drug to market had quadrupled to $802 million (DiMasi *et al.*, 2003). Interestingly, the number of new drugs approved in the last 20 years has not dramatically increased despite improvements in regulatory review time (Reichert, 2003) and initiatives to involve drug metabolism optimization earlier in the drug design stage rather than in later lead stages (Roberts, 2003). Drug development attrition remains especially high when pursuing novel targets, largely due to incomplete information about novel signaling pathways, unpredictable safety issues, continued gaps in preclinical to clinical modeling and skyrocketing development costs. In theory, targeted proteomic approaches could alleviate some of these hurdles by providing information on protein-protein interactions within individual targeted pathways, providing protein "profiles" or signatures that could flag safety issues early in the development, creating links between preclinical and clinical models by examining identical proteins affected by a drug in both models and streamlining clinical trial design by providing more quantitative measures of outcome, and by identifying patients at earlier stages of disease. The following treatise discusses recent advances in proteomic techniques and highlights a "profiling" approach to identify early markers of disease state and disease progression in Alzheimer's disease (AD).

B. Overview of Proteomic Approaches

Current proteomic strategies are actually quite diverse but often focus on rather narrow scientific questions. Indeed, the most successful approaches tailor scientific studies to the strengths of specific proteomic technologies. Today, most approaches can be separated into two basic categories—profiling approaches and functional approaches—with a few methods capable of exploring both protein abundance and functional interactions issues. The following discussion provides a brief overview of existing technologies and in no way does justice to the complexity of the current proteomic field. The overview is meant to survey the field and highlight one example of proteomic technology used in drug discovery and development.

Traditional proteomic approaches have centered on profiling strategies. Profiling approaches include two-dimensional gel electrophoresis (*2DE*) combined with mass spectrometry (*MS*), liquid chromatography separation combined with mass spectrometry (LC-MS), protein affinity microarrays, metabonomics and matrix-assisted laser desorption ionization (MALDI) based imaging. 2DE is the oldest approach and remains the most common tool to examine changes in protein expression (Gygi *et al.*, 2000; Klose, 1975; O'Farrell *et al.*, 1977). In 2DE, proteins are separated first via isoelectric focusing, followed by standard polyacrylamide sodium dodecyl sulfate gel electrophoresis. Although recent advances have made the approach more high throughput (Bandara *et al.*, 2003; Harris *et al.*, 2002; Page *et al.*, 1999), the technology is not optimized for examining proteins with extreme pH and molecular weight ranges, and the approach is not well suited for analysis of membrane proteins or proteins in low abundance (Gygi *et al.*, 2000). Nevertheless, the technique, in combination with advances in peptide sequencing technology, has provided significant advances in specific matrix or organelle sub types, including plasma or serum proteomes (Lathrop *et al.*, 2003; Pieper *et al.*, 2003), bacterial proteomes (VanBogelen, 1999), and cellular subregions (Jang and Hanash, 2003; Li *et al.*, 2003). Were it not for 2DE approaches, scientists would not have appreciated the fact that a single protein could be represented by as many as 100 (or more) different isoforms due to proteolytic cleavage, alternative splicing, and post-translational modification events. Thus early 2DE initiatives led scientists from a rather naïve and simplistic view of protein interactions to alternate technologies capable of addressing gaps not amenable to 2DE approaches.

An alternative separation approach to 2DE is liquid chromatography followed by MS analysis. Hunt and colleagues (1992) first pioneered LC-based approaches to examine peptides bound to major histocompability complex molecules. The basic protocol has since been expanded to examining proteolytic fragments of proteins, with improvements enabling more quantitative MS analysis. Quantitative LC-MS methods are better suited for low-molecular weight and membrane proteins (Gygi *et al.*, 1999; Lill, 2003; Link *et al.*, 1999; Wu and Yates, 2003). As a result, LC-MS approaches are often complementary to standard 2DE technologies. Quantitative LC-MS–based approaches have been used to compare genomic to proteomic changes in expression following system perturbations, to follow changes associated with disease state or with developmental differentiation, and to address more functional questions aimed at protein-protein interaction and post-translational modifications (Aebersold, 2003). Although the technology has been applied to questions central to drug discovery and development, existing disadvantages including incomplete bioinformatics software, problems with internal standard tags, and sensitivity issues, have impeded routine implementation. As a result, alternative approaches continue to be used.

Microarray technology shares some properties with LC-MS–based technology, as both can selectively screen for specific proteins based on covalent or ligand specific interactions. In theory, microarray technology can also be used as a functional method if the protein under study is well characterized. Microarrays utilize ligands such as proteins, peptides, antibodies, antigens, allergens, and other ligand-specific physiochemical properties (e.g., hydrophobicity, metal) to capture proteins of interest (Espina *et al.*, 2003; Grubb *et al.*, 2003; Tang *et al.*, 2004; Templin *et al.*, 2003). Detection of the ligand-protein interaction can vary from immunobased techniques to surface-enhanced laser desorption ionization (SELDI) mass spectrometry (Espina *et al.*, 2003; Grubb *et al.*, 2003; Haab, 2003; Tang *et al.*, 2004; Templin *et al.*, 2003). Although the subset of proteins capable of being analyzed at any one time is limited in microarray approaches, microarrays offer a more focused approach to profiling and are able to screen for specific types of post-translational modifications. Similar to other types of profiling approaches, microarrays have been most useful as screening tools in identifying proteins associated with a particular disease state (Haab, 2003; Hanash, 2003).

Another application for proteomic profiling is metabolic characterization, long used by the pharmaceutical industry to assess drug metabolite profiles. Only recently has the analysis of metabolites been extended into the proteomics arena. Large-scale analysis of metabolites, known as metabolomics or metabonomics, typically employs traditional LC/MS or more recent advances in ^{1}H NMR spectroscopy to examine the metabolic profile associated with cellular and pathological processes (Griffin, 2003; Watkins and German, 2002). Types of metabolic profiles can include drug metabolites, lipids (Brindle *et al.*, 2003), amino acids (Griffin *et al.*, 2003), or urinary metabolites (Robertson *et al.*, 2001). Metabonomics is sometimes characterized as a functional approach, and it can be when the metabolites under study are well defined. However, a number of the more recent NMR-based approaches look at complex matrices including plasma and urine to generate "metabolic profiles" that are largely descriptive in nature and may or may not shed insights into the underlying biological processes. Nevertheless, the technology lends itself well to personalized medicine, because subjects at risk of disease development or who may respond differentially to drug treatment could possibly be identified solely on the basis of a metabolic profile (Brindle *et al.*, 2002; Griffin, 2003; Watkins and German, 2002). The current impediments to clinical application include the development of sophisticated bioinformatics algorithms, slow turnaround time in data analysis, and the high cost of existing technology. Despite these hurdles, metabonomics offers several advantages to existing technologies and can be applied to matrices that are easily accessible in the clinic.

The last "profiling" technology, MS-based imaging, is yet another result of further advancements in mass spectrometry technology. Imaging-based profiling takes advantage of MALDI or secondary ion mass spectrometry (SIMS) to profile and map proteins in thin tissue sections (Chaurand *et al.*, 2002, 2003; Stoeckli *et al.*, 2001, 2002; Todd *et al.*, 2001). Individual cells isolated by laser capture microdissection, or simply, sections of tissues are amenable to the technology. Recent advances in the technology have achieved a spatial resolution of up to 50 μm. However, sensitivity in comparison to antibody approaches remains an issue, and quantitation problems have not yet been fully resolved. The technology has been used to examine aberrant expression of amyloid beta (Abeta) peptides in the brain, (Stoeckli *et al.*, 2002) as well as to examine localization of drug and metabolites within various tissues (Todd *et al.*, 2001). Mass spectrometry imaging is unique in that it offers cellular localization in addition to profiling. As a result, it is a technology that will likely yield useful and functional, as well as protein abundance, information.

Whereas profiling approaches tend to focus on expression patterns and relative changes in protein abundance, functional proteomic strategies focus on defining protein-protein interactions, enzymatic activity, downstream activation of signaling cascades, and post-translational modifications. Although functional proteomics can be performed in a high throughput fashion, delineating the relevance of biological interactions often requires further assay development and extensive bioinformatic infrastructure. As a result, functional approaches have yet to reach their full potential in terms of delivering assays that can be used in drug discovery and development. Nevertheless, understanding the function behind protein-protein interactions is the basic tenet to most drug discovery programs, and functional proteomics can provide insights into what were perceived as previously intractable scientific problems. Functional approaches are quite diverse and include identifying protein-binding interactions (e.g., yeast two-hybrid systems, phage display, fluorescence resonance energy transfer ([FRET]-like assays, and subtypes of protein microarrays) or identifying downstream components of activated systems via chemical tagging or activity-based profiling.

The yeast two-hybrid system has been in use for more than a decade to study protein-protein interactions (Fields and Song, 1989). Yeast two-hybrid technology is a direct outgrowth of the genomics explosion and uses genetic approaches to express hybrid proteins in yeast systems. In brief, fusion proteins are expressed in yeast systems that are capable of binding to each other and resulting in detectable signals. The original format expressed a protein fused to a DNA-binding protein (the bait) in combination with other proteins fused to an activation domain of a transcription factor (screen candidates). Binding typically occurred in the nucleus and resulted in either the expression of a protein that would yield a color product or would enable positive colonies to survive in metabolically deficient environments. Screen candidates can be representative of proteins from an entire genome and have been applied to characterizing whole genome protein interactions in *Saccharomyces cerevisiae, Caenorhabditis elegans* (Uetz *et al.*, 2000; Walhout *et al.*, 2000), *Escherichia coli* (Bartel *et al.*, 1996), hepatitis C virus (Flajolet *et al.*, 2000), Vaccinia virus (McCraith *et al.*, 2000), and *Helicobacter pylori* (Rain *et al.*, 2001). Yeast two-hybrid approaches are prone to high false positive and false negative rates. In addition, the approach is not applicable for membrane proteins, nor for proteins that require extensive folding and post-translational modifications. Furthermore, binding is often out of biological context. Despite limitations in the technology, yeast two-hybrid systems have yielded a number of significant insights into protein-protein interactions (Uetz, 2002).

Phage display is yet another technology suitable for studying peptide recognition domains (Sidhu *et al.*, 2003) and is complementary to yeast two-hybrid systems. Phage display genetically engineers bacteriophage particles so that the peptide or protein of interest is expressed as a fusion surface protein to bacteriophage capsid or coat protein. The exposed "bait" protein can then be used to capture potential binding partners expressed by phage particles. The method is, in theory, more applicable than yeast two-hybrid systems to transcription factor interactions and has been successfully applied to elucidate binding partners of the PDZ domains   (Fuh *et al.*, 2000; Skelton *et al.*, 2003). Interestingly, peptides against PDZ domains were then shown to be suitable targets for ischemic stroke (Aarts *et al.*, 2002). Phage display has also proved useful in mapping out signal-transduction pathways for EGF, hormone receptors, antibody generation, and other immunogenic signaling cascades (Chang *et al.*, 2003; Hoogenboom *et al.*, 1998; Hufton *et al.*, 1999; Zozulya *et al.*, 1999).

Other functional technologies have taken advantage of advances in fluorophore technology to examine protein binding. These include (FRET) and fluorophore fusion tagging (Sekar and Periasamy, 2003; Wouters *et al.*, 2001; Zeytun *et al.*, 2003). FRET is typically used on a microscopic platform to measure the nonradioactive energy transfer from an excited donor fluorophore to another acceptor fluorophore that is within 10–100 angstroms in proximity (Sekar and Periasamy, 2003; Wouters *et al.*, 2001). Although the method is primarily applied in high throughput screening to examine intracellular interactions of known fluorophore fusion-proteins, it is capable of screening unknown binding interactions, as well as post-translational modifications, by using antibodies that recognize specific modifications (Sekar and Periasamy, 2003; Wouters *et al.*, 2001) or binding domains (Zeytun *et al.*, 2003). Fluorophore epitope tagging also has utility in delineating intracellular localization. Thus fluorophore and related FRET-based technologies have great utility in functional proteomics.

Fluorophore tagging has been extended to activity-based technologies that use chemical matter as probes (Adam *et al.*, 2002a; Kozarich, 2003). In brief, chemical probes designed to recognize a conserved catalytic/functional/structural motif in target proteins are labeled with a chemical or fluorescent detection tag. The tagged chemical probe then covalently interacts with active targets within biological relevant matrices. Covalently tagged complexes can then be analyzed and quantitated by standard gel electrophoresis (or other LC separation techniques), followed by MS identification. Information garnered from the assay is really based on the detection of active proteins rather than on quantifying total amounts of protein (e.g., both active and inactive forms). Activity-based profiling is particularly useful in identifying mechanistic markers that signal drug interaction with target proteins. Although original formats utilized biotinylated fluorophosphonates to irreversibly inactivate serine proteases in a complex biological homogenate (Liu *et al.*, 1999), later improvements used more sensitive fluorophore labeling and chemical matter that allowed reversible interactions with target proteins (Adam *et al.*, 2002a; Kozarich, 2003; Patricelli *et al.*, 2001). The technique has been successfully applied to examining enzyme activity profiles in malignant cancer (Jessani *et al.*, 2002), as well as in profiling deubiquitinating (Borodovsky *et al.*, 2002) and tyrosine phosphates activities in complex mixtures (Lo *et al.*, 2002). With the appropriate chemical matter on hand, the technique could be quite powerful in addressing fundamental, functional questions central to drug development programs.

C. Summary

To date, no one technology is capable of fully examining all aspects of the proteomic spectrum. As a result, many different technologies are in use, each with individualized strengths and weaknesses. In drug development and discovery, "browsing" or profiling approaches are more suited for specific development issues related to predicting safety or identifying subjects at risk of developing a disease or exhibiting differential responses to a drug. Profiling approaches may or may not shed light onto the underlying biological mechanism of disease, but they do serve as useful predictive tools of outcome and efficacy, which enables early decision making in the drug development process. Unfortunately, the steps required to validate information obtained from profiling studies have impeded easy transition into the clinic. Nevertheless, profiling information tends to be more disease specific and therefore applicable across a variety of different programs targeted at a single indication.

The issues facing early drug discovery are highly dependent on understanding the functional relationship between proteins and signaling pathways. Proteomic profiling is sometimes difficult to apply to early drug discovery because exploratory proteomic profiling may or may not provide insights into signaling pathways and disease processes. Functional proteomics, on the other hand, is particularly suited for drug discovery issues but has not yet fully matured as an independent field. Nevertheless, rapid advances in functional proteomics are proving complementary to existing technologies within genomic and pharmaceutical fields. The challenge will be in translating evolving technologies into assays that can deliver information central to understanding a drug's modulatory effect on protein function and ultimately on pathological processes.

Clearly each proteomic approach exhibits specific strengths and weaknesses, and the majority of successful studies have addressed relatively narrow questions using the most appropriate technology. In the following section, a case study is presented that shows how 2DE-MS profiling approaches can be applied to one type of issue central to drug discovery and development—the ability to identify subjects at risk or in the early stages of disease.

II. Using Proteomics to Identify Biomarkers of Alzheimer's Disease: A Case Study

A. BACKGROUND

Approximately 4 million people suffer from Alzheimer's disease in the United States, with prevalence expected to quadruple in the next 50 years (Brookmeyer and Gray, 2000). Indeed, AD is the most common neurodegenerative disease afflicting the U.S. population over the age of 60. The economic impact of AD is estimated at more than $100 billion per year in the United States alone, with health care costs rising as the number of elderly increases. Current clinical trials rely on cognitive assessments as the primary endpoint, which can make a clear assessment of efficacy difficult given that international standards vary considerably and many cognitive test scales fail to fully capture changes in the very early and very late stages of the disease. In addition, the rate in cognitive decline within the AD population is not constant and can occur over several years. Although many patients exhibit relatively steady cognitive decline throughout the disease progression, there are many others who experience plateaus before declining further, and still others can plateau for well over a decade before declining further

(Doody *et al.*, 2001). Natural history studies suggest the reasons underlying such heterogeneity are pleitropic and can be attributed to: (1) true differences in progression rates, (2) floor and ceiling effects of cognitive indices, (3) differences in progression endpoints chosen, (4) genetic heterogeneity, and (5) differences in patient care and medical comorbidities. The unpredictable nature of disease progression and the difficulty in identifying subjects in the very early stages of AD increase the difficulty of running effective clinical trials.

AD is currently diagnosed by changes in cognitive symptoms presumed to be associated with the deposition of amyloid plaques and the formation of neurofibrillary tangles in the brain. Although recent pharmacological efforts have yielded temporary symptomatic relief, current approaches have failed to effectively halt the onslaught of progressive neurodegeneration. As a result, current therapeutic initiatives have focused primarily on disease modification strategies. Successful disease modification intervention will likely depend on effective treatment during the early or even prodromal stages of the disease. Unfortunately, early clinical signs of AD can be subtle and conclusive diagnosis difficult. Nevertheless, emerging evidence suggests that alterations in pathology occur much earlier than symptomatic manifestation, suggesting that biochemical changes can be detected prior to significant cognitive deterioration.

The current study describes an initiative to use a 2DE-MS based proteomic approach to identify proteins that are differentially expressed in the cerebrospinal fluid (CSF) of AD patients and normal controls. It is hypothesized that use of one or more of these differentially expressed proteins will provide tools to successfully: (1) differentiate AD patients from non-AD patients, (2) identify "at risk" patients who will go on to develop AD or are in the very early stages of the disease, and (3) correlate with disease progression, thereby providing more quantitative measures of disease modification therapeutic strategies.

B. Experimental Design and Methods

1. Overview of Experimental Design

Longitudinal samples were collected from patients with dementia of the Alzheimer's type (AD, N = 219), normal control patients with a first-degree relative (NCF, N = 108), and normal control patients (NCO, N = 56). CSF was immunodepleted of high abundant proteins (see Section on immunodepletion later in the chapter) and subjected to 2DE. Prior studies had already characterized the identity of more than 1400 spots within the CSF gels by mass spectrometry. Resultant gels were imaged, and normalized volumes of individual spots were compared for differences in protein expression between AD and control subjects.

2. Subjects Population and Demographics

All AD subjects in the present study were diagnosed according to the National Institute of Neurological and Communicative Disorders and Stroke-Alzheimer's Disease and Related Disorders Association (NINCDS-ADRDA) criteria (McKhann *et al.*, 1984). AD and control CSF samples were obtained from Dr. Trey Sunderland from the National Institute of Mental Health (NIMH; 336 subjects), Dr. Stephen; Ferris from New York University (NYU; 23 subjects), Lampire Biologicals (20 subjects), and Impath (21 subjects). Evaluation of subjects from NIMH and NYU included a complete medical screening, neurocognitive profile, apolipoprotein epsilon (APO ε) genotyping, lumbar puncture for CSF examination, and behavioral observations for at least 1–2 weeks. Medical evaluations for all subjects involved a physical examination, a routine electrocardiogram, and blood tests to eliminate other known contributors to memory impairment. Routine magnetic resonance imaging (MRI) or computed tomographic (CT) scans were also performed to exclude subjects with overt cerebrovascular disease. A subset of NIMH AD subjects were autopsy confirmed (N = 24). Medical evaluation of control subjects was performed to exclude serious medical illnesses, including type 1 diabetes mellitus, significant hypertension, or cardiovascular disease. All normal control subjects with a first-degree AD relative were tested longitudinally on specialized cognitive tests designed to detect subtle alterations in memory (Rosen *et al.*, 2002). Normal controls from the NIMH sample set were also cognitively screened for subtle memory impairment. Trained inpatient staff administered clinical dementia ratings (CDR), global deterioration scale (GDS), and the Mini-Mental State Examination (MMSE). All cognitive tests were performed within 1 month of lumbar puncture. Medical evaluation of subjects obtained from commercial sources included a routine MRI or CT scan to exclude cerebrovascular disease, medical screening, APO ε genotyping, and clinical MMSE assessments. In addition, CSF measurements of Abeta 1–42, Abeta 1–40, and total tau were obtained in samples from the NIMH and Impath. CDR in all AD subjects ranged from 0.5 to 3.0. Disease onset, duration, and demographics were recorded for all subjects.

The AD proteomic study included analysis of 772 CSF samples run on 772 separate 2D gels. Of the 772 gels, 485 were from subjects with AD, 165 from control subjects with a first-degree relative (NCF), 79 from normal controls (NCO), 11 from mild cognitive impairment (MCI), 8 from normal controls ages 20–40, and 24 quality control gels. In general, longitudinal samples were obtained both from AD and from normal controls ranging over a period of 3–72 months in AD patients and from 3–48 months in controls. Although patients were matched by gender, the controls were on average 10 years younger than the AD set, and subsequent statistical analysis included age corrections. Within the AD group, 167 patients were obtained from the NIMH sample bank and 52 from independent sources, including 20 from Steve Ferris at NYU and 31 from commercial sources. All NCF patient samples were obtained from NIMH. Within the NCO group, 51 patients were from the NIMH sample bank and 5 from commercial sources. Finally, quality control (QC) samples (aliquots of pooled CSF) were submitted to enable quality control checks of the technology.

3. Lumbar Puncture

Lumbar puncture for CSF was performed early in the morning while the patient was in the lateral decubitus or a sitting position. Following application of local 1–2% lidocaine anesthetic, a lumbar puncture was performed in the L3–4 or L4–5 interspace using a 4-cm long 20- or 22-gauge needle. A 25-gauge Whitacre spinal point needle was then inserted into the 20- or 22-gauge needle and connected to a polypropylene line and 10-ml syringe (Linker *et al.*, 2002). CSF sample was withdrawn at a rate of 2 ml per minute. After collection, patients reclined for approximately 15–20 minutes before resuming normal activities. Samples were immediately frozen on dry ice and transferred to $-70\,^{\circ}C$ for long-term storage.

4. Immunodepletion and Sample Loading Protocol

Total protein content for each CSF sample was determined through the use of protein assay kits (e.g., Pierce). CSF (3–5 ml) was then subjected to immuno-depletion of high abundant proteins. In brief, polyclonal antibodies against albumin, alpha-2 macroglobulin, haptoglobin, transferrin, and alpha-1 antitryp-sin were coupled to protein-G sepharose on "Hi-Trap" (Pharmacia) columns. Two such columns were then placed in tandem with a third protein G column for removal of immunoglobulin G. CSF was passed through columns using an auto-mated AKTA fast protein liquid chromatography (FPLC) system, and proteins were eluted with Immuno Pure Ag/Ab elution buffer (Pierce). The eluate was desalted and concentrated by centrifugal ultrafiltration and total protein recovery determined. A subset of the gels was loaded based on constant volume of CSF immunodepletion such that total protein loaded varied between 30–980 μg per gel. The remaining gels were loaded with constant 100 μg, of protein. All solutions were resuspended in 10% SDS, 65 millimolar (mM) DTT, 8 M urea, 4% CHAPS, and 2% resolytes 3.5–10, then subjected to 3–10 pH isoelectric focusing using an Immobline DryStrip kit (Pharmacia) per manufacturer's directions and focused overnight (70 KvH, 20C), as described previously (Sanchez *et al.*, 1997). Resultant strips were then subjected to standardized SDS-PAGE, as described previously (Amess and Tolkovsky, 1995). After electrophoresis, gels were fixed with 40% ethanol, 10% acetic acid, and 50% ddH$_2$O overnight and then primed with 7.5% acetic acid, 0.05% SDS, and 92.5% ddH$_2$O for 30 minutes. Gels were then stained with 1.2 mg per liter of pyridinium, 4[2-[4[(dipentylamino)-2-trifluoromethylphenyl]ethenyl]-1-(sulfobutyl)] salt prepared in 7.5% acetic acid.

Gels were scanned with Apollo II scanners to obtain 16-bit monochrome
fluorescence images at 200 μm resolution (Oxford GlycoSciences, UK). Data
was processed using MELANIE III analysis software (BioRad, US). One gel image
was generated for each sample. Individual resolved protein spots (features) were
enumerated and quantified based on fluorescence intensity. The pI and molecular
weight of each feature were calculated by bilinear interpolation, as described in
detail (Page *et al.*, 1999). Images from individual gels were mapped to a common
master gel, and coordinates and intensities for the dataset were entered into the
protein expression matrix, as described previously (Page *et al.*, 1999). All analyses
were based on using percentage volume (%Vol) measurements rather than absolute volume of individual spots. The percentage volume was the ratio of a single
feature's volume divided by the summation of the volume of all features (spots)
per gel. Differential analysis was performed using either proprietary software
(ROSETTA, Oxford GlycoSciences) or as described in the following section on
statistical analysis. A pooled CSF sample was used as a quality control sample to
assess interassay and intraassay precision.

5. *CSF Proteome*

Approximately 7000 unique spots were identified in the CSF proteome. Of
the 7000 spots, Oxford GlycoSciences had identified and sequenced approximately 1400 spots that were utilized in the current analysis. Protein features were
excised from gel and sequenced as described previously (Page *et al.*, 1999).

6. *Statistical Analysis*

For the initial analysis, both univariate and multivariate approaches were
applied to identify top candidates. Case subjects (i.e., patients with Alzheimer's
disease) were categorized by three different methods: (1) by autopsy confirmed,
(2) by disease duration, and (3) by CDR. One CSF sample per patient was utilized
in statistical analysis. Longitudinal CSF samples were used to examine patterns of
expression of individual features over time. Data were corrected for age and
gender, and comparisons were done with missing values either excluded (null) or
set to zero. In addition, only features that were present in at least 60% of the gels
were analyzed. For univariate analysis, both parametric student t tests and nonparametric Wilcoxon rank tests were used to rank the top candidates based on
p values. Univariate analysis were performed separately on data obtained from the
NIMH sample set. Once the top candidates from the NIMH dataset were identified, univariate analysis was applied to independent datasets of 20 NYU samples
plus 39 commercial samples. Top biomarker candidate lists were generated from
the independent datasets using student's t-test and Wilcoxon rank test with age and
gender as covariates. These candidates were then compared to the original NIMH
dataset and a finalized top candidate list generated. Only candidates that appeared
on all lists were included in the top candidate biomarker list.

From the final individual feature list, groups of proteins were categorized into related families and multivariate approaches applied. The primary multivariate analysis used in the present study was linear discriminant analysis (LDA). LDA was performed using features that included all known members of a single protein family (e.g., all complements or all secretogranins). LDA generated a score for each sample based on a linear function that weighted the summations of individual spots (i.e., score $= C_1*spot_1 + C_2*spot_2 + \cdots C_K*spot_K$). The coefficients (weights) were determined using a subset of predefined samples (the training samples) such that the LDA score would best discriminate between cases and controls. LDA scores obtained from analysis including related family members were used to assess correlation with disease progression as assessed by MMSE scores.

C. RESULTS

Figure 1 illustrates the clinical information associated with the NIMH dataset. Information for NIMH included age at time of CSF draw, age at disease onset, date of CSF draw, visit number, disease duration, APO ϵ allele status, MMSE, CDR, GDS, handedness, education level, and CSF biomarker data, including total tau, Abeta 1–42 and Abeta 1–40 levels. A subset of patients had additional information on total brain and hippocampal volume, as well as responses to scopolamine challenge tests. Age and gender were used as covariates in the statistical modeling. Some analyses were also performed that segregated

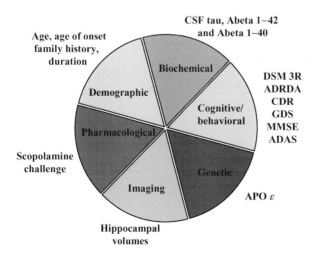

FIG. 1. Overview of clinical characteristics of NIMH dataset. (See Color Insert.)

AD subjects based on disease duration, MMSE, CDR, APO ϵ allele status or biomarker levels (data not presented). In general there were more women than men in the proteomic dataset and patients with Alzheimer's disease were older than controls by approximately 10 years (Table I). As a result, all statistical analyses corrected for age discrepancies. Based on the MMSE, there was an even distribution of patients during early, progressive, and late stages of AD (see Table I).

One technological challenge of 2DE profiling is that variations in protein expression can be as great as 10,000-fold. As a result, abundant protein expression dominates proteomic profiles. In CSF, albumin, alpha-2 macroglobulin, haptoglobin, transferrin, and alpha-1 antitrypsin were some of the most highly expressed proteins, and 2DE analysis of straight CSF was dominated by these species (Fig. 2B). To address abundant protein masking difficulties, an immunodepletion step was introduced to remove abundant proteins. Figure 2 illustrates the procedure for immunodepletion. In brief, CSF was passed through immunodepletion columns to remove albumin, alpha-2 macroglobulin, haptoglobin, transferrin, alpha-1 antitrypsin, and immunoglobulin G (Fig. 2A). The resultant eluate was run on 2D gels (See Fig. 2A). Figure 2B shows examples of 2D gels following loading of untreated CSF, of fraction bound by immunodepletion columns, and of resultant CSF eluate. Note improved resolution of CSF eluate following removal of abundant proteins (See Fig. 2B).

After electrophoresis and staining, the gels were imaged using an Apollo II scanner and images aligned to a single master gel (Fig. 3A). During batch runs, quality control samples were run to assess the variability associated with inter-assay precision. QC samples consisted of a pooled CSF sample aliquoted into 5-ml aliquots, which were used to test reproducibility of immunodepletion and gel runs. Features that appeared in 70% of the QC gels were assessed for coefficient of variability (CV) and a variability map generated (Fig. 3B). For most regions of the gel, CVs averaged between 25% and 35%. However, there were certain regions of the gel that were prone to extremely poor test retest analysis

TABLE I
PATIENT DEMOGRAPHICS IN AD PROTEOMICS DATASET

	AD	Controls NCF	Controls NCO	All Controls
Gender (M/F)	96/123	36/70	32/24	68/94
Age yrs (Mean ± STD)	71±9.6	56 ± 9.9	64 ± 11.2	59 ± 10
MMSE < 8[a]	7	–	–	–
8 < MMSE ≤ 15	60	–	–	–
15 < MMSE ≤ 22	61	–	–	–
22 < MMSE	87	–	–	–

[a]MMSE range based on first visit per patient.

A   CSF   Affinity columns   Fractions

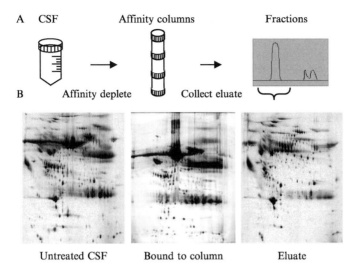

B   Affinity deplete   Collect eluate

        Untreated CSF   Bound to column   Eluate

Fig. 2. Affinity depletion of high abundant proteins. (A) CSF was passed through depletion columns designed to capture high abundant proteins. (B) These images show representative 2DE gels loaded with either untreated CSF, fraction bound by depletion columns, or immunodepleted fraction (eluate). Note improved resolution of lower abundance proteins upon removal of high abundant proteins.

(See Fig. 3B; CVs greater than 50%). Features that were localized in highly variable regions were excluded from subsequent statistical analysis.

Another difficulty associated with 2D gel approaches involves the complexity of differential processing and post-translational modifications. As a result, one protein can be represented by many different features (Gygi and Aebersold, 2000). Figure 4 provides an example of one family of proteins, the complements, which exemplifies the complexity of proteomic profiling approaches. In the CSF proteome a small protein-like complement C3 can be represented by more than 70 different spots on the gel with variations in pH and size due primarily to proteolytic processing. As a result, multivariate analysis was initiated to include multiple isoforms of the same protein in addition to inclusion of related protein family members.

Preliminary univariate analysis involved parametric and nonparametric t-tests between AD and control subjects. AD subjects were subdivided based on disease duration, CDR, MMSE, and whether subjects had been autopsy confirmed. Comparisons were also made between AD and NCO, AD and NCF, and AD versus a combined NCO/NCF group. For each comparison a top candidate list was generated based on consistent fold change (e.g., increased in all comparisons) and on p value significance level by t-tests (with lower p values ranked highest). Comparisons were corrected for age and gender. In cases in which multiple samples were available from the same patient the first sample

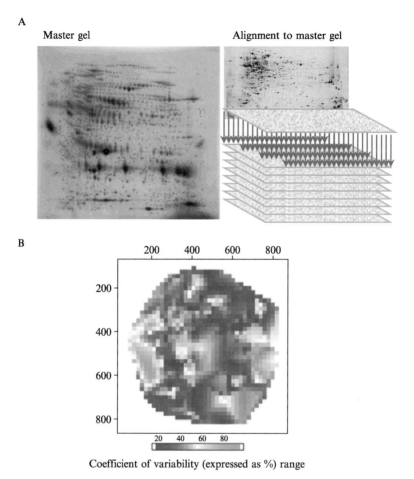

A

Master gel   Alignment to master gel

B

Coefficient of variability (expressed as %) range

Fig. 3. Gel alignments and test retest variability. (A) One master gel was created, and gels containing experimental samples were all mapped to coordinates defined by one single master gel. (B) Assessment of test retest variability as measured by coefficient of variation of individual features from aliquots of a pooled CSF sample (quality control) run multiple times. Only features that appeared on 70% of the gels were included in the analysis. Note variability changed throughout the spatial map. (See Color Insert.)

from the subject was typically used in the analysis. Table II summarizes those proteins that consistently appeared in the top 100 rankings of the various comparisons between case (AD) and control. In general the majority of the candidates showed decreased levels in AD when compared to controls, with the exception of gelsolin and hemopexin (See Table II). In some instances different proteolytic fragments of proteins were increasing while others were decreasing. Some examples of differential process included the complements and pigment

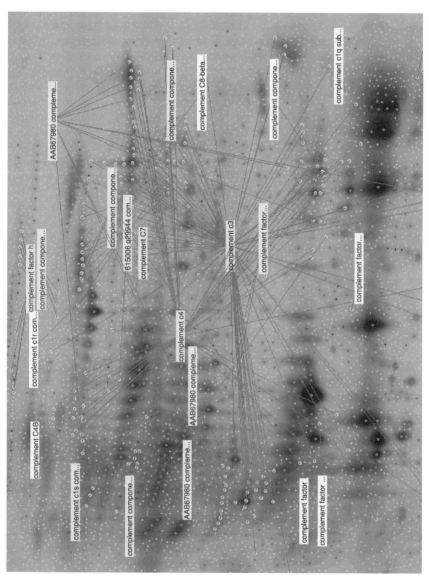

complement C4B

complement c1r com...

complement factor h

complement compone...

AAB67980 compleme...

complement c1s com...

complement compone...

complement compone...

615006 q29944 com...

complement C7

complement C8-beta...

complement c4

AAB67980 compleme...

AAB67980 compleme...

complement c3

complement compone...

complement factor...

complement factor...

complement factor

complement factor ...

complement c1q sub...

FIG. 4. The complexity of the CSF proteome as exemplified by the complement cascade. (See Color Insert.)

TABLE II

Top CSF Candidate Biomarkers Using Univariate Approaches

NCAMs	Secretogranins
Complement	ApoE/Transthyretin
Cystatin C	*Gelsolin*
Neuron-specific enolase	**Neuronal pentraxin/dynein**
Prostaglandin H2 isomerases	**Acetylcholinesterase membrane anchor protein**
Superoxide Dismutase	Angiotensinogen
KIAAA0911	**Zinc glycoproteins**
PEDF	**Malate dehydrogenases**
Kallikreins/kinins	Exostosin/acetylglucosaminyl transferases
Hemopexin	PAMs

Proteins that were decreased in Alzheimer's disease are highlighted in bold are italicized; proteins that were increased in AD; Multiple isoforms that were either increasing or decreasing depending on the isoform are shaded.

epithelial derived factor. Although some isoforms of apolipoprotein were identified as being differentially expressed, many of the apolipoproteins were in regions of the gel that showed poor test retest reproducibility. In some cases there were multiple isoforms of the protein, but only a few of the isoforms changed in Alzheimer's compared to controls. An example of this included the neural cell adhesion molecule (NCAM)s in which some isoforms were decreased, but not all isoforms.

One of the more interesting candidates identified were members of the secretogranin family. Figure 5A shows seven secretogranin family members identified as being differentially expressed in AD subjects compared to controls. Using percentage volume as a normalized measure of abundance, one of the seven members was profiled based on disease duration (Fig. 5B). In general, patients with AD had significantly lower levels of this particular secretogranin in comparison to control subjects (NCO) and control subjects with a first-degree relative with Alzheimer's disease (NCF). However, there were overlaps between the AD and control groups. In addition, univariate comparisons did not fully capture the complexity or contribution of changes associated with related family members. As a result, multivariate LDA approaches were employed to analyze differences in all secretogranin expression in Alzheimer's disease.

Linear discriminant analysis utilizes an iterative process with known AD and control samples to calculate coefficients that are best suited at discriminating between case and control. In Fig. 6, 80 AD samples and 128 control samples were used to train the LDA model. Cutoff levels were set such that misclassification rate for AD was 22% and misclassification rate for controls was 37% (See Fig. 6). The final model was then tested on ability to discriminate between AD and control patients using a subset of samples from the NIMH dataset (Fig. 7A and B), as well as independent samples obtained from NYU (Fig. 7C) and from

A

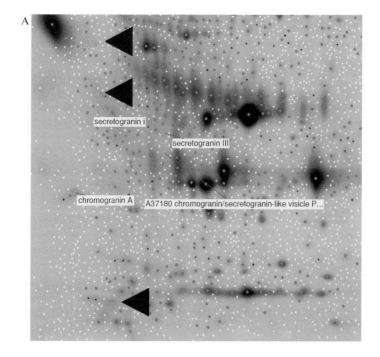

secretogranin i

secretogranin III

chromogranin A   A37180 chromogranin/secretogranin-like visicle P...

B

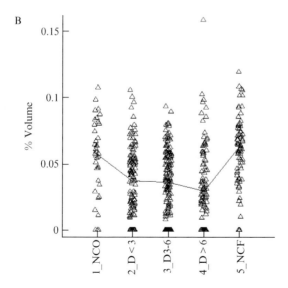

Secretogranin, app. err. rate = 0.312, CV err. rate = 0.378

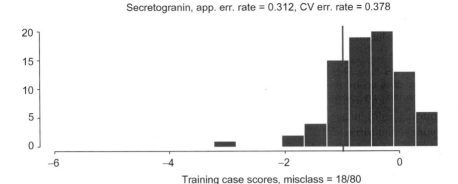

Training case scores, misclass = 18/80

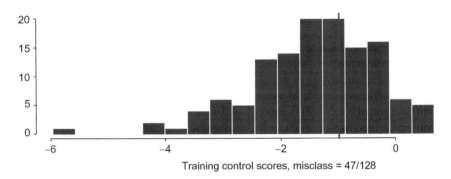

Training control scores, misclass = 47/128

FIG. 6. Linear discriminant analysis (LDA) using all seven secretogranin members in model to delineate between case (AD) and control (NCO and NCF) in the training model. Cutoffs were set with a misclassification rate of 22% for case (specificity of 78%) and 37% for controls (sensitivity of 63%).

Lampire Biologicals (Fig. 7D). Figure 7 shows that in general the model could differentiate AD patients with a misclassification rate ranging from 14% to 35%. Misclassification rates (false positive rate) were 39% for the controls.

Finally, an analysis was performed to determine whether multivariate analysis of the secretogranin family correlated with disease severity as assessed by MMSE. Figure 8 shows results from the analysis. LDA scores based on use of all seven

---

FIG. 5. The secretogranin family. (A) Region of gel showing the seven secretogranin proteins identified in CSF proteome. (B) Expression of one of the secretogranin proteins in AD versus control patients. AD subjects were subdivided by disease duration. D < 3-disease duration of less than 3 years. D3-6-disease duration between 3–6 years. D > 6-disease duration of greater than 6 years. NCO-normal controls. NCF-normal controls with first degree AD relative. Note that levels of the secretogranin protein are decreased in AD versus normal controls. (See Color Insert.)

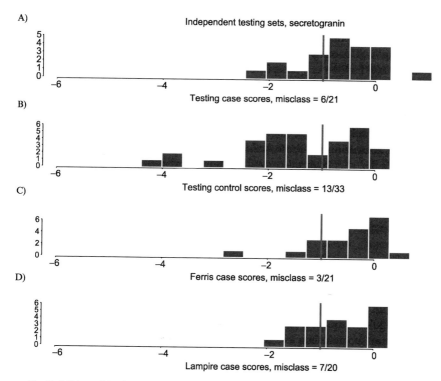

Fig. 7. LDA model using all seven secretogranins in the testing model. Model was used to test accuracy of differentiating between case (AD) and controls from NIMH, NYU, and commercial datasets. (A) AD samples from NIMH dataset. (B) Control samples from NIMH dataset. (C) AD samples from NYU dataset. (D) AD samples from Lampire dataset. Note misclassification rates for AD NIMH was 29%, for NYU 14%, for Lampire 35%, and for controls 39%.

secretogranin family members correlated with disease severity as assessed by MMSE.

D. Discussion and Summary

In summary, 2DE proteomic approaches can be used to successfully identify changes in CSF protein expression in patients with Alzheimer's disease. Several modifications were made to enable examination of low abundant proteins as well as improve comparisons across samples. Specifically, CSF was immunodepleted of high abundant proteins, including albumin, haptoglobulin, transferrin, alpha-2 macroglobulin, and immunoglobulin. In addition, there were regions of the gel that were excluded from the analysis as a result of poor test retest reproducibility.

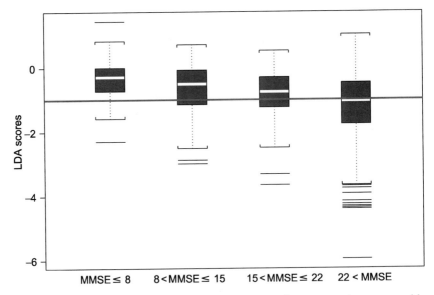

FIG. 8. Comparison of secretogranin family LDA scores to disease progression, as assessed by MMSE. Note LDA scores showed correlation with MMSE.

Following a number of univariate approaches that involved comparison of AD versus controls based on different classifications of the AD, it was found that specific families of proteins were consistently and repeatedly altered in subjects with AD. Multivariate LDA identified protein families that correlated with disease state and progression. Sensitivity and specificity of the markers was even better when multiple proteins within individual families were analyzed as a composite group.

Many of the proteins identified have been previously implicated in AD pathological processes. For example, there are numerous reports to suggest that the complement cascade is activated through the classical pathway by Abeta interactions with C1q (Emmerling *et al.*, 2000; Shen and Meri, 2003). Furthermore, pigment epithelial derived factor (PEDF) has been identified in other AD proteomic screens as a potential biomarker in dementia (Davidsson *et al.*, 2002). Thus the technology appears capable of identifying biologically relevant players in AD pathological processes.

Although univariate approaches could identify proteins that were differentially expressed in AD versus control patients, univariate approaches often failed to capture the full complexity of the proteome, and multivariate approaches using related family members were employed. One of the protein families examined by the multivariate LDA was the secretogranin family. Linear discriminant analyses were able to discriminate AD from controls with a diagnostic accuracy not too different from existing CSF Abeta and tau approaches to differentiate between AD and controls (Jensen *et al.*, 1999; Kanai *et al.*, 1998; Sunderland *et al.*, 2003; Tapiola *et al.*, 2000). Furthermore, LDA showed correlation with disease progression as assessed by MMSE, which is a relatively rare finding for AD biomarkers.

The secretogranins are a unique group of acidic, soluble secretory proteins typically located in dense core vesicles of the neuroendocrine system (Taupenot *et al.*, 2003). The granins are proproteins with multiple recognition sites for endopeptidases. Peptides derived from the proteolytic processing of granins have autocrine, paracrine, and endocrine activities (Taupenot *et al.*, 2003). Preliminary functional studies suggest that granins are essential for the formation of dense core vesicles (Kim *et al.*, 2003). In addition, peptides generated from the granin profamily appear to have modulatory activity on catecholaminergic systems. For example, secretoneurin derived from secretogranin II has been demonstrated to stimulate dopaminergic release from nigrostriatal neurons (Wiedermann, 2000). Furthermore, many of the granins have been localized to vesicles within synaptic regions of the hippocampus, and a number of the granins have been reported to be down-regulated in both hippocampus and CSF of patients with Alzheimer's disease (Blennow *et al.*, 1995; Kaufmann *et al.*, 1998; Marksteiner *et al.*, 2000, 2002). Thus identification of alterations in the secretogranin family in the present study is perhaps not surprising. However, correlation with disease progression is a relatively rare finding, and the secretogranins could serve as useful clinical endpoints in tracking disease modulatory effects as well as in identifying patients in the early stages of disease.

Despite the success in identifying biologically relevant proteins, there were technological difficulties. For example, introduction of the immunodepletion step may have depleted proteins relevant to Alzheimer's disease. Specifically, some amyloid beta peptides were likely to have been immunodepleted, because they are known to interact with high abundant albumin proteins. In addition, membrane-bound proteins could not be examined and proteins that were in very low abundance or were at the extreme ranges of pH and molecular weight could not be examined. Indeed, proteins known to change in AD, which should have been detected on the gel (e.g., tau, S100B), were not identified. The CSF proteome has not yet been fully characterized because only 1400 of the total 7000 spots had been sequenced by mass spectrometry. Thus it is possible that S100B and tau have yet to be mapped onto the current proteome. Nevertheless, incomplete characterization of proteomes is one of the disadvantages facing current profiling approaches. Finally, there was a high degree of noise associated with the technology (e.g., CVs of features in most regions of the gel averaged between 25–40%) and some regions of the gel showed very poor test retest performance (CVs greater than 50%). Nevertheless, the technology proved useful in determining which isoforms of known proteolytically cleaved proteins alter with disease. Furthermore, the technology was particularly useful for delineating possible post-translational modifications of individual protein isoforms that were most relevant to the disease state. In summary, 2DE profiling provided a starting point for developing more sensitive quantitative assays capable of differentiating AD from control subjects and of identifying tools that may correlate with disease progression and identification of subjects in the early stages of disease.

III. Future Challenges and Conclusions

The proteome is significantly more complex than the genome, because the inherent biochemical nature of proteins depend on more complicated building blocks (e.g., amino acids, sugars, and carbohydrates rather than four nucleotides). Furthermore, intracellular localization, proteolytic processing, post-translational modification, and protein-protein interactions add greatly to protein complexity. As a result, there is no one technological format capable of addressing all aspects of protein dynamics in the context of disease state and disease progression. Nevertheless, each type of technological platform yields distinct and often times nonoverlapping advantages in addressing proteomic-related questions. For example, 2DE approaches may be better suited to identify patterns of expression associated with a particular disease state, whereas activity-based approaches are more suitable for functional questions related to drug-target interactions. Thus, success in proteomic initiatives will depend on asking well-defined questions and choosing the most appropriate technology format best suited for the scientific question under study. One significant challenge that remains is developing more powerful informatics tools to handle the extremely large amounts of data associated with proteomic initiatives. In addition, developing more quantitative and robust assay formats using MS-based approaches remains a technological hurdle. However, recent advances in mass spectrometry instrumentation and immuno-based multiplexing technology have improved the feasibility of quantitating multiple proteins in a single assay.

From a drug discovery and development perspective, the greatest challenge remains translating the information garnered from proteomic initiatives into quantitative, sensitive, and specific assays capable of delivering information about a drug's effect on the target and whether the drug can effectively alter the disease in a clinically beneficial manner. Although proteomics may provide information about new targets, one of the major hurdles in early drug discovery is to demonstrate that the drug has bound specifically to target and produced a *biological*, meaningful activity both *in vitro* and *in vivo*. In theory, evolving functional proteomic approaches are capable of providing answers to these types of functional questions. In addition, profiling proteomic approaches can be used to predict whether a drug will be safe in the clinic and improve clinical study design by identifying placebo responders or patients at risk of disease or in the very early stages of disease (i.e., those most likely to benefit from disease modification strategies). In the current case study a profiling approach was used to identify proteins that correlate with disease progression and could potentially be used to identify patients in the early stages of disease. However, translating these early findings into an assay that satisfies the rigorous regulatory requirements of drug development programs remains a challenge that is common to most proteomic approaches being developed. Despite existing challenges, proteomic technologies offer powerful tools to sometimes difficult scientific questions and is certainly a path to the future for more efficient drug discovery and development.

References

Aarts, M., Liu, Y., Liu, L., Besshoh, S., Arundine, M., Gurd, J. W., Wang, Y. T., Salter, M. W., and Tymianski, M. (2002). Treatment of ischemic brain damage by perturbing NMDA receptor-PSD-95 protein interactions. *Science* **298**(5594), 846–850.

Adam, G. C., Sorensen, E. J., and Cravatt, B. F. (2002a). Chemical strategies for functional proteomics. *Mol. Cell Proteomics* **1**(10), 781–790.

Adam, G. C., Sorensen, E. J., and Cravatt, B. F. (2002b). Proteomic profiling of mechanistically distinct enzyme classes using a common chemotype. *Nat. Biotechnol.* **20**(8), 805–809.

Aebersold, R. (2003). A mass spectrometric journey into protein and proteome research. *J. Am. Soc. Mass. Spectrom.* **14**, 685–695.

Amess, B., and Tolkovsky, A. M. (1995). *Electrophoresis* **16,** 1255–1267.

Bandara, L. R., Kelly, M. D., Lock, E. A., and Kennedy, S. (2003). A correlation between a proteomic evaluation and conventional measurements in the assessment of renal proximal tubular toxicity. *Toxicol. Sci.* **73**(1), 195–206.

Bartel, P. L., Roecklein, J. A., SenGupta, D., and Fields, S. (1996). A protein linkage map of Escherichia coli bacteriophage T7. *Nat. Genet.* **12**(1), 72–77.

Blennow, K., Davidsson, P., Wallin, A., and Ekman, R. (1995). Chromogranin A in cerebrospinal fluid: A biochemical marker for synaptic degeneration in Alzheimer's disease? *Dementia* **6**(6), 306–311.

Boguski, M. S., and McIntosh, M. W. (2003). Biomedical informatics for proteomics. *Nature* **422**(6928), 233–237.

Borodovsky, A., Ovaa, H., Kolli, N., Gan-Erdene, T., Wilkinson, K. D., Ploegh, H. L., and Kessler, B. M. (2002). Chemistry-based functional proteomics reveals novel members of the deubiquitinating enzyme family. *Chem. Biol.* **9**(10), 1149–1159.

Brindle, J. T., Antti, H., Holmes, E., Tranter, G., Nicholson, J. K., Bethell, H. W., Clarke, S., Schofield, P. M., McKilligin, E., Mosedale, D. E., and Grainger, D. J. (2002). Rapid and noninvasive diagnosis of the presence and severity of coronary heart disease using 1H-NMR-based metabonomics. *Nat. Med.* **8**(12), 1439–1444.

Brindle, J. T., Nicholson, J. K., Schofield, P. M., Grainger, D. J., and Holmes, E. (2003). Application of chemometrics to 1H NMR spectroscopic data to investigate a relationship between human serum metabolic profiles and hypertension. *Analyst* **128**(1), 32–36.

Brookmeyer, R., and Gray, S. (2000). Methods for projecting the incidence and prevalence of chronic diseases in aging populations: Application to Alzheimer's disease. *Stat. Med.* **19**(11–12), 1481–1493.

Chakravarti, D. N., Chakravarti, B., and Moutsatsos, I. (2002). Informatic tools for proteome profiling. *Biotechniques* (Suppl.), 4–10, 12–15.

Chang, C. Y., Norris, J. D., Jansen, M., Huang, H. J., and McDonnell, D. P. (2003). Application of random peptide phage display to the study of nuclear hormone receptors. *Methods Enzymol.* **364,** 118–142.

Chaurand, P., Fouchecourt, S., DaGue, B. B., Xu, B. J., Reyzer, M. L., Orgebin-Crist, M. C., and Caprioli, R. M. (2003). Profiling and imaging proteins in the mouse epididymis by imaging mass spectrometry. *Proteomics* **3**(11), 2221–2239.

Chaurand, P., Schwartz, S. A., and Caprioli, R. M. (2002). Imaging mass spectrometry. A new tool to investigate the spatial organization of peptides and proteins in mammalian tissue sections. *Curr. Opin. Chem. Biol.* **6**(5), 676–681.

Clark, B. F. (1981). Towards a total human protein map. *Nature* **292**(5823), 491–492.

Davidsson, P., Sjogren, M., Andreasen, N., Lindbjer, M., Nilsson, C. L., Westman-Brinkmalm, A., and Blennow, K. (2002). Studies of the pathophysiological mechanisms in frontotemporal dementia by proteome analysis of CSF proteins. *Brain Res. Mol. Brain Res.* **109**(1–2), 128–133.

DiMasi, J. A., Hansen, R. W., and Grabowski, H. G. (2003). The price of innovation: New estimates of drug development costs. *J. Health Econ.* **22**(2), 151–185.

DiMasi, J. A., Hansen, R. W., Grabowski, H. G., and Lasagna, L. (1991). Cost of innovation in the pharmaceutical industry. *J. Health Econ.* **10**(2), 107–142.

Doody, R. S., Massman, P., and Dunn, J. K. (2001). A method for estimating progression rates in Alzheimer disease. *Arch. Neurol.* **58**(3), 449–454.

Emmerling, M. R., Watson, M. D., Raby, C. A., and Spiegel, K. (2000). The role of complement in Alzheimer's disease pathology. *Biochim. Biophys. Acta.* **1502**(1), 158–171.

Espina, V., Mehta, A. I., Winters, M. E., Calvert, V., Wulfkuhle, J., Petricoin, E. F., III, and Liotta, L. A. (2003). Protein microarrays: Molecular profiling technologies for clinical specimens. *Proteomics* **3**(11), 2091–2100.

Fenyo, D., and Beavis, R. C. (2002). Informatics and data management in proteomics. *Trends Biotechnol.* **20**(Suppl. 12), S35–S38.

Fields, S., and Song, O. (1989). A novel genetic system to detect protein-protein interactions. *Nature* **340**(6230), 245–246.

Flajolet, M., Rotondo, G., Daviet, L., Bergametti, F., Inchauspe, G., Tiollais, P., Transy, C., and Legrain, P. (2000). A genomic approach of the hepatitis C virus generates a protein interaction map. *Gene* **242**(1–2), 369–379.

Fuh, G., Pisabarro, M. T., Li, Y., Quan, C., Lasky, L. A., and Sidhu, S. S. (2000). Analysis of PDZ domain-ligand interactions using carboxyl-terminal phage display. *J. Biol. Chem.* **275**(28), 21486–21491.

Gerlt, J. A. (2002). "Fishing" for the functional proteome *Nat. Biotechnol.* **20**(8), 786–787.

Griffin, J. L. (2003). Metabonomics: NMR spectroscopy and pattern recognition analysis of body fluids and tissues for characterisation of xenobiotic toxicity and disease diagnosis. *Curr. Opin. Chem. Biol.* **7**(5), 648–654.

Griffin, J. L., Cemal, C. K., and Pook, M. A. (2003). Defining a metabolic phenotype in the brain of a transgenic mouse model of spinocerebellar ataxia 3. *Physiol. Genomics.* **16**, 16.

Grubb, R. L., Calvert, V. S., Wulkuhle, J. D., Paweletz, C. P., Linehan, W. M., Phillips, J. L., Chuaqui, R., Valasco, A., Gillespie, J., Emmert-Buck, M., Liotta, L. A., and Petricoin, E. F.

(2003). Signal pathway profiling of prostate cancer using reverse phase protein arrays. *Proteomics* **3**(11), 2142–2146.

Gygi, S. P., and Aebersold, R. (2000). Mass spectrometry and proteomics. *Curr. Opin. Chem. Biol.* **4**(5), 489–494.

Gygi, S. P., Corthals, G. L., Zhang, Y., Rochon, Y., and Aebersold, R. (2000). Evaluation of two-dimensional gel electrophoresis-based proteome analysis technology. *Proc. Natl. Acad. Sci. USA* **97**(17), 9390–9395.

Gygi, S. P., Rist, B., Gerber, S. A., Turecek, F., Gelb, M. H., and Aebersold, R. (1999). Quantitative analysis of complex protein mixtures using isotope-coded affinity tags. *Nat. Biotechnol.* **17**(10), 994–999.

Haab, B. B. (2003). Methods and applications of antibody microarrays in cancer research. *Proteomics* **3**(11), 2116–2122.

Hagenstein, M. C., Mussgnug, J. H., Lotte, K., Plessow, R., Brockhinke, A., Kruse, O., and Sewald, N. (2003). Affinity-based tagging of protein families with reversible inhibitors: A concept for functional proteomics. *Angew Chem. Int. Ed. Eng.* **42**(45), 5635–5638.

Hanash, S. (2003). The emerging field of protein microarrays. *Proteomics* **3**(11), 2075.

Harris, R. A., Yang, A., Stein, R. C., Lucy, K., Brusten, L., Herath, A., Parekh, R., Waterfield, M. D., O'Hare, M. J., Neville, M. A., Page, M. J., and Zvelebil, M. J. (2002). Cluster analysis of an extensive human breast cancer cell line protein expression map database. *Proteomics* **2**(2), 212–223.

Hoogenboom, H. R., de Bruine, A. P., Hufton, S. E., Hoet, R. M., Arends, J. W., and Roovers, R. C. (1998). Antibody phage display technology and its applications. *Immunotechnology* **4**(1), 1–20.

Hufton, S. E., Moerkerk, P. T., Meulemans, E. V., de Bruine, A., Arends, J. W., and Hoogenboom, H. R. (1999). Phage display of cDNA repertoires: The pVI display system and its applications for the selection of immunogenic ligands. *J. Immunol. Methods* **231**(1–2), 39–51.

Hunt, D. F., Henderson, R. A., Shabanowitz, J., Sakaguchi, K., Michel, H., Sevilir, N., Cox, A. L., Appella, E., and Engelhard, V. H. (1992). Characterization of peptides bound to the class I MHC molecule HLA-A2.1 by mass spectrometry. *Science* **255**(5049), 1261–1263.

Jang, J. H., and Hanash, S. (2003). Profiling of the cell surface proteome. *Proteomics* **3**(10), 1947–1954.

Jarvik, J. W., Fisher, G. W., Shi, C., Hennen, L., Hauser, C., Adler, S., and Berget, P. B. (2002). In vivo functional proteomics: Mammalian genome annotation using CD-tagging. *Biotechniques* **33**(4), 852–854, 856, 858–860 passim.

Jensen, M., Schroder, J., Blomberg, M., Engvall, B., Pantel, J., Ida, N., Basun, H., Wahlund, L. O., Werle, E., Jauss, M., Beyreuther, K., Lannfelt, L., and Hartmann, T. (1999). Cerebrospinal fluid A beta42 is increased early in sporadic Alzheimer's disease and declines with disease progression. *Ann. Neurol.* **45**(4), 504–511.

Jessani, N., Liu, Y., Humphrey, M., and Cravatt, B. F. (2002). Enzyme activity profiles of the secreted and membrane proteome that depict cancer cell invasiveness. *Proc. Natl. Acad. Sci. USA* **99**(16), 10335–10340.

Kanai, M., Matsubara, E., Isoe, K., Urakami, K., Nakashima, K., Arai, H., Sasaki, H., Abe, K., Iwatsubo, T., Kosaka, T., Watanabe, M., Tomidokoro, Y., Shizuka, M., Mizushima, K., Nakamura, T., Igeta, Y., Ikeda, Y., Amari, M., Kawarabayashi, T., Ishiguro, K., Harigaya, Y., Wakabayashi, K., Okamoto, K., Hirai, S., and Shoji, M. (1998). Longitudinal study of cerebrospinal fluid levels of tau, A beta1-40, and A beta1-42(43) in Alzheimer's disease: A study in Japan. *Ann. Neurol.* **44**(1), 17–26.

Kaufmann, W. A., Barnas, U., Humpel, C., Nowakowski, K., DeCol, C., Gurka, P., Ransmayr, G., Hinterhuber, H., Winkler, H., and Marksteiner, J. (1998). Synaptic loss reflected by secretoneurin-like immunoreactivity in the human hippocampus in Alzheimer's disease. *Eur. J. Neurosci.* **10**(3), 1084–1094.

Kenyon, G. L., DeMarini, D. M., Fuchs, E., Galas, D. J., Kirsch, J. F., Leyh, T. S., Moos, W. H., Petsko, G. A., Ringe, D., Rubin, G. M., and Sheahan, L. C. (2002). Defining the mandate of proteomics in the post-genomics era: Workshop report. *Mol. Cell Proteomics* **1**(10), 763–780.

Kim, T., Tao-Cheng, J. H., Eiden, L. E., and Peng Loh, Y. (2003). The role of chromogranin A and the control of secretory granule genesis and maturation. *Trends Endocrinol. Metab.* **14**(2), 56–57.

Klose, J. (1975). Protein mapping by combined isoelectric focusing and electrophoresis of mouse tissues. A novel approach to testing for induced point mutations in mammals. *Humangenetik* **26**(3), 231–243.

Kozarich, J. W. (2003). Activity-based proteomics: Enzyme chemistry redux. *Curr. Opin. Chem. Biol.* **7**(1), 78–83.

Lathrop, J. T., Anderson, N. L., Anderson, N. G., and Hammond, D. J. (2003). Therapeutic potential of the plasma proteome. *Curr. Opin. Mol. Ther.* **5**(3), 250–257.

Le Blanc, J. C., Hager, J. W., Ilisiu, A. M., Hunter, C., Zhong, F., and Chu, I. (2003). Unique scanning capabilities of a new hybrid linear ion trap mass spectrometer (Q TRAP) used for high sensitivity proteomics applications. *Proteomics* **3**(6), 859–869.

Li Kw, K., Hornshaw, M. P., Van Der Schors, R. C., Watson, R., Tate, S., Casetta, B., Jimenez, C. R., Gouwenberg, Y., Gundelfinger, E. D., Smalla, K. H., and Smit, A. B. (2003). Proteomics analysis of rat brain postsynaptic density: Implications of the diverse protein functional groups for the integration of synaptic physiology. *J. Biol. Chem.* **7,** 7.

Lill, J. (2003). Proteomic tools for quantitation by mass spectrometry. *Mass. Spectrom. Rev.* **22**(3), 182–194.

Lin, D., Tabb, D. L., and Yates, J. R., III (2003). Large-scale protein identification using mass spectrometry. *Biochim. Biophys. Acta.* **1646**, 1–10.

Link, A. J., Eng, J., Schieltz, D. M., Carmack, E., Mize, G. J., Morris, D. R., Garvik, B. M., and Yates, J. R., III (1999). Direct analysis of protein complexes using mass spectrometry. *Nat. Biotechnol.* **17**(7), 676–682.

Linker, G., Mirza, N., Meyer, M., Putnam, K. T., and Sunderland, T. (2002). Fine-needle, negative-pressure lumbar puncture: A safe technique for collecting CSF. *Neurology* **59**(12), 2008–2009.

Liu, Y., Patricelli, M. P., and Cravatt, B. F. (1999). Activity-based protein profiling: The serine hydrolases. *Proc. Natl. Acad. Sci. USA* **96**, 14964–14699.

Lo, L. C., Pang, T. L., Kuo, C. H., Chiang, Y. L., Wang, H. Y., and Lin, J. J. (2002). Design and synthesis of class-selective activity probes for protein tyrosine phosphatases. *J. Proteome Res.* **1**(1), 35–40.

Marksteiner, J., Kaufmann, W. A., Gurka, P., and Humpel, C. (2002). Synaptic proteins in Alzheimer's disease. *J. Mol. Neurosci.* **18**(1–2), 53–63.

Marksteiner, J., Lechner, T., Kaufmann, W. A., Gurka, P., Humpel, C., Nowakowski, C., Maier, H., and Jellinger, K. A. (2000). Distribution of chromogranin B-like immunoreactivity in the human hippocampus and its changes in Alzheimer's disease. *Acta. Neuropathol. (Berl)* **100**(2), 205–212.

McCraith, S., Holtzman, T., Moss, B., and Fields, S. (2000). Genome-wide analysis of vaccinia virus protein-protein interactions. *Proc. Natl. Acad. Sci. USA* **97**(9), 4879–4884.

McKhann, G., Drachman, D., Folstein, M., Katzman, R., Price, D., and Stadlan, E. M. (1984). Clinical diagnosis of Alzheimer's disease: Report of the NINCDS-ADRDA Work Group under the auspices of Department of Health and Human Services Task Force on Alzheimer's Disease. *Neurology* **34**(7), 939–944.

O'Farrell, P. Z., Goodman, H. M., and O'Farrell, P. H. (1977). High resolution two-dimensional electrophoresis of basic as well as acidic proteins. *Cell* **12**(4), 1133–1141.

Ong, S. E., Foster, L. J., and Mann, M. (2003). Mass spectrometric-based approaches in quantitative proteomics. *Methods* **29**, 124–130.

Page, M. J., Amess, B., Townsend, R. R., Parekh, R., Herath, A., Brusten, L., Zvelebil, M. J., Stein, R. C., Waterfield, M. D., Davies, S. C., and O'Hare, M. J. (1999). Proteomic definition of normal human luminal and myoepithelial breast cells purified from reduction mammoplasties. *Proc. Natl. Acad. Sci. USA* **96**(22), 12589–12594.

Patricelli, M. P., Giang, D. K., Stamp, L. M., and Burbaum, J. J. (2001). Direct visualization of serine hydrolase activities in complex proteomes using fluorescent active stie-directed probes. *Proteomics* **1,** 1067–1071.

Pieper, R., Gatlin, C. L., Makusky, A. J., Russo, P. S., Schatz, C. R., Miller, S. S., Su, Q., McGrath, A. M., Estock, M. A., Parmar, P. P., Zhao, M., Huang, S. T., Zhou, J., Wang, F., Esquer-Blasco, R., Anderson, N. L., Taylor, J., and Steiner, S. (2003). The human serum proteome: Display of nearly 3700 chromatographically separated protein spots on two-dimensional electrophoresis gels and identification of 325 distinct proteins. *Proteomics* **3**(7), 1345–1364.

Rain, J. C., Selig, L., De Reuse, H., Battaglia, V., Reverdy, C., Simon, S., Lenzen, G., Petel, F., Wojcik, J., Schachter, V., Chemama, Y., Labigne, A., and Legrain, P. (2001). The protein-protein interaction map of Helicobacter pylori. *Nature* **409**(6817), 211–215.

Reichert, J. M. (2003). Trends in development and approval times for new therapeutics in the United States. *Nat. Rev. Drug Discov.* **2**(9), 695–702.

Roberts, S. A. (2003). Drug metabolism and pharmacokinetics in drug discovery. *Curr. Opin. Drug Discov. Devel.* **6**(1), 66–80.

Robertson, D. G., Reily, M. D., Albbassam, M., and Dethloff, L. A. (2001). Metabonomic assessment of vasculitis in rats. *Cardiovasc. Toxicol.* **1**(1), 7–19.

Rosen, V. M., Bergeson, J. L., Putnam, K., Harwell, A., and Sunderland, T. (2002). Working memory and apolipoprotein E: What's the connection? *Neuropsychologia* **40**(13), 2226–2233.

Sanchez, J. C., Rouge, V., Pisteur, M., Ravier, F., Tonella, L., Moosmayer, M., Wilkins, M. R., and D.F., H. (1997). *Electrophoresis* **18,** 324–327.

Sekar, R. B., and Periasamy, A. (2003). Fluorescence resonance energy transfer (FRET) microscopy imaging of live cell protein localizations. *J. Cell Biol.* **160**(5), 629–633.

Shen, Y., and Meri, S. (2003). Yin and Yang: Complement activation and regulation in Alzheimer's disease. *Prog. Neurobiol.* **70**(6), 463–472.

Sidhu, S. S., Bader, G. D., and Boone, C. (2003). Functional genomics of intracellular peptide recognition domains with combinatorial biology methods. *Curr. Opin. Chem. Biol.* **7**(1), 97–102.

Skelton, N. J., Koehler, M. F., Zobel, K., Wong, W. L., Yeh, S., Pisabarro, M. T., Yin, J. P., Lasky, L. A., and Sidhu, S. S. (2003). Origins of PDZ domain ligand specificity. Structure determination and mutagenesis of the Erbin PDZ domain. *J. Biol. Chem.* **278**(9), 7645–7654.

Smith, R. D. (2002). Trends in mass spectrometry instrumentation for proteomics. *Trends Biotechnol.* **20**(Suppl. 12), S3–S7.

Stoeckli, M., Chaurand, P., Hallahan, D. E., and Caprioli, R. M. (2001). Imaging mass spectrometry: A new technology for the analysis of protein expression in mammalian tissues. *Nat. Med.* **7**(4), 493–496.

Stoeckli, M., Staab, D., Staufenbiel, M., Wiederhold, K. H., and Signor, L. (2002). Molecular imaging of amyloid beta peptides in mouse brain sections using mass spectrometry. *Anal. Biochem.* **311**(1), 33–39.

Stupka, E. (2002). Large-scale open bioinformatics data resources. *Curr. Opin. Mol. Ther.* **4**(3), 265–274.

Sunderland, T., Linker, G., Mirza, N., Putnam, K. T., Friedman, D. L., Kimmel, L. H., Bergeson, J., Manetti, G. J., Zimmermann, M., Tang, B., Bartko, J. J., and Cohen, R. M. (2003). Decreased beta-amyloid1-42 and increased tau levels in cerebrospinal fluid of patients with Alzheimer disease. *JAMA* **289**(16), 2094–2103.

Tang, N., Tornatore, P., and Weinberger, S. R. (2004). Current developments in SELDI affinity technology. *Mass. Spectrom. Rev.* **23**(1), 34–44.

Tapiola, T., Pirttila, T., Mikkonen, M., Mehta, P. D., Alafuzoff, I., Koivisto, K., and Soininen, H. (2000). Three-year follow-up of cerebrospinal fluid tau, beta-amyloid 42 and 40 concentrations in Alzheimer's disease. *Neurosci. Lett.* **280**(2), 119–122.

Taupenot, L., Harper, K. L., and O'Connor, D. T. (2003). The chromogranin-secretogranin family. *N. Engl. J. Med.* **348**(12), 1134–1149.

Taylor, C. F., Paton, N. W., Garwood, K. L., Kirby, P. D., Stead, D. A., Yin, Z., Deutsch, E. W., Selway, L., Walker, J., Riba-Garcia, I., Mohammed, S., Deery, M. J., Howard, J. A., Dunkley, T., Aebersold, R., Kell, D. B., Lilley, K. S., Roepstorff, P., Yates, J. R., 3rd, Brass, A., Brown, A. J., Cash, P., Gaskell, S. J., Hubbard, S. J., and Oliver, S. G. (2003). A systematic approach to modeling, capturing, and disseminating proteomics experimental data. *Nat. Biotechnol.* **21**(3), 247–254.

Templin, M. F., Stoll, D., Schwenk, J. M., Potz, O., Kramer, S., and Joos, T. O. (2003). Protein microarrays: Promising tools for proteomic research. *Proteomics* **3**(11), 2155–2166.

Todd, P. J., Schaaf, T. G., Chaurand, P., and Caprioli, R. M. (2001). Organic ion imaging of biological tissue with secondary ion mass spectrometry and matrix-assisted laser desorption/ionization. *J. Mass. Spectrom.* **36**(4), 355–369.

Uetz, P. (2002). Two-hybrid arrays. *Curr. Opin. Chem. Biol.* **6**(1), 57–62.

Uetz, P., Giot, L., Cagney, G., Mansfield, T. A., Judson, R. S., Knight, J. R., Lockshon, D., Narayan, V., Srinivasan, M., Pochart, P., Qureshi-Emili, A., Li, Y., Godwin, B., Conover, D., Kalbfleisch, T., Vijayadamodar, G., Yang, M., Johnston, M., Fields, S., and Rothberg, J. M. (2000). A comprehensive analysis of protein-protein interactions in Saccharomyces cerevisiae. *Nature* **403**(6770), 623–627.

VanBogelen, R. A. (1999). Generating a bacterial genome inventory. Identifying 2-D spots by comigrating products of the genome on 2-D gels. *Methods Mol. Biol.* **112,** 423–429.

Walhout, A. J., Boulton, S. J., and Vidal, M. (2000). Yeast two-hybrid systems and protein interaction mapping projects for yeast and worm. *Yeast* **17**(2), 88–94.

Watkins, S. M., and German, J. B. (2002). Metabolomics and biochemical profiling in drug discovery and development. *Curr. Opin. Mol. Ther.* **4**(3), 224–228.

Wiedermann, C. J. (2000). Secretoneurin: A functional neuropeptide in health and disease. *Peptides* **21**(8), 1289–1298.

Wouters, F. S., Verveer, P. J., and Bastiaens, P. I. (2001). Imaging biochemistry inside cells. *Trends Cell Biol.* **11**(5), 203–211.

Wu, C. C., and Yates, J. R., 3rd (2003). The application of mass spectrometry to membrane proteomics. *Nat. Biotechnol.* **21**(3), 262–267.

Zeytun, A., Jeromin, A., Scalettar, B. A., Waldo, G. S., and Bradbury, A. R. (2003). Fluorobodies combine GFP fluorescence with the binding characteristics of antibodies. *Nat. Biotechnol.* **21**(12), 1473–1479.

Zozulya, S., Lioubin, M., Hill, R. J., Abram, C., and Gishizky, M. L. (1999). Mapping signal transduction pathways by phage display. *Nat. Biotechnol.* **17**(12), 1193–1198.

SECTION III
INFORMATICS

PROTEOMIC INFORMATICS

Steven A. Russell,* William Old,† Katheryn A. Resing,† and Lawrence Hunter*

*Center for Computational Pharmacology, University of Colorado Health Sciences Center
Aurora, Colorado 80045
†Department of Chemistry and Biochemistry, University of Colorado, Boulder, Colorado 80309

I. What Is Proteomics?

Proteomics is the study of the protein composition of a complex, an organelle, a cell, or even an entire organism. Proteomic characterizations provide crucially important information about the structure and function of cells and more complex biological systems. Although protein sequences and many regulatory signals are encoded in DNA, aspects of the protein composition of a cell, such as expression levels, splice variants, and post-translational modifications (e.g., cleavages or covalent chemical modifications), are not so encoded. Indeed

129

these aspects of protein composition fluctuate rapidly and over an enormous range; such fluctuations play a variety of critical roles in biological processes. Sensitive and accurate assays of relevant aspects of complex protein mixtures are needed to fully understand and influence these processes. Such assays are rapidly improving along a variety of dimensions, including the number of proteins that can be characterized simultaneously, the aspects of these proteins that can be assayed, and the cost of doing such characterizations. As proteomics technology continues to improve, it is likely that it will play an increasingly important role in basic research, medical applications, and the development of biotechnology.

Spurred by the availability of whole genomic sequences, advances in mass spectrometry, and the development of relevant informatics techniques, proteomics research is growing rapidly from a trickle to a flood. Integration of this burgeoning class of information with other global surveys, such as metabolomics and mRNA profiling, helped spawn the new field of systems biology (Kitano, 2002).[1] The promise of these tools includes the potential of development of personalized and preventive medicine at the molecular level, as well as many other applications. However, before these methods can reach their potential, proteomics assays must become more informative, more reliable, and less dependent on extensive expertise of the operators.

A set of ultimate goals for shotgun proteomic technology can be clearly stated. Ideally, proteomics should be able to do the following:

- Identify all of the proteins present in a complex mixture, such as whole cell lysates, ideally with sufficient sensitivity to find proteins present in single molecule per cell concentrations;
- Identify and characterize all of the isoforms of all proteins in a mixture, including splice variants, cleavage products, and post-translational covalent modifications; and
- Quantify the concentration of each protein and all of its isoforms.

Of course the current state of the art is only partially able to fulfill these goals, but technical progress is rapid, and the existing technology already has had tremendous scientific impact. The informatics methods reviewed in this chapter play a key role in the ability to transform mass spectra data into information addressing the aforementioned goals. Although instruments or methods other than mass spectrometry (e.g., antibody or aptamer arrays) show some potential for addressing these goals, because of their relative immaturity, the informatics methods relevant to them will not be reviewed.

---

[1]Loosely speaking, systems biology is the characterization of biological systems by enumeration of a comprehensive list of components, their structure, and their dynamics.

II. Proteomic Informatics

Proteomics at present is a field that is in an exhilarating yet frustrating phase, with new ideas emerging almost daily, but with far less clarity regarding how the field will ultimately evolve. However, it is clear that this research will result in the production of thousands or even hundreds of thousands of mass spectra per day in many proteomics laboratories. Extracting the maximum scientific value from this activity depends crucially on informatics at many stages, from managing the instruments to analyzing the resulting spectra. The purpose of this review is to describe the myriad roles that informatics plays in the field, to identify some of the informatics challenges that remain to be resolved, and to suggest some future directions that proteomics informatics is likely to take. Our focus will be on informatics relevant to high-throughput, or "shotgun," proteomics efforts.

III. Mass Spectrometry and Shotgun Proteomics

Although proteomic profiling was first carried out in 1975 using two-dimensional polyacrylamic gel electrophoresis (2D-PAGE; also called two-dimensional gel electrophoresis or 2DE) (O'Farrell, 1975), the development of new mass spectrometry (MS) methods has generated a renewed interest in such profiling. Early studies used blotting to membranes, followed by Edman sequencing to identify the proteins one amino acid at a time. An important methodological improvement involves a technique whereby protein "spots"[2] from 2D gels are identified by excising the spots and carrying out in-gel proteolytic digests. The digest is an enzymatic fragmentation of the purified protein into a set of peptides. The peptides are recovered and analyzed by MS to obtain mass and sequence information, which can in turn be used to infer the protein in the original spot by matching the observed peptide masses and sequences to expected values calculated for each protein that could potentially have been present in the original sample (usually defined by a protein database derived from an organism's genomic sequence).

The recent increase in interest in proteomics was stimulated in 1996 when Matthias Mann's laboratory published the application of this method to the analysis of proteins in yeast extracts resolved by 2D-PAGE (Shevchenko et al., 1996). However, this method is limited by the difficulties of 2D gels (e.g., limited dynamic range and the fact that basic and membrane proteins are poorly detected). Furthermore, 2D-PAGE does not lend itself to high-throughput

[2]Isolated regions of a gel that putatively contain a single, purified protein isoform.

analysis. These problems have led to the recent introduction of an approach that eliminates the use of gels altogether, sometimes referred to as shotgun proteomics (Yao *et al.*, 2001). In this approach all of the proteins in a sample are simultaneously digested with a protease, and then the large collection of peptides is analyzed to identify all of the proteins in the original sample. Typically the peptides are resolved into several fractions by ion exchange (IE) chromatography, and then the peptides in each IE fraction are analyzed by a reverse phase column directly coupled to a liquid chromatography mass spectrometer (LC-MS). This MudPIT (multiple-dimension protein identification technology; Washburn *et al.*, 2001) procedure allows the sequencing of a large number of peptides in one experiment. Computational methods then analyze all this peptide sequence information to identify the list of the proteins in the original sample. Using this approach, more than 1500 proteins from a given sample can be identified in one MudPIT analysis (Jacobs *et al.*, 2004; Peng *et al.*, 2003). This is sufficient for bacterial proteomics, but is inadequate for higher eukaryotes. Although the size of the eukaryotic proteome is unknown, it is likely to be on the order of 12,000–20,000 proteins. Thus the proteome must be prefractionated. A recent study using fractionation of the soluble proteins by gel filtration revealed slightly more than 5000 proteins from the soluble extract of a mammalian cell line (Resing *et al.*, 2004) but required hundreds of individual LC-MS analyses. In addition to capacity, difficulties remain in sensitivity (dynamic range), resolving all of the protein isoforms, and in quantification, but innovations in instrument capabilities and protocols continue to move the state of the art forward at a rapid pace.

A. Brief Overview of Spectrometers and Spectrometry

To understand the informatics issues, it is important to have a sense of the instruments and procedures that generate the data. The biological sample is first separated into component fractions by physical and chemical means. Each fraction has fewer constituents than the original sample, and hence is easier to analyze; however, then the many individual analyses must be recombined in some manner.

As a typical example, the proteins in a given sample can be cleaved into short segments of 1–200 amino acids by a protease such as trypsin, which cleaves at a specific peptide bond (lysine or arginine). However, this cleavage is not perfect due to steric, hydrophobic, and other influences of adjacent amino acid residues. This is an example of the importance of understanding the underlying processes; protein identification algorithms have to model this cleavage step, and approaches that incorporate these variations in detail perform significantly better than those that assume perfect cleavage.

Two-dimensional gel electrophoresis allows the creation of protein fractions that have a specific isoelectric point and molecular weight; this is often enough to isolate a specific isoform of a single protein from a complex mixture. The isolated protein spots are either physically cut out of the gel and digested, or digested in place and then removed. The digested fractions are generally analyzed using matrix-assisted laser desorption ionization time-of-flight (MALDI-TOF) mass spectrometry.

However, as previously described, 2D gels are being supplanted by higher-throughput methods of separating complex mixtures into fractions without electrophoretic separation. MudPIT involves enzymatic digestion of the entire complex mixture, followed by other fractionation steps. After enzymatic digestion, resulting peptides can be fractionated according to charge using strong cation exchange (SCX) chromatography. A reverse phase (RP) filtration step will further separate the peptides based on hydrophobicity. In either fractionation (as in many others), molecules with identical properties do not all flow through the chromatography medium at exactly the same rate but elute in a "peak," with a variance due to diffusion or heterogeneous interaction with the chromatography medium. Using the actual variances and other characteristics of the fractionation method in subsequent computation, rather than an unrealistically simple model, can lead to better performance in a variety of respects.

Fractions containing peptides are then introduced into the mass spectrometer (via a spray or laser vaporization process) and accelerated by electric and magnetic fields that act on the charged residues on each peptide. Excitation of the peptide ions may be employed using either a collision gas or high electric potentials at the mass spectrometer orifice to induce fragmentation of the peptide ion, providing useful information about the peptide sequence. The spectrometer's fields are tuned to measure the time that a species takes to traverse a given distance in a given trajectory before being detected, or the peptides are trapped in a circulating pattern until a chosen time when molecules with specific properties are released for measurement. Of course even with highly precise instruments, noise occurs (as in any physical or electrical process) from imperfect equipment, chemical impurities, and human error.

Spectrometers effectively measure the mass to charge (m/z) ratio, because that is what determines the acceleration of the molecules. The instrument reports the spectrum of intensities of the signal over a given m/z range. During the ionization process, a peptide can acquire or lose an additional hydrogen atom (a unit of charge), so a population of molecules of the same peptide will distribute over multiple charge states, each with a unique m/z. Using charge deconvolution algorithms, the mass of the peptides may be calculated from the measured m/z values.

Tandem MS, or MS/MS uses two connected sequential spectrometers. Peptides are separated by m/z in the first spectrometer, then subjected to fragmentation and sent to a second spectrometer. The second spectrum provides information about each individual peptide, which can be used to determine its amino acid sequence. Shotgun proteomics methods often combine the LC-MS fractionation approach with the MS/MS peptide sequencing approach in a method called LC-MS/MS.

Recall that the goals of these proteomics efforts are: (1) to identify all the proteins in a complex mixture; (2) to determine the presence of protein isoforms such as post-translational modifications or splice variants; and (3) to quantify the concentrations of each protein or isoform. The inference of the answers to these questions from the kinds of a forementioned spectra is the task of informatics.

IV. Identifying Proteins

Both qualitative (identification only) and quantitative (identification and determination of abundance) proteomics require that the masses detected by the spectrometer be converted into information about the proteins in the original mixture. It is generally the case that information from the spectra is used to characterize the peptides that resulted from the enzymatic digestion; this characterization is in turn used to determine which proteins produced those peptides.

There are two broad approaches to the task of peptide characterization: database-driven techniques and *de novo* sequencing. The database method matches observed peptide masses with calculations of the masses of peptides that would theoretically be produced by enzymatic digestion of all of the protein sequences from the organism under study. These theoretical calculations depend both on a model of the cleavage properties of the digestion enzyme and on a database that contains the complete set of sequences of the proteins in the organism (generally derived from the sequenced genome). *De novo* algorithms infer a peptide sequence from the spectra alone. For organisms whose genomes are not sequenced, *de novo* methods are the only option for proteomic analysis. This approach could also be used in identifying unexpected modifications.

A. DATABASE METHODS FOR PEPTIDE CHARACTERIZATION

The database-searching algorithms in turn include three dominant approaches: (1) peptide mass fingerprinting, (2) sequence tag identification, (3) and MS/MS identification. Mass fingerprinting involves matching peptide masses to theoretical digests calculated on the proteins in the database. Sequence tag identification involves generating a partial amino acid sequence from MS/MS fragmentation spectra and searching based on that partial sequence (and peptide mass information). The MS/MS full sequencing approach correlates experimentally derived fragmentation spectra with theoretical fragmentation patterns derived from a protein sequence database. We will now consider specific algorithms for each of these methods.

Peptide mass fingerprinting (PMF; also sometimes called protein mass mapping) is the mainstay technique for protein identification in gel-based proteomics, in which 2DE is used to separate proteins by isoelectric point and molecular weight prior to the MS analysis. The isolated protein spots are cut out of the gel and digested, after which the peptides are eluted and analyzed using MALDI-TOF mass spectrometry, providing a "mass fingerprint" of the peptides. In PMF methods, peptides are characterized only by their masses, and the main algorithmic task is to match the set of masses to database protein sequences that could have generated them.

Successful identification depends on high mass accuracy for the peptides, complete resolution of the proteins in the gel to avoid getting peptides from multiple proteins in a sample, and sufficient detection of peptides by the spectrometer. The procedure is only practical when the peptides were digested with highly specific enzymes such as trypsin. The peptide masses are then compared with the theoretical masses calculated for each protein in the database and a score is calculated representing the degree of matching. For a variety of reasons, it is always the case that some predicted masses will be missing from the spectrum and other unexpected masses will be present. For example, a covalent modification of the protein will cause the theoretical mass of a peptide to be missing, and an unexpected mass (with the additional mass from the modification) will be present. Contaminants are usually present, generating unexpected masses, or chemical processes can mask certain peptide signals. Most algorithms use a rudimentary matching score, which represents the overlap between expected and observed masses, such as PepSea (Henzel *et al.*, 1993), MS-Fit (Clauser *et al.*, 1999), PepFrag (Fenyo *et al.*, 1998), and PepIdent (Wilkins and Williams, 1997). Others incorporate probabilistic models to account for the nonuniform distribution in peptide and protein molecular weights; these include (MOWSE) (Pappin *et al.*, 1993) and ProFound (Zhang and Chait, 2000). These algorithms are generally packaged with organism-specific protein sequence databases and are sometimes referred to as "search engines," because they search a database for proteins that would produce the observed spectra. ProteinScape (Chamrad *et al.*, 2003) is a meta-method that performs automated calibration and peak filtering and searches across multiple PMF search engines (currently Mascot, MS-Fit, and ProFound). ProteinScape combines the results into a single score and calculates a statistical significance, using an expectation based on simulations. The tool FindPept (Gattiker *et al.*, 2002) can be used to identify unmatched masses present in these spectra due to chemical noise, matrix peaks, and modifications of the peptides introduced through sample handling and contaminating proteins.

The other two peptide characterization techniques rely on MS/MS fragmentation analysis of peptides, using peptide sequence tags or correlating the MS/MS spectra with theoretical spectra calculated from sequence databases. Peptide sequence tag queries involve generating a partial amino acid sequence from the fragmentation spectra, followed by searching the sequence database with this partial sequence and an associated mass. Search programs using theoretical spectra score the experimentally derived fragmentation spectra by measuring the correlation of its theoretical fragmentation pattern with the experimental spectrum. The sequence tag and theoretical spectra searching techniques are better suited for analysis of complex mixtures than PMF. These methods can be applied to proteases or chemical methods with nonspecific cleavage, because they generate information about the sequence of the peptides, not just the masses.

The first publically available tool available for sequence tag searching was PeptideSearch (Mann and Wilm, 1994; Mann et al., 1993) from Matthias Mann, which was designed primarily for lower-resolution data from triple quadrupole mass spectrometers, and allows searching with short sequences derived from ion ladders in peptide fragmentation spectra. More recent tools for this task include MS-Tag (Clauser et al., 1999), TagIdent (Wilkins et al., 1998), and GutenTag (http://fields.scripps.edu/GutenTag/index.html). When searching sequence tags for organisms with incomplete or unsequenced genomes, MultiTag (Sunyaev et al., 2003) may be useful, because it identifies homologous proteins from the genomes of related organisms.

The spectrum of programs and algorithms for peptide identification using MS/MS spectra is quite large and constantly changing, from simple scoring algorithms to integrative systems built on top of the basic scoring methods. One of the most widely used scoring algorithms is SEQUEST's XCorr (Yates et al., 1995), which uses cross-correlation to calculate a score between the experimental and theoretical spectrum for each peptide in the database within a user-specified tolerance of the parent mass. The result is a list of candidate peptides sorted by score. The top scoring peptide is chosen as the correct identification if it scores above a certain threshold, the level of which is somewhat subjective, because the score distributions vary according to mass of the parent peptide and charge state, as well as database size. To address the mass dependence, MacCoss et al. (2002) developed SEQUEST-Norm, which is normalized to be independent of peptide mass and protein database. Another popular program is MASCOT (Perkins et al., 1999), which is based on the MOWSE (Pappin et al., 1993) algorithm by incorporating probability based scoring and prebuilt peptide indexes.

Currently SEQUEST and MASCOT are the most popular approaches to MS/MS spectra analysis, although neither is ideal. Both SEQUEST and MASCOT are distributed commercially, so the source code is not generally available. This makes it difficult to know exactly what the programs are doing, to track changes from release to release, and to test all aspects of each approach independently. A recently developed open source software program for MS/MS identification, X! Tandem (Craig and Beavis, 2003), matches peptide sequences with MS/MS spectra and identifies modifications using an iterative approach, in which the likely candidates are identified first from the total databases, followed by a search on the refined, smaller list of proteins to search for modifications. In a comparison of X! Tandem, Sonar MS/MS, and MASCOT, all three packages identified the same set of peptides, although with different scores and expectation values (Craig and Beavis, 2003).

Several probability based scoring algorithms have emerged recently, such as SCOPE (Bafna and Edwards, 2001), ProbID (Zhang *et al.*, 2002), and OLAV (Colinge *et al.*, 2003), all of which use stochastic models to improve the separation of correct from incorrect or random matches of expected to observed MS/MS spectra. SCOPE employs a two-stage stochastic model for matching spectra to peptides sequences. The first step involves the generation of fragment ions from a precursor peptide using fragment ion probabilities derived empirically from a training set of expert-curated MS/MS spectra. The second step incorporates a model of instrument measurement error. OLAV, an algorithm based on signal detection theory, calculates a likelihood ratio score based on the degree of matching between experimental and theoretical spectra, and incorporates additional information about the match, such as parent mass and charge state. When compared to MASCOT using receiver operating characteristic analysis, OLAV demonstrated higher discrimination between correct and random matches (Colinge *et al.*, 2003). As part of the RADARS (Field *et al.*, 2002) package from Genomic Solutions (Ann Arbor, MI), developed by Beavis and co-workers, Sonar MS/MS (Field *et al.*, 2002) calculates a correlation score using the inner product of the experimental and theoretical spectra, and incorporates expectation values in the calculation of a confidence score.

Meta-methods are useful in this context too. The simple approach of comparing SEQUEST and MASCOT peptide identifications, and requiring a reasonable level of agreement between them, can be useful for improving confidence in identifications, and is generally used in our laboratory. SpectrumMill is a web-based workbench type of environment for extracting, searching, and visualizing LC-MS/MS data, compatible with mass spectrometers from multiple vendors. It was developed by Karl Clauser at Millennium Pharmaceuticals and is marketed by Agilent Technologies (www.chem.agilent.com). Qscore (Moore *et al.*, 2002) and PeptideProphet (Keller *et al.*, 2002) are probabilistic systems built on top of other scoring systems and are designed to improve the separation of positive and negative identifications. Qscore was designed for SEQUEST score evaluation and is based on a model of random peptide matching, incorporating the fraction of distinct tryptic peptides matched in the database that are present in the identified protein. Keller and co-workers from the Institute for Systems

Biology (Seattle WA) designed PeptideProphet to distinguish correct from incorrect peptide assignments from SEQUEST searches using a machine learning approach called discriminant analysis, trained on a known set of validated MS/MS spectra. Similarly, Anderson *et al.* use a machine learning algorithm, called a support vector machine, trained on a set of validated identifications, using as input multiple scoring values from SEQUEST searches.

Kislinger *et al.* (2003) developed PRISM, which is a systems approach rather than an algorithm, and addresses every step in the process, from subcellular fractionation and extraction of proteins to the clustering and annotation of the final protein list. Associated with the PRISM process is an algorithm called STATQUEST, which postprocesses the output of SEQUEST. STATQUEST performs a statistical analysis of peptide identification scores to estimate the accuracy of identifications, using an empirically derived probabilistic model that applies specifically to the PRISM process.

Visualization and filtering programs are often used to aid in the manual interpretation of results or initial filtering of spectra prior to processing. CHOMPER, developed by Eddes *et al.* (2002) as well as DTAselect and Contrast, developed by Yates and co-workers (Tabb *et al.*, 2002), aid in the validation of SEQUEST results by human experts, using a series of HTML-based output windows. These programs display the sequences of automatically identified peptides alongside the underlying MS/MS spectra, allowing experts to assess the reliability of the identification by eye. INTERACT (Han *et al.*, 2001) is a similar tool developed by Jimmy Eng to collect and organize the large number of MS/MS spectra generated from large shotgun proteomics experiments. It is open source and freely available.

B. *De Novo* Peptide Characterization

There are fewer options for *de novo* (non database) peptide sequencing from MS/MS spectra. Most algorithms enumerate and score sequence ladders made from the mass differences of the peaks, which should correspond to combinations of amino acid masses. Lutefisk (Taylor and Johnson, 1997) uses a graph algorithm to enumerate all possible paths through the MS/MS peaks and scores the candidates using cross-correlation and an intensity based score. A *de novo* sequencing algorithm based on supervised machine learning, SHERENGA (Dancik *et al.*, 1999), uses a set of validated test spectra and learns the relative intensities of ion types, which will be specific to the type of mass spectrometer; it can handle data from triple quadrupole, quadruple time of flight (QTOF), and ion trap instruments. Using this information, a list of ranked and scored sequences is generated for the set of unknown spectra. CIDentify (Taylor and Johnson, 2001) is a hybrid approach that takes as input the identified sequence candidates from Lutefisk and performs a homology-based database search. This approach is applicable to source organisms without sequenced genomes, so long as sequence from a related organism is available.

C. From Peptides to Proteins

Recall that mass fingerprinting methods attempt to map from collections of proteolytic peptide masses to the particular proteins that could have contained them. The addition of sequence information makes this problem more tractable and less subject to error. However, the protein identification from peptide data is still potentially ambiguous, and all existing algorithms make at least some errors in this step. In general the programs that do MS/MS identification of peptides also provide database-driven matching of identified sets of peptides to specific proteins. These programs function much the same way that the mass finger-printing programs do, and are often derived from them. A small number of peptides (sometimes only one) can be enough to uniquely identify a particular protein, and these programs make protein identification calls even when the majority of peptides that are predicted from the digestion of that protein are not found.

ProteinProphet from Institute of Systems Biology, performs such a task, assembling peptide identifications with associated probabilities into protein identifications and derived probabilities. One difficulty in this task arises because of the large abundance of alternative splicing, protein isoforms, and database redundancies. Identified peptides may belong to more than one related protein. Generally the aforementioned programs integrate this step into their processing. ProteinProphet is unusual in that it is a stand-alone program that takes the peptide identification output of MASCOT, SEQUEST, or another program as its input, and only does protein identification. Isoform Resolver is a similar program, but it assigns the protein identification from the peptide sequence, independent of the search program assignment (Resing et al., 2004).

V. Post-hoc Validation of Protein Identification Program Output

The most popular approaches to protein identification (SEQUEST and MASCOT) both have fairly high false-positive and false-negative rates (MacCoss et al., 2002; Moore et al., 2002). In recent studies, manual analysis and direct spectral comparison have shown that, at their high confidence cutoffs, SEQUEST and MASCOT both miss at least half of potentially identifiable MS/MS spectra. Furthermore, even at these high confidence cutoffs, they make incorrect assignments 29–45% of the time (Keller et al., 2002; MacCoss et al.,

2002; Resing *et al.*, 2004). Because the peptide assignments are so noisy, protein identification is also suspect when based on a small number of peptide assignments. Validation of the peptide and protein assignments, and characterization of the types of errors existing programs make, is an important problem under active research by several groups. The significant problems with automated methods drive many laboratories to validate peptide assignments for MS/MS spectra by experts to confirm that the fragmentation is chemically plausible. Typically this focuses only on those cases in which a protein identification is supported by 1–3 peptides (for other cases, misidentification of 1–2 peptides does not throw out the protein identification). For example, this approach allowed detection of 25% of the total ORFs (open reading frames) in a yeast extract (approximately 1500 proteins) (Washburn *et al.*, 2001), all with high confidence.

In higher eukaryotes, greater sensitivity is required to sample the whole proteome because there are larger numbers of proteins in the proteome, proteins are larger, and the range of protein concentrations is broader. A useful way to increase sensitivity is to carry out repeated LC-MS analyses using narrow overlapping mass ranges during data collection (often called gas phase fractionation; Spahr *et al.*, 2001; Yi *et al.*, 2002), which allows the MS to collect data on the weak ions but greatly increases the amount of data collected. Furthermore, with large databases, such as for human samples, the number of candidate peptide matches to an MS/MS spectrum can be very high (in the thousands). Manual analysis becomes a daunting task with substantial error; therefore better post-hoc validation methods are needed that can be implemented computationally.

As described previously in the meta-analysis discussion, there have been recent attempts to postprocess the scores generated by SEQUEST (Anderson *et al.*, 2003; Keller *et al.*, 2002; Nesvizhskii *et al.*, 2002) in order to improve the confidence of sequence assignments, using linear discriminant analysis or machine learning algorithms. Alternative methods have used peptide properties other than the fragmentation pattern, such as exact mass measurements (Smith *et al.*, 2002), to validate the peptide assignments. Exact mass measurements are powerful, but the approach requires more expensive FTICR-MS (Fourier transform ion cyclotron resonance) instrumentation, which is inaccessible to most MS laboratories. The most successful method for validating peptides with lower resolution MS instruments has used a multi-information approach. This method minimizes false negative peptide assignments by requiring consensus between two separate search programs (generally SEQUEST and MASCOT) and requiring that the peptide assignment agrees with SCX elution and charge properties in order to exclude false positive assignments (Resing *et al.*, 2004). It is possible to envision extending this approach to other properties of the peptides and processing in order to improve validation, including hydophobicity of the peptide and consistency of pI (isoelectric point) with observed distribution of charge forms (ratio of singly, doubly, and triply charged ions).

VI. Quantification

Quantifying changes in protein abundance among samples is a key goal when surveying proteins on a global scale, but accomplishing the comparisons is still an unsolved problem. Although the peak intensity at the detector is assayed through a m/z spectrum, the relationship between that intensity and the abundance of the protein or peptide being assayed is unclear. Most processing ignores the intensity, except to set a cutoff for the presence of true peak versus noise. Current methods for quantitative shotgun proteomics are primarily based on isotope and/or mass tag labeling of peptides, in which two samples to be compared are labeled with different covalent chemical groups. The samples are mixed, and relative quantitation is determined from the ratio of intensities between the differentially labeled peaks. One method often used is isotope coded affinity tagging (ICAT), in which proteins from two samples are reacted with ^{1}H- versus ^{2}H- or ^{12}C- versus ^{13}C-labeled biotin functional groups, through Cys alkylation (Gygi $et\ al.$, 2002; Ong $et\ al.$, 2002; Shen $et\ al.$, 2003). In this case, Cys-containing peptides are enriched by streptavidin chromatography before linker cleavage and removal of the biotin group, thus simplifying the peptide mixture. A similar strategy using stable isotope labeling of amino acids in cell culture (Ong $et\ al.$, 2002) involves metabolic labeling of proteins by growing cells in media containing ^{2}C- versus ^{13}C- or ^{14}N- versus ^{15}N-enriched amino acids, or feeding animals isotopically enriched food. XPRESS (Han $et\ al.$, 2001), developed by Eng and co-workers at the Institute for Systems Biology, is software for relative quantitation of proteins from isotope-labeling–based LC-MS/MS experiments. It interfaces with the INTERACT software for doing ICAT in large shotgun proteomics experiments. However, only a few studies have carefully validated ICAT in these larger datasets (Patton $et\ al.$, 2002; Shiio $et\ al.$, 2002). Of course, feeding humans isotopically enriched foods is unethical.

It is currently unclear whether mass tag labeling methods can achieve high sensitivity in mammalian systems. For example, most of the proteins detected by ICAT methods in recent publications are high abundance proteins (Patton $et\ al.$, 2002; Shiio $et\ al.$, 2002). This suggests that for mammalian systems, in which proteins are expressed over a large concentration range, the method does not sample proteins that are present in low copy number. Another important drawback is the cost of labeling the protein amounts required for high sensitivity. Even with complete recovery, 20 mg of protein (from approximately 10^8 cells) is needed to observe peptides derived from proteins that are present at 200 copies per cell, using a mass spectrometer that is sensitive to 25 femtomoles. The cost of the ^{12}C- and ^{13}C-labeled ICAT reagents needed for a single experiment comparing two sample conditions is currently almost \$15,000. In addition, samples must be assayed in combinations, and deciding how best to normalize many samples to one another is a critical issue that is not often considered. Thus there are limitations because of low sequence coverage, low sensitivity, and scaling to large number of samples. Alternative methods for label-free protein quantitation are sorely needed.

The ability to transform directly observed peak intensities into estimates of peptide abundance would obviate the limitations of ICAT, such as limited sequence coverage and cost. Two groups have reported encouraging results demonstrating correlations between mass spectral peak intensities of peptide ions and protein abundances. Linearity in the correlations was observed with both standard mixtures and with more complex biological samples. Bondarenko *et al.* (2002) demonstrated linear responses of peptide ion peak areas from 10 to 1000 fmol for myoglobin spiked into human plasma, with a relative standard deviation of less than 11%. Likewise, Wang and co-workers (Wang *et al.*, 2003) published similar results with protein standards spiked into serum. They also introduced a matching algorithm called dynamic time warping, which pairs parent ions into two different datasets based on m/z and elution time, regardless of sequence assignment. For nearly 3400 ions from 25 replicates of one sample, they found the median relative standard deviation of peak intensity ratios to be 25.7%.

Two objections often cited against the use of peak intensity methods are nonlinearity of signal intensity and ion suppression during ionization in the MS source (King *et al.*, 2003; Muller *et al.*, 2002). Indeed, Wang *et al.* (2003) observed ion suppression, lowering the overall intensity of myoglobin peptides in serum compared with a simple protein mixture. However, they argued that ion suppression did not significantly alter the linear relationship between normalized intensities and analyte concentration, suggesting that the effects of differential ion suppression are minimal when comparing samples of similar complexity. What was missing from both studies was a systematic, statistical analysis of the quantitation results to identify and characterize peptide reproducibility within complex samples. Nevertheless, the findings suggest that with careful controls, label-free quantitation from measured ion intensities should eventually be successful. Informatics methods to compensate for the nonlinearities and other confounding phenomenon are likely to be important in these efforts.

VII. Detection of Protein Isoforms

Most proteins, particularly in eukaryotes, naturally occur in a variety of isoforms, which leads to significant challenges to proteomics informatics. Some of these isoforms lead to ambiguous protein identification from peptides, whereas others (e.g., covalent post-translational modifications) need to be detected by proteomics methods because they are of great biological importance, and other assays (e.g., gene expression arrays) do not detect them.

The identification ambiguity problem arises from gene duplications or paralogs that are common in eukaryotes. For example, there are seven distinct isoforms of human hemoglobin, which have very high sequence similarity to each other. It is generally the case that even detection of several MS/MS sequenced peptides will not reliably discriminate among these isoforms. How this ambiguity is reported (or even whether it is noted at all) varies among the different programs, making postprocessing difficult. There is currently no reliable, automated method for distinguishing between low-confidence assignments and ones that are ambiguous only with respect to other gene family members. This is an important area for the development of new informatics methods.

Another source of ambiguity comes from the importance of post-translational cleavages. Many proteins (e.g., polyproteins and signal peptides) are inactive until cleaved into two or more pieces. The nature of the MS proteomics process makes distinguishing between cleaved and uncleaved forms of a protein difficult. Similarly, the alternative splicing of genes in eukaryotes is becoming more fully appreciated; recent reports suggest between 40% and 60% of genes are alternatively spliced in mammals. Splice variants pose similar problems for protein identification through MS. One approach to distinguish among these ambiguous forms (as well as among gene family members) uses nonspecific proteases for the initial digest in MS/MS experiments, then aligns the overlapping sequenced peptides (Wu et al., 2003). Although unique peptides could be diagnostic for these cases, shotgun proteomics samples only a portion of the sequence. Top-down proteomics is a new approach that does not use proteases but rather analyzes proteins directly (Bergquist et al., 2003; Ge et al., 2004). In this approach, new instrumentation allows direct sequencing of intact proteins. When combined with resolution of proteins in multidimensional chromatography, a significant portion of the proteome can be analyzed in this manner. It also allows analysis of covariation of modifications at individual sites in a protein, areas that cannot be addressed by shotgun proteomics.

Extensive work has been applied to identifying covalently modified proteins in shotgun proteomics. A modified protein has the same amino acid sequence as the parent protein but has some small chemical change in one or more amino acids, such as the addition of a phosphate group to a serine residue. There are more than 30 post-translational modifications that have been reported in the literature, including the addition of phosphate, sugars, alcohols, and other moieties, as well as the addition and loss of specific protons. For instance, one review of glycomics has been recently published (Zaia et al., 2004). Each of these modifications changes the mass of the peptide, and in principle is detectable by MS. On the other hand, these mass changes also interfere with many of the peptide and protein identification methods previously described, particularly those that rely on theoretical calculations based on database sequence information. Each modification increases the number of theoretical masses that a database of sequences might generate, contributing to potential ambiguities among mass matches; combinations of modifications greatly exacerbate this problem.

Several programs have been published to address these issues. Designed for PMF data, FindMod (Wilkins *et al.*, 1999) searches for unaccounted masses in the mass map of a previously identified protein for matches to user specified modifications. The rules for modification patterns are built from the annotated Swiss-Prot database. The MS/MS peptide identification algorithms, MS-CONVOLUTION and MS-ALIGNMENT (Pevzner *et al.*, 2001), circumvent the problem of increased "virtual" database size and false positive rate encountered by other approaches when searching for post-translational modifications. By using a spectral convolution between the experimental and theoretical spectra, modifications present in the experimental spectrum may be found without exhaustive search of all combinations of modifications.

A. DETECTION OF PROTEIN PHOSPHORYLATION

The identification of global patterns of phosphorylation is important for understanding how signaling processes affect the cell system. Phosphorylation is probably the best studied protein modification and certainly the most common. Assuming that a typical mammalian cell expresses approximately 15,000 proteins, as suggested by measurements of mRNA complexity (Hastie and Bishop, 1976), and assuming that a third of those are phosphorylated, an average cell may contain approximately 5000 phosphoproteins. If an average phosphoprotein contains two tryptic phosphopeptides (arising from multisite phosphorylation, a conservative estimate), then a tryptic digest of an "average" mammalian cell extract should generate more than 10,000 phosphopeptides. Although many analyses of phosphorylation by MS have been carried out, this is not necessarily a routine method. Some sites are easily identified; however, other sites are difficult to detect, let alone characterize. In a 2003 ABRF (Association of Biomolecular Resource Facilities) survey of MS core facilities, most labs identified one of two phosphopeptides present in a sample containing two proteins, but only three of 54 labs successfully identified the second phosphopeptide (Arnott *et al.*, 2003). Many phosphoproteins are also present at low abundance within the cell, because only a small percentage may be phosphorylated at any one time. Another difficulty is that ionization of phosphopeptides is often suppressed due to the electronegativity of the phosphoryl groups (Kratzer *et al.*, 1998; Liao *et al.*, 1994; Mann *et al.*, 2002), charge competition, or formation of salt interactions with basic peptides.

Because of these problems, global analysis of the phosphoproteome has employed affinity methods to first isolate and enrich phosphopeptides from crude cell extracts, and then establish their identity by MS. For example, Chait and co-workers (Oda *et al.*, 2001) developed a method that replaces the phosphate groups of Ser and Thr phosphopeptides with a biotin tag, followed by avidin-affinity chromatography. An approach developed by the Aebersold lab chemically modifies phosphate groups, replacing them with sulfhydryl groups. Phosphopeptides are then recovered by reaction with immobilized iodoacetyl moieties (Zhou *et al.*, 2001). However, both methods are limited by inefficient derivatization, lengthy chemistry, and poor reproducibility. Thus an analysis of *Saccharomyces cerevisiae* revealed only 12 phosphoproteins, far fewer than expected (Zhou *et al.*, 2001).

A method used for many years in this research involves enrichment of phosphopeptides using immobilized metal affinity chromatography (IMAC) (Andersson and Porath, 1986). IMAC isolates phosphopeptides by electrostatic attraction of the phosphate group to metals, primarily with Fe^{3+}, and as such has a tendency to nonspecifically isolate peptides containing high levels of Glu or Asp. Thus the selectivity of IMAC for phosphopeptide adsorption is limited. Recently a simple method of methylesterification prior to enrichment by IMAC was published, along with identification of 383 phosphorylation sites in the *S. cerevisiae* phosphoproteome, of which only 18 had been characterized previously (Ficarro *et al.*, 2002). A flurry of excitement went through the mass spectrometry community; however, no lab has been able to reproduce this result. What happened? Besides the difficulty of reproducing the analytical method itself, a close examination of the search results from this type of experiment reveals the presence of the identification ambiguity problem that arises from allowing multiple modifications, as previously described. Allowing the phosphorylation of all serine, threonine, and tyrosine residues in the protein sequences increases the number of theoretically matching masses approximately tenfold, because each theoretically calculated mass can be increased by any of several multiples of the mass of the phosphate group. This increase in the number of theoretically expected masses means that the chance of an observed mass matching a calculated mass simply by chance is greatly increased and, consequently, the statistical discrimination power of the search programs is markedly reduced. The original publication does not provide sufficient information to assess the significance of the peptide identifications, but it is likely that many of the identifications are incorrect.

As is clear from this section, the issues of protein isoform ambiguity remain daunting. The post-translational modification ambiguity problem resulting from the combinatorial explosion of theoretical masses remains a key to opening the problem in both PMF and MS/MS informatics. By putting limits or assigning probabilities to various combinations of modifications, this problem may be ameliorated. However, any shotgun proteomics approach to detecting modified proteins will have higher ambiguity than identifying the unmodified peptides from these proteins and cannot address combinatorial signaling between different sites or different types of modifications in a protein. It is likely that top-down proteomics will be required to adequately address this aspect of proteins. Furthermore, informatics approaches to the cleavage and gene family isoform problems have barely begun.

VIII. Systems and Workflow Issues

Proteomics is maturing from manual biochemical analyses to ever more automated workflows. Instruments are increasingly computer controlled and generally deposit the data collected directly into computer files or (better) database tables. This tight connection between instruments and analytical computer systems makes automated process monitoring, quality control, and workflow scripting increasingly practical. Although not yet used in proteomics, a closed-loop experimental design, execution, and hypothesis generation computer system was recently reported (King *et al.*, 2004). Also, the precedent of computerized workflow and quality control software in managing large collections of robotic DNA sequencers at genome sequencing centers suggests that similar approaches will prove useful in high-throughput proteomics.

Although these systems-level informatics tasks will become increasingly important as proteomics matures, there are not any software packages to support the entire pipeline, nor many publications on the issues involved. One exception is the aforementioned PRISM approach (Kislinger *et al.*, 2003). Our survey is necessarily subjective, and reflects our perceptions and experiences.

It is not even always the case that computer-controlled instruments are available. The equipment facilities in academic settings are sometimes standalone units with minimal network interconnections. Tracking experimental information often requires manual entry or merging in order to be integrated. Even with such equipment, automated planning and scheduling algorithms can help improve efficiency.

Fortunately the biochemical equipment for controlling sample fractionation and MS runs is increasingly computer accessible. Instruments allow for external computer control of settings and timing, and laboratory robotics can control the passing of samples automatically from step to step. With increasing potential for automation come increasing requirements for automated quality assurance and monitoring of the processes and resulting data. Such improvements also make possible increased automation in scheduling, such as allowing the automatic rescheduling of runs with results that did not meet quality control (QC) guidelines. Laboratory information management systems (LIMS) can include sample tracking (generally through bar codes), scheduling optimization, instrument control, and quality control subsystems to organize larger laboratories. Smaller laboratories can use project scheduling and tracking systems to ensure the high-quality flow of work and reliable resulting data. Although generic laboratory control software is available, we are not aware of publications or commercial software specifically tuned to the needs of high-throughput proteomics.

Because equipment can be costly and can require careful setup steps by trained personnel, the matter of scheduling machines and people for a set of diverse experiments can be a difficult matter in itself. For samples that are reused, or when steps are separated by any length of time, the tracking before, during, and after the experiment is an added concern. Beginning-to-end computerized tracking of all samples and activities, from collection, through analysis and QC to the final interpretations of the analyzed data, is the ultimate goal of LIMS—although proteomics laboratories, unlike genome sequencing centers, have not generally found it cost effective to invest in the design and implementation of such systems.

The data produced by spectrometers are often output as a large set of flat (ASCII-format) files that require individual naming, storage, and management. However, a single experiment can produce tens of thousands of distinct datasets. That many files are difficult to even name uniquely and meaningfully for organized storage. Thereafter, there are problems in routinely accessing this large number of files for integrated and comparative analyses. When problems arise from experimental errors, such as equipment malfunctions, the troublesome file may not be detected among a host of similar files until many days after the experiment was run—too late to easily correct. Most laboratories develop naming and data storage procedures to link related spectra and annotate information about samples, protocols, and other relevant information. Using a computer's file system as a database (and file names as identifiers) has many pitfalls, yet the more appropriate use of databases to manage such information has yet to find widespread acceptance.

To the degree that more systematic approaches have been developed, including automatic loading of instrument data into a defined database schema, automated quality control calculations on data as it comes in, and user interfaces for annotation, they exist mostly as unpublished, ad hoc computer "scripts" in some of the larger laboratories. Because the particular needs of each laboratory vary with the instrumentation and protocols used, general purpose systems may be hard to develop, or require extensive local configuration to be useful. The optimal design of informatics tools for this task remains an open problem.

Quality control checks, particularly at the point of data capture from the instruments, can improve the efficiency and outcome of the entire process. It is possible to check for missing values, impossible or unlikely values, consistency of various kinds (e.g., between fraction characteristics and protein identifications), for adherence to expected ranges, or even to match computer models that simulate the experiment and its likely outcomes. This data can also be used to automatically monitor instruments for consistency and reliability, particularly when experiments are designed to include known control samples.

Another systems issue is ensuring that the protocol used in the analysis of the data is captured so that it can be reported, reproduced, and shared. It may also be possible to enforce consistency, check for reasonableness, or give automated advice about various decisions necessary in doing the analyses. Decisions about parameter settings of the identification programs (e.g., SEQUEST), the choice of post processing validations, and even the sequence databases used for the theoretical calculations all have a large effect on the final results.

An example of the difficulties that arise in trying to manually manage these decisions can be found in the choice of protein (or genome) sequence databases used by the search programs. Two commonly used protein datasets are the nonredundant database available from the National Center for Biotechnology Information (NCBI)[3] and the International Protein Index (IPI.)[4] Theoretical digests (e.g., by trypsin) of all of the proteins in a reference database are provided by some of the database suppliers (e.g., SwissProt's Peptide Cutter program)[5] These databases contain information including structures, taxonomies, and links to species-specific databases of proteins and peptides. They are quite large databases, so proteomics laboratories generally download local copies from the source websites. However, these databases are different from each other, and they are constantly updated, changing accession numbers, and adding new variants. Day-to-day changes (which accumulate rapidly over time) mean that a set of protein identifications generated one day using one version of the database will generally have some differences from the exact same data run using a different version of the database. Ideally it is possible to resolve the ambiguities caused by these changes by some translation procedure, but there is no automated tool to do this. Nor is it the case that the specific database version and other parameters relevant to the identification process are always captured and stored, which can lead to conflicts among laboratories and even informatics-related difficulty reproducing published results.

Another problem relates to how the different identification methods handle ambiguity among protein isoforms. In both SEQUEST and MASCOT, fairly arbitrary choices appear to be made about which among several ambiguous isoforms is reported, meaning that two search programs may "pick" different accession numbers for what is essentially the same identification. This also leads to ambiguity when comparing results between laboratories. Eventually, standardization of the isoform-related methods will eliminate these problems, but at this stage the best method is not clear. To commit the field to standards at this point could stifle creativity and codify problems into the system in a way that will be difficult to correct later. A better alternative is to capture and report all the information relevant to the workflow.

Graphical user interfaces can present available information in formats that highlight important results and reduce the chances of errors or oversights. In the area of proteomics, interfaces could be designed to present information about instruments, spectra, and analyses in order to emphasize trends, outliers, out-of-

[3]www.ncbi.nlm.nih.gov/entrez/query.fcgi?db=Protein.
[4]www.ebi.ac.uk/IPI/IPIhelp.html
[5]http://ca.expasy.org/tools/peptidecutter/peptidecutter_enzymes.html

spec values, and other concerns that might require human attention. Other than the user interfaces on commercial software associated with particular instruments, we are not aware of any publications regarding the sort of user interfaces best suited for proteomics. Generally, large labs will design reports or triggers based on scripts or (when available) database queries to meet their specific needs. There is, of course, a large, general literature in computer science related to user interfaces (Galitz, 2002), and even some in related scientific areas such as protein crystallography (McPhillips et al., 2002). Appropriate graphical displays and other monitoring tools for high-throughput proteomics facilities are another relatively unexplored area of proteomics informatics.

A. Data Exchange, Sharing, and Privacy Issues

Data sharing and concomitant data exchange standards are becoming an increasingly important aspect of high-throughput molecular biology. Two recently developed XML standards for proteomics and MS data are mzXML Schema and Tools by Patrick Pedrioli at ISB (www.systemsbiology.org), and MIAPE (minimum information to describe a proteomics experiment) by Stephen Oliver's group (Taylor et al., 2003).

Another effort, PROXIML (http://xml.coverpages.org/proximl.html) appears to be moribund. Unlike macromolecular sequence, structure, or expression array data, there is no widely accepted public repository for proteomics data, nor do journals generally require deposition of raw data as a condition for publication. Standardized vocabularies or more formal ontologies for the description of proteomics experiments is similarly undeveloped. There are nascent efforts among experts in the proteomics field to address these issues, such as the effort by the Human Proteome Organisation (www.hupo.org/) to support a Proteomics Standards Initiative (http://psidev.sourceforge.net/) to develop community-based standards.

There are a few areas related to proteomics informatics in which government regulation plays a role. When proteomics information is gathered about samples from human beings, Health Insurance Portability and Accountability Act (HIPAA) privacy regulations may require that specific computer security, auditing, and other standards be met (Adler, 2003). When proteomics information is used in research supporting drug discovery, (Food and Drug Administration (FDA) requirements for good laboratory practices require the collection of quality assurance and audit trail information (Turner and Bolton, 2001). Most proteomics laboratories and informaticians either will not confront these issues, or will do so in the context of a larger institutional effort to meet these requirements.

IX. Conclusion

Informatics plays a crucial role in high-throughput proteomics. In this chapter we reviewed the contributions of dozens of individual computer programs and systems, which are listed topically in an appendix. We also described more generally the computational requirements of modern shotgun proteomics. Despite the central role of informatics, there are many areas in which open problems exist and informatics-driven improvements in the state of the art are desirable. Such improvements are possible in algorithms, systems, databases, sample tracking, user interfaces, and a variety of other areas. We hope that this chapter spurs the informatics and proteomics communities to systematically address these issues, bringing proteomics technology closer to its ideal as a source of information about the identity, isoforms, and abundances of proteins in living systems.

X. Appendix: List of Mentioned Algorithms by Topic

A. IDENTIFICATION ALGORITHMS FOR MS/MS DATABASE CORRELATION

SEQUEST (Yates *et al.*, 1995)—One of the most widely used algorithms for matching MS/MS data to a sequence database. Uses cross-correlation between the experimental and theoretical spectrum for each peptide within a user specified tolerance of the parent mass.

SEQUEST-Norm (MacCoss *et al.*, 2002)—This version of SEQUEST attempts to remove the dependence of the SEQUEST XCorr score and molecular weight of the protein.

MASCOT (Perkins *et al.*, 1999)—MASCOT builds on the MOWSE algorithm by incorporating probability based scoring and removal of prebuilt indexes.

PepFrag (Fenyo and Chait, 1998; Qin *et al.*, 1997)—An early search program.

SpectrumMill—A workbench type of environment for extracting, searching, and visualizing LC-MS/MS data, compatible with multiple mass spectrometers: www.chem.agilent.com.

SonarMS/MS (Field *et al.*, 2002)—Part of the RADARS package from Genomic Solutions, this algorithm originally developed by Beavis and coworkers. It calculates a correlation score using the inner product of the experimental and theoretical spectra, and incorporates the use of expectation values in the calculation of a confidence score.

SCOPE (Bafna and Edwards, 2001)—Two-stage stochastic model for matching MS/MS spectra to peptide sequences that incorporates fragment ion probabilities, noisy spectra, and instrument measurement error.

Popitam (Hernandez *et al.*, 2003)—Uses a graph algorithm similar to those used in *de novo* sequencing to identify a list of candidate peptide sequences ranked by their correlation.

ProbID (Zhang *et al.*, 2002)—A Bayesian probabilistic algorithm inspired by the approach developed for the ProFound algorithm.

OLAV (Colinge *et al.*, 2003)—Based on signal detection theory, this algorithm calculates a likelihood ratio score based on the degree of matching between the experimental and theoretical spectra, as well as incorporating additional information about the match.

PeptideProphet (Keller *et al.*, 2002)—Designed to distinguish correct from incorrectly assigned peptides from SEQUEST searches using a machine learning approach applied to a known set of validated MS/MS spectra.

ProteinProphet—Combines scores from peptide assignments from MS/MS search into a protein identification score. Addresses the problem that many peptides in the database are degenerate.

Qscore (Moore *et al.*, 2002)—Probabilistic SEQUEST validation algorithm based on a model of random peptide matching. It incorporates the fraction of distinct tryptic peptides matched in the database that are also present in the protein, and generates a protein identification score, like ProteinProphet.

SVM-based filtering (Anderson *et al.*, 2003)—In the same manner that PeptideProphet uses discriminate analysis, Anderson et al. use a machine learning algorithm, support vector machine to maximize the discrimination between correct and incorrect identifications, based on multiple scoring values from SEQUEST searches.

PRISM (Kislinger *et al.*, 2003)—A system or approach, rather than an algorithm, that encompasses every step from subcellular fractionation and extraction of proteins to MudPIT/SEQUEST analysis to the clustering of the final protein list. After MudPIT analysis, statistical analysis of peptide identification scores is performed by their STATQUEST algorithm to estimate the accuracy of identifications, which uses an empirically derived probabilistic model. This is followed by clustering and functional annotation of the protein list using GOClust, which groups proteins based on shared annotations from the GO schema (Ashburner *et al.*, 2000). X! Tandem (Craig and Beavis, 2003)—Open source software from Manitoba Centre for Proteomics. Matches peptide sequences with MS/MS spectra and identifies modifications using an iterative approach, where the likely candidates are identified first from the total database, followed by a search on the refined, smaller list of proteins to search for modifications. When compared to Sonar MS/MS and Mascot, all three packages identified the same set of peptides, although with different scores and expectation values.

B. Filtering and Visualization Tools

CHOMPER (Eddes *et al.*, 2002)—Displays MS data for validation.
DTAselect (Tabb *et al.*, 2002)—Filtering and visualization of SEQUEST results.
INTERACT (Han *et al.*, 2001)—A tool developed by Jimmy Eng to collect and organize the large number of MS/MS spectra generated from large shotgun proteomics experiments. Freely available.
VEMS (Matthiesen *et al.*, 2003)—Interpretation and annotation of MS/MS spectra and database searching.

C. Peptide Mass Fingerprinting

PepSea (Henzel *et al.*, 1993)—The first web based search algorithm.
MS-Fit (Clauser *et al.*, 1999)—An early search program, currently available at http://prospector.ucsf.edu
MOWSE (Pappin *et al.*, 1993)—The original probability based search algorithm that is now part of MASCOT.
FindPept (Gattiker *et al.*, 2002)—Identifies unmatched masses.
ProFound (Zhang and Chait, 2000)—A sophisticated PMF protein identification algorithm that uses bayesian theory to calculate a probability score.
ProteinScape (Chamrad *et al.*, 2003)—Performs automated calibration and peak filtering and searches across multiple PMF search engines. Combines the results from into a single score, the significance of which is determined through simulations and calculation of an expectation score. Currently uses MASCOT, MS-Fit, and ProFound.

D. Sequence Tag ID

MS-Tag (Clauser *et al.*, 1999)—Part of the ProteinProspector suite of programs; searches sequence databases with sequence tag data.
PeptideSearch (Mann *et al.*, 2002)—One of the first search programs that was downloadable.
TagIdent (Wilkins *et al.*, 1998)—Identification of proteins using pI and MW, as well as short sequence tags up to six amino acids.
MultiTag (Sunyaev *et al.*, 2003)—Designed for sequence tag searches of organisms with unsequenced genomes. Identifies homologous proteins from related organisms.
GutenTag—A recent program developed by the Yates laboratory, available at http://fields.scripps.edu/GutenTag/index.html

E. *De Novo*

Lutefisk (Taylor and Johnson, 1997)—*De novo* sequencing program that uses a graph algorithm to enumerate all possible paths through the MS/MS peaks, and scores the candidates using cross-correlation and an intensity-based score. Recently modified to handle data from triple quad, QTOF, and ion trap instruments.

CIDentify (Taylor and Johnson, 2001)—Takes as input the identified sequence candidates from Lutefisk and performs a homology based sequence search for cases in which the proteins of interest are not sequenced.

SHERENGA (Dancik *et al.*, 1999)—A supervised learning based *de novo* sequencing algorithm. Using a set of validated test spectra, the algorithm learns the relative intensities of ion types, which will be specific to the type of mass spectrometer. Using this information, a list of ranked and scored sequences is generated for the set of unknown spectra.

F. Post-Translational Modification Identification

FindMod (Williams *et al.*, 1999)—Designed for PMF data, FindMod searches for unaccounted masses in the mass map of a previously identified protein for matches to user specified modifications. The rules for modification patterns are built from the annotated Swiss-Prot database.

MS-CONVOLUTION, MS-ALIGNMENT (Pevzner *et al.*, 2001)—These MS/MS peptide identification algorithms circumvent the problem of increased "virtual" database size and false positive rate encountered by other approaches when searching for post-translational modifications. By using a spectral convolution between the experimental and theoretical spectra, modifications present in the experimental spectrum may be found without exhaustive search of all combinations of modifications.

G. Other

MS2Assign (Schilling *et al.*, 2003)—Analysis of cross-linked peptides for studying 3D structure.

H. Analysis Systems (LIMS)

RADARS (Field *et al.*, 2002)—A LIMS type of system for storage and analysis of high-throughput mass spectrometry data. Integrates the Sonar MS/MS and ProFound algorithms.

Commercialized by Genomic Solutions (Ann Arbor, MI).

I. QUANTITATIVE SOFTWARE

XPRESS (Han *et al.*, 2001)—Software for relative quantitation of proteins from isotope-labeling based LC-MS/MS experiments. Interfaces with the INTERACT software.

References

Adler, M. P. (2003). The final security rule. Compliance begins with risk analysis. *Healthcare Informatics* **20**(10), 74–76.

Anderson, D. C., *et al.* (2003). A new algorithm for the evaluation of shotgun peptide sequencing in proteomics: Support vector machine classification of peptide MS/MS spectra and SEQUEST scores. *J. Proteome Res.* **2**(2), 137–146.

Andersson, L., and Porath, J. (1986). Isolation of phosphoproteins by immobilized metal (Fe3+) affinity chromatography. *Anal. Biochem.* **154**(1), 250–254.

Arnott, D., *et al.* (2003). ABRF-PRG03: Phosphorylation site determination. *J. Biomol. Tech.* **14**(3), 205–215.

Ashburner, M., *et al.* (2000). Gene ontology: Tool for the unification of biology. The Gene Ontology Consortium. *Nat. Genet.* **25**(1), 25–29.

Bafna, V., and Edwards, N. (2001). SCOPE: A probabilistic model for scoring tandem mass spectra against a peptide database. *Bioinformatics* **17**(Suppl. 1), S13–S21.

Bergquist, J. (2003). FTICR mass spectrometry in proteomics. *Curr. Opin. Mol. Ther.* **5**(3), 310–314.

Bondarenko, P. V., Chelius, D., and Shaler, T. A. (2002). Identification and relative quantitation of protein mixtures by enzymatic digestion followed by capillary reversed-phase liquid chromatography-tandem mass spectrometry. *Anal. Chem.* **74**(18), 4741–4749.

Chamrad, D. C., *et al.* (2003). Interpretation of mass spectrometry data for high-throughput proteomics. *Anal. Bioanal. Chem.* **376**(7), 1014–1022.

Clauser, K. R., Baker, P., and Burlingame, A. L. (1999). Role of accurate mass measurement (+/−10 ppm) in protein identification strategies employing MS or MS/MS and database searching. *Anal. Chem.* **71**(14), 2871–2882.

Colinge, J., *et al.* (2003). OLAV: Towards high-throughput tandem mass spectrometry data identification. *Proteomics* **3**(8), 1454–1463.

Craig, R., and Beavis, R. C. (2003). A method for reducing the time required to match protein sequences with tandem mass spectra. *Rapid Commun. Mass Spectrom.* **17**(20), 2310–2316.

Dancik, V., *et al.* (1999). De novo peptide sequencing via tandem mass spectrometry. *J. Comput. Biol.* **6**(3–4), 327–342.

Eddes, J. S., *et al.* (2002). CHOMPER: A bioinformatic tool for rapid validation of tandem mass spectrometry search results associated with high-throughput proteomic strategies. *Proteomics* **2**(9), 1097–1103.

Fenyo, D., Qin, J., and Chait, B. T. (1998). Protein identification using mass spectrometric information. *Electrophoresis* **19**(6), 998–1005.

Ficarro, S. B., *et al.* (2002). Phosphoproteome analysis by mass spectrometry and its application to Saccharomyces cerevisiae. *Nat. Biotechnol.* **20**(3), 301–305.

Field, H. I., Fenyo, D., and Beavis, R. C. (2002). RADARS, a bioinformatics solution that automates proteome mass spectral analysis, optimises protein identification, and archives data in a relational database. *Proteomics* **2**(1), 36–47.

Galitz, W. O. (2002). "The Essential Guide to User Interface Design," ed 2. John Wiley & Sons, Indianapolis, IN.

Gattiker, A., et al. (2002). FindPept, a tool to identify unmatched masses in peptide mass fingerprinting protein identification. Proteomics 2(10), 1435–1444.

Ge, Y., et al. (2002). Top down characterization of larger proteins (45 kDa) by electron capture dissociation mass spectrometry. J. Am. Chem. Soc. 124(4), 672–678.

Gygi, S. P., et al. (2002). Proteome analysis of low-abundance proteins using multidimensional chromatography and isotope-coded affinity tags. J. Proteome Res. 1(1), 47–54.

Han, D. K., et al. (2001). Quantitative profiling of differentiation-induced microsomal proteins using isotope-coded affinity tags and mass spectrometry. Nat. Biotechnol. 19(10), 946–951.

Hastie, N. D., and Bishop, J. O. (1976). The expression of three abundance classes of messenger RNA in mouse tissues. Cell 9(4 PT 2), 761–774.

Henzel, W. J., et al. (1993). Identifying proteins from two-dimensional gels by molecular mass searching of peptide fragments in protein sequence databases. Proc. Natl. Acad. Sci. USA 90(11), 5011–5015.

Hernandez, P., et al. (2003). Popitam: Towards new heuristic strategies to improve protein identification from tandem mass spectrometry data. Proteomics 3(6), 870–878.

Jacobs, J. M., et al. (2004). Multidimensional proteome analysis of human mammary epithelial cells. J. Proteome Res. 3(1), 68–75.

Keller, A., et al. (2002). Empirical statistical model to estimate the accuracy of peptide identifications made by MS/MS and database search. Annal. Chem. 74(20), 5383–5392.

King, R. D., et al. (2004). Functional genomic hypothesis generation and experimentation by a robot scientist. Nature 427(6971), 247–252.

King, R., et al. (2003). Mechanistic investigation of ionization suppression in electrospray ionization. J. Am. Soc. Mass Spectrom. 11(11), 942–950.

Kislinger, T., et al. (2003). PRISM, a generic large scale proteomic investigation strategy for mammals. Mol. Cell Proteomics 2(2), 96–106.

Kitano, H. (2002). Systems biology: A brief overview. Science 295(5560), 1662–1664.

Kratzer, R., et al. (1998). Suppression effects in enzymatic peptide ladder sequencing using ultraviolet—matrix assisted laser desorption/ionization—mass spectrometry. Electrophoresis 19(11), 1910–1919.

Liao, P. C., et al. (1994). An approach to locate phosphorylation sites in a phosphoprotein: Mass mapping by combining specific enzymatic degradation with matrix-assisted laser desorption/ionization mass spectrometry. Anal. Biochem. 219(1), 9–20.

MacCoss, M. J., Wu, C. C., and Yates, J. R., III (2002). Probability-based validation of protein identifications using a modified SEQUEST algorithm. Anal. Chem. 74(21), 5593–5599.

Mann, M., Hojrup, P., and Roepstorff, P. (1993). Use of mass spectrometric molecular weight information to identify proteins in sequence databases. Biol. Mass Spectrom. 22(6), 338–345.

Mann, M., et al. (2002). Analysis of protein phosphorylation using mass spectrometry: Deciphering the phosphoproteome. Trends Biotechnol. 20(6), 261–268.

Mann, M., and Wilm, M. (1994). Error-tolerant identification of peptides in sequence databases by peptide sequence tags. Anal. Chem. 66(24), 4390–4399.

Matthiesen, R., et al. (2003). Interpreting peptide mass spectra by VEMS. Bioinformatics 19(6), 792–793.

McPhillips, T. M., et al. (2002). Blu-Ice and the distributed control system: Software for data acquisition and instrument control at macromolecular crystallography beamlines. J. Synchrotron. Radiat. 9(Pt 6), 401–406.

Moore, R. E., Young, M. K., and Lee, T. D. (2002). Qscore: An algorithm for evaluating SEQUEST database search results. J. Am. Soc. Mass Spectrom. 13(4), 378–386.

Muller, C., et al. (2002). Ion suppression effects in liquid chromatography-electrospray-ionisation transport-region collision induced dissociation mass spectrometry with different serum extraction methods for systematic toxicological analysis with mass spectra libraries. *J. Chromatogr. B. Analyt. Technol. Biomed. Life Sci.* **773**(1), 47–52.

Nesvizhskii, A. I., *et al.* (2002). A statistical model for identifying proteins by tandem mass spectrometry. *Anal. Chem.* **75**, 4646–4658.

O'Farrell, P. H. (1975). High resolution two-dimensional electrophoresis of proteins. *J. Biol. Chem.* **250**(10), 4007–4021.

Oda, Y., Nagasu, T., and Chait, B. T. (2001). Enrichment analysis of phosphorylated proteins as a tool for probing the phosphoproteome. *Nat. Biotechnol.* **19**(4), 379–382.

Ong, S. E., *et al.* (2002). Stable isotope labeling by amino acids in cell culture, SILAC, as a simple and accurate approach to expression proteomics. *Mol. Cell Proteomics* **1**(5), 376–386.

Patton, W. F., Schulenberg, B., and Steinberg, T. H. (2002). Two-dimensional gel electrophoresis; better than a poke in the ICAT? *Curr. Opin. Biotechnol.* **13**(4), 321–328.

Pappin, D. J. C., Hojrup, P., and Bleasby, A. J. (1993). Rapid identification of proteins by peptide mass fingerprinting. *Curr. Biol.* **3**, 327–332.

Peng, J., *et al.* (2003). Evaluation of multidimensional chromatography coupled with tandem mass spectrometry (LC/LC-MS/MS) for large-scale protein analysis: The yeast proteome. *J. Proteome Res.* **2**(1), 43–50.

Perkins, D. N., *et al.* (1999). Probability-based protein identification by searching sequence databases using mass spectrometry data. *Electrophoresis* **20**(18), 3551–3567.

Pevzner, P. A., *et al.* (2001). Efficiency of database search for identification of mutated and modified proteins via mass spectrometry. *Genome Res.* **11**(2), 290–299.

Qin, J., *et al.* (1997). A strategy for rapid, high-confidence protein identification. *Anal. Chem.* **69**(19), 3995–4001.

Resing, K. A., *et al.* (2004). Improving reproducibility and sensitivity in identifying human proteins by shotgun proteomics. *Anal. Chem.* **76**(13), 3556–3568.

Schilling, B., *et al.* (2003). MS2Assign, automated assignment and nomenclature of tandem mass spectra of chemically crosslinked peptides. *J. Am. Soc. Mass Spectrom.* **14**(8), 834–850.

Shen, M., *et al.* (2003). Isolation and isotope labeling of cysteine- and methionine-containing tryptic peptides: Application to the study of cell surface proteolysis. *Mol. Cell Proteomics* **2**(5), 315–324.

Shevchenko, A., *et al.* (1996). Linking genome and proteome by mass spectrometry: Large-scale identification of yeast proteins from two dimensional gels. *Proc. Natl. Acad. Sci. USA* **93**(25), 14440–14445.

Shiio, Y., *et al.* (2002). Quantitative proteomic analysis of Myc oncoprotein function. *EMBO J.* **21**(19), 5088–5096.

Smith, R. D., *et al.* (2002). An accurate mass tag strategy for quantitative and high-throughput proteome measurements. *Proteomics* **2**(5), 513–523.

Spahr, C. S., *et al.* (2001). Towards defining the urinary proteome using liquid chromatography-tandem mass spectrometry. I. Profiling an unfractionated tryptic digest. *Proteomics* **1**(1), 93–107.

Sunyaev, S., *et al.* (2003). MultiTag: Multiple error-tolerant sequence tag search for the sequence-similarity identification of proteins by mass spectrometry. *Anal. Chem.* **75**(6), 1307–1315.

Tabb, D. L., McDonald, W. H., and Yates, J. R., III (2002). DTASelect and Contrast: Tools for assembling and comparing protein identifications from shotgun proteomics. *J. Proteome Res.* **1**(1), 21–26.

Taylor, C. F., *et al.* (2003). A systematic approach to modeling, capturing, and disseminating proteomics experimental data. *Nat. Biotechnol.* **21**(3), 247–254.

Taylor, J. A., and Johnson, R. S. (1997). Sequence database searches via *de novo* peptide sequencing by tandem mass spectrometry. *Rapid Commun. Mass Spectrom.* **11**(9), 1067–1075.

Taylor, J. A., and Johnson, R. S. (2001). Implementation and uses of automated *de novo* peptide sequencing by tandem mass spectrometry. *Anal. Chem.* **73**(11), 2594–2604.

Turner, E., and Bolton, J. (2001). Required steps for the validation of a laboratory information management system. *Qual. Assur.* **9**(3–4), 217–224.

Wang, W., *et al.* (2003). Quantification of proteins and metabolites by mass spectrometry without isotopic labeling or spiked standards. *Anal. Chem.* **75**(18), 4818–4826.

Washburn, M. P., Wolters, D., and Yates, J. R., III (2001). Large-scale analysis of the yeast proteome by multidimensional protein identification technology. *Nat. Biotechnol.* **19**(3), 242–247.

Wilkins, M. R., *et al.* (1999). High-throughput mass spectrometric discovery of protein post-translational modifications. *J. Mol. Biol.* **289**(3), 645–657.

Wilkins, M. R., and Williams, K. L. (1997). Cross-species protein identification using amino acid composition, peptide mass fingerprinting, isoelectric point and molecular mass: A theoretical evaluation. *J. Theor. Biol.* **186**(1), 7–15.

Wilkins, M. R., *et al.* (1998). Multiple parameter cross-species protein identification using MultiIdent—a world-wide web accessible tool. *Electrophoresis* **19**(18), 3199–3206.

Wilkins, M. R., *et al.* (1998). Protein identification with N and C-terminal sequence tags in proteome projects. *J. Mol. Biol.* **278**(3), 599–608.

Wu, C. C., *et al.* (2003). A method for the comprehensive proteomic analysis of membrane proteins. *Nat. Biotechnol.* **21**(5), 532–538.

Yao, X., *et al.* (2001). Proteolytic 18O labeling for comparative proteomics: Model studies with two serotypes of adenovirus. *Anal. Chem.* **73**(13), 2836–2842.

Yates, J. R., III, *et al.* (1995). Method to correlate tandem mass spectra of modified peptides to amino acid sequences in the protein database. *Anal. Chem.* **67**(8), 1426–1436.

Yi, E. C., *et al.* (2002). Approaching complete peroxisome characterization by gas-phase fractionation. *Electrophoresis* **23**(18), 3205–3216.

Zaia, J. (2004). Mass spectrometry of oligosaccharides. *Mass. Spectrom. Rev.* **23**(3), 161–227.

Zhang, N., Aebersold, R., and Schwikowski, B. (2002). ProbID: A probabilistic algorithm to identify peptides through sequence database searching using tandem mass spectral data. *Proteomics* **2**(10), 1406–1412.

Zhang, W., and Chait, B. T. (2000). ProFound: An expert system for protein identification using mass spectrometric peptide mapping information. *Anal. Chem.* **72**(11), 2482–2489.

Zhou, H., Watts, J. D., and Aebersold, R. (2001). A systematic approach to the analysis of protein phosphorylation. *Nat. Biotechnol.* **19**(4), 375–378.

SECTION IV
CHANGES IN THE PROTEOME BY DISEASE

PROTEOMICS ANALYSIS IN ALZHEIMER'S DISEASE: NEW INSIGHTS INTO MECHANISMS OF NEURODEGENERATION

D. Allan Butterfield*,† and Debra Boyd-Kimball*

*Department of Chemistry, Center of Membrane Sciences
University of Kentucky, Lexington, Kentucky 40506
†Sanders-Brown Center on Aging, University of Kentucky
Lexington, Kentucky 40506

I. Introduction

Alzheimer's disease (AD) is a progressive, age-related neurodegenerative disorder associated with cognitive decline and aging that is estimated to affect more than 5 million Americans and more than 15 million people worldwide (Katzman and Saitoh, 1991). Oxidative stress is associated with the pathogenesis of the disease (Markesbery, 1997). Protein carbonyl formation, lipid peroxidation, 3-nitrotyrosine (3-NT), and DNA oxidation are among the oxidative stress markers reported for AD (Butterfield, 2002; Butterfield and Lauderback, 2002; Castegna et al., 2003; Lovell et al., 2001; Smith et al., 1997).

Amyloid β-peptide (1-42) (Aβ[1-42]) has been implicated as a causative agent in AD. Evidence supporting a central role for Aβ(1-42) in the pathogenesis of AD has been provided by the genetic mutations resulting in overexpression of this peptide in cases of familial Alzheimer's disease (FAD). For example, mutations of presenillin-1(PS1), presenillin-2 (PS2), and amyloid precursor protein (APP) result in overexpression of Aβ(1-42) and subsequent inheritance of AD. APP, the transmembrane glycoprotein from which Aβ(1-42) is proteolytically cleaved, is

161

encoded by chromosome 21. Consequently, individuals with Down syndrome, or trisomy 21, who have three copies of chromosome 21, typically have an increased load of $A\beta(1\text{-}42)$ and will develop AD if they live long enough. Likewise, in rodent models of AD, overexpression of human APP and tau lead to the development of plaques prior to neurofibrillar deposits (Selkoe, 2001a,b; Selkoe and Podlisny, 2002). $A\beta(1\text{-}42)$ induces protein carbonylation, lipid peroxidation, and formation of 3-NT (Butterfield, 2003; Butterfield and Lauderback, 2002; Butterfield *et al.*, 2002). Such $A\beta(1\text{-}42)$-induced oxidative stress is inhibited by antioxidants (Yatin *et al.*, 2000). Taken together, these findings suggest that $A\beta(1\text{-}42)$ plays a primary role in the oxidative damage evident in AD.

Consistent with this notion, protein oxidation in AD occurs in $A\beta$-rich brain regions such as the hippocampus and cortex, but not in $A\beta$-poor regions such as the cerebellum (Hensley *et al.*, 1995). Until recently the ability to determine which proteins were specifically oxidized has been limited to immunoprecipitation techniques, which requires an educated guess as to the identity of the protein and readily available antibodies. These procedures are lengthy and laborious. Fortunately the coupling of two-dimensional gel electrophoresis and improvement of mass spectrometry (MS) techniques has allowed for the rapid screening and identification of proteins.

In this review we discuss the tools that have made proteomics possible, as well as their application to AD. Results thus far have offered invaluable insight into the pathogenesis of the disease. The implications of these results with respect to the pathological and biochemical abnormalities that have been reported for AD will be discussed, as well as our opinion of the future direction of proteomics studies in AD.

II. Proteomics Tools

A. Two-Dimensional Polyacrylamide Gel Electrophoresis

Two-dimensional polyacrylamide gel electrophoresis (2D-PAGE) of biological samples involves the separation of proteins based on their properties of isoelectric point and size. The first step in the technique is isoelectric focusing (IEF), in which the proteins are focused within a pH gradient by an applied electric field to their isoelectric point, or the point at which the net charge on the protein is zero. The second step is sodium dodecyl sulfate polyacrylamide gel electrophoresis (SDS-PAGE), in which the proteins are further purified based on their migration within an applied electric field according to molecular size. The result is a two-dimensional map in which there exists a high probability that each individual spot represents an individual protein. Ultimately, the two-dimensional map provides an expression profile of the proteins present in a given sample. Computer-assisted comparison of such profiles, or maps, allows for the determination of differences in the expression of proteins between different states (i.e., diseased versus control). Additionally, 2D-PAGE maps have enabled development of databases, which catalog the proteins (Gauss *et al.*, 1999). One of the advantages of 2D-PAGE is the ability to separate a large number of proteins from a given sample at one time. This allows for the screening of thousands of proteins at once and provides information on post-translational modifications, which result in changes in total protein charge (i.e., shift in the position of the protein spot on the gel).

Several techniques have been developed to improve and expand on the capabilities of 2D-PAGE, resulting in the evolution of a reliable and reproducible method. The introduction of immobilized pH gradient (IPG) strips to replace the tube gels with ampholytes has eliminated "cathodic drift" during IEF, resulting in an increase in reproducibility between samples (Molloy, 2000). Additionally, the development of narrow pH ranges (e.g., 4–7, 5–8) within the IPG strips has allowed for the separation of proteins that are close in isoelectric point and may not have resolved well on the more traditional 3–10 broad pH range strips. Solubilization of proteins has been the so-called stumbling block of proteomics. Because IEF does not allow induction of charge, which can interfere with the focusing process, ionic detergents such as SDS cannot be used to solubilize lipidated proteins (e.g., transmembrane proteins). The use of SDS has been reported, but the samples must be dialyzed before IEF. This produces a further limitation when working with precious biological samples that can potentially be lost in the process. As a result, chaotropic agents such as urea and thiourea (Rabilloud, 1998), coupled with nonionic or zwitterionic detergents such as CHAPS, have been used to prevent the precipitation of proteins during IEF and SDS-PAGE (Herbert, 1999). Tributyl phosphine also has been used as a reducing agent in place of dithiothreitol (Herbert *et al.*, 1998). Regardless of the improvements that have been made in the methods of 2D-PAGE, several obstacles and limitations remain. Solubilization techniques are still mainly limited to cytosolic proteins, resulting in difficulties in obtaining gel maps of membrane proteins and lipidated proteins. Maps of membrane proteins have been reported (Friso and Wikstrom, 1999; Molloy *et al.*, 1998; Pasquali *et al.*, 1997; Santoni *et al.*, 2000); however, further investigation is necessary in order to develop a method that is reliable and reproducible. Additional limitations include the resolution of very basic proteins, although IPG strips have recently been developed to address this issue (Hoving *et al.*, 2002). Finally, low-abundance proteins are typically undetectable on a gel map and thus remain elusive. This is particularly important when low-abundance proteins may play a role in the pathogenesis of a disease but are virtually silent.

The proteomics techniques of our laboratory have revolved around the identification of specifically, oxidatively modified proteins (Butterfield, 2004;

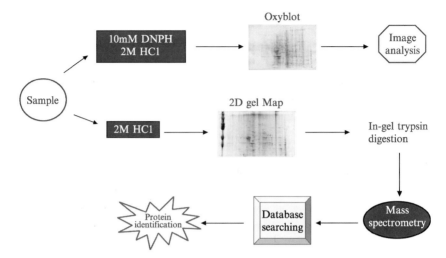

Fɪɢ. 1. Summary of procedure for parallel analysis of 2D gel maps and 2D oxyblots. (See Color Insert.)

Butterfield and Castegna, 2003a,b,c; Castegna *et al.*, 2002a,b, 2003, 2004). We used a parallel analysis in which the 2D gel map is coupled with immunochemical detection of protein carbonyls derivatized by 2,4-dinitrophenylhydrazine (DNPH), followed by MS analysis to identify proteins of particular interest. Immunochemical detection of protein carbonyls is carried out by transfer of DNPH-derivatized protein from the gel to a membrane, which is developed with specific antibodies to create a 2D oxyblot (Fig. 1). The 2D oxyblots and 2D gel maps are matched, and the immunoreactivity is normalized to the actual protein content as measured by the intensity of a protein stain such as colloidal Coomassie blue or SYPRO ruby. Such parallel analysis allows the comparison of oxidation levels of individual brain proteins in AD versus control.

B. New Techniques/Nontraditional Proteomics

Alternative techniques that do not use 2D-PAGE have also been developed (Ferguson and Smith, 2003). These methods reflect the growing technology that addresses and circumvents the disadvantages and obstacles present in the traditional 2D-PAGE method associated with proteomics analyses. It should be noted, however, that no single technique is ideal and the methodology of proteomics is constantly expanding and evolving.

1. *2D-HPLC*

High-performance liquid chromatography (HPLC) has been used to separate the peptides produced from the tryptic digestion of a protein solution. To accomplish separation of complex peptide mixtures for mass spectrometry analysis, a series of columns that separate the peptides based on different chemical and physical properties is used (Wang and Hanash, 2003). This technique is referred to as 2D-HPLC and commonly utilizes a strong cation-exchange (SCX) column, coupled with a reverse-phase (RP) column (Stevens *et al.*, 2003; Wagner *et al.*, 2003). HPLC is typically tied to a nanoelectrospray inlet mass spectrometer. This technique has also been referred to as multidimensional protein identification technology (MudPIT) (Washburn *et al.*, 2001). An ion exchange column and a size-exclusion column can be used to separate peptides based on the same principles as 2D-PAGE (Issaq *et al.*, 2002).

2. *Isotope-Coded Affinity Tags*

The technique referred to as isotope-coded affinity tags (ICAT) is one that circumvents the challenges and shortcomings of 2D-PAGE, such as problems with solubility of membrane proteins and proteins that fall outside of the *pI* and molecular weight range commonly used. ICAT uses tags that consist of three functional moieties, including a cysteine reactive site, a linker containing either 8 hydrogen atoms or 8 deuterium atoms, and a biotin affinity tag. The cysteine reactive moiety forms a chemical bond to the reduced cysteine residue of the protein, while the biotin label allows for the isolation of the iosotopically tagged peptide fragment following separation on an avidin affinity column. In this manner the isotopic label allows for quantitation of the spectra generated by MS analysis between two different cellular states by a difference of 8 Da (Gygi *et al.*, 1999). Although ICAT provides a variety of advantages over the traditional methods of protein separation and mapping based on 2D-PAGE, these advantages are accompanied by a variety of disadvantages, including the fact that the method only tags proteins with cysteine residues that are available for reaction with the isotope-coded affinity tag (Moseley, 2001).

3. *Protein Phosphorylation*

Protein phosphorylation is an important post-translational modification involved in cellular signaling and regulation (Butterfield and Stadtman, 1997). Consequently, the phosphorylation state of proteins under specific cellular conditions is of great interest; however, such studies typically involve immunoprecipitation and probing with specific phosphoprotein antibodies. Proteomics has provided the basic tools for high-throughput screening of phosphoproteins. In spite of this advance, screening of 2D gel maps transferred to membranes with antibodies has proved unsuccessful because of the lack of specific phosphoantibodies (e.g., antibodies to phosphotyrosine, phosphothreonine, and phosphoserine). As a result, a number of methods have been used to detect differences in phosphorylated proteins. In cell culture ^{32}P or ^{33}P, radiolabeling can be used to visualize phosphorylated protein separated in a 2D gel. This method has been utilized in conjunction with desalting to concentrate and purify the peptides generated from in-gel digestion of phosphoproteins with various proteases, resulting in an increase in identification of phosphorylated proteins (Larsen et al., 2001). Phosphospecific gel stains (Steinberg et al., 2003) have also been developed for 2D-PAGE to be used in conjunction with SYPRO ruby protein stain (Berggren et al., 2002), allowing detection of phosphoproteins and total expression in the same gel. Additionally, enzymatic dephosphorylation of the phosphopeptides with alkaline phosphatase was coupled with peptide mass mapping to determine the amino acid site of phosphorylation (Larsen et al., 2001).

An alternative method was developed independently by two different groups (Goshe et al., 2001; Oda et al., 2001), which involved the β-elimination of the phosphate moiety from phosphothreonine and phosphoserine residues, followed by Michael addition of 1,2-ethanedithiol (EDT), biotinylation, and separation on an avidin affinity column. This method did not prove ideal because of problems with isolating the peptides based on the biotin/avidin affinity. A modification of the Goshe et al. (2001) study was proposed by Qian et al. (2003). The method, referred to as phosphoprotein isotope-coded solid-phase tag (PhIST), varies from the previously reported phosphoprotein isotope-coded affinity tag (PhIAT) by reaction of the EDT thiolate moiety with either light (six ^{12}C and one ^{14}N) or heavy (six ^{13}C and one ^{15}N) leucine isotope-coded beads rather than a biotin affinity tag. The captured peptides are released from the beads by photocleavage of the linker from the solid support, resulting in transfer of the leucine isotope-coded linker to the EDT-modified peptides, thereby generating the PhIST peptides. The mass of serine and threonine residues is increased by 246.08 Da or 253.10 Da for the light and heavy tags, respectively. The improved method boasts approximately 80% recovery and requires considerably less protein ($<$100 μg) (Qian et al., 2003).

Another method for the detection and mapping of protein phosphorylation sites was recently reported (Knight et al., 2003). This method uses chemical modification of the site of phosphorylation to specifically target the site for proteolytic cleavage. Such a technique would result in hydrolysis of the amide bond adjacent to the site of phosphorylation, allowing detection of the site based on the cleavage of the peptide rather than the sequence itself, because the phosphoaminoacid would always be the carboxy-terminal amino acid. The method is specific for phosphoserine and phosphothreonine and relies on β-elimination of the phosphate group to produce dehydroalanine and β-methyl-dehydroalanine, respectively, followed by reaction via Michael addition with cysteamine to generate aminoethylcysteine and β-methylaminoethylcysteine.

Aminoethylcysteine is isosteric to lysine; therefore proteases that cleave with respect to lysine residues will cleave proteins at the aminoethylcysteine residue and, consequently, at the site of phosphorylation. Trypsin was found to cleave at the β-methylaminoethylcysteine residue less efficiently than at the aminoethylcysteine; however, the protease Lys-C was found to cleave both aminoethylcysteine and β-methylaminoethylcysteine efficiently (Knight *et al.*, 2003). This method provides an efficient and effective means of identifying the specific site of protein phosphorylation that is often a limitation of current techniques; nevertheless, this method does not provide quantitative information regarding differences in the extent of phosphorylation of a protein, with the exception of the number of phosphorylated residues, and would need to be coupled to techniques such as 2D-PAGE and autoradiography.

4. Membrane Proteins: High pH and Proteinase K

Membrane proteins have been difficult to study because of their low solubility in the buffers typically used in 2D-PAGE. A method using high pH and proteinase K (hpPK) was recently described for the study of both membrane and soluble proteins (Wu *et al.*, 2003). The high pH disrupts the membrane structures and favors the formation of membrane sheets, allowing for the cleavage of the hydrophilic domains of membrane proteins that are exposed by proteinase K without disrupting or solubilizing the lipid bilayer. These experimental conditions coupled with MudPIT allow for the cleavage and identification of integral membrane proteins (Wu *et al.*, 2003).

C. Mass Spectrometry

1. MALDI and ESI LC-MS

Once protein spots of particular interest have been detected, the protein must be eluted from the gel to undergo MS analysis. Most often the spot(s) corresponding to the protein(s) of particular interest are excised from the gel and undergo a series of manipulations and chemical modifications of the protein in order to facilitate the cleavage of the protein by a protease into several peptides. This procedure, more commonly referred to as in-gel digestion, has several advantages, including higher recovery, because the protein is cleaved into many smaller peptides that result from sequence-specific proteolysis, which is an important means of identifying the protein of interest. These smaller peptides constitute mass fingerprints that are characteristic of a particular protein, and the molecular weight of each peptide is determined by MS. Peptide mass fingerprinting, as the process is known, requires the use of MS analysis to determine the experimental masses. Database searching, in which the experimental masses are compared and matched to protein-specific mass fingerprints generated by the *in silico* "digestion" of proteins, is used to identify the protein of interest based on the quality of peptide matches (Aebersold and Goodlet, 2001).

Mass spectrometry is an invaluable tool for the identification and study of proteins without which proteomic analysis would be relatively unknown. Before the evolution of "softer" ionization techniques that prevent or lessen the extent of fragmentation of ions generated by polypeptides, proteins were identified by the use of specific antibodies, which requires a well-educated guess based on the knowledge of the molecular weight and *pI* of the protein of interest, or by Edman degradation and protein sequencing. These are both long and laborious processes, and Edman degradation also requires the use of database searching.

The two techniques most commonly used for MS analysis of proteins are matrix-assisted laser desorption ionization (MALDI) and electrospray ionization (ESI). MALDI requires the mixing of the analyte with a matrix (commonly α-cyano-4-hydroxycinnamic acid) and crystallization of the mixture on a plate that is subjected to a laser radiation. The matrix absorbs the energy from the laser and transfers the energy in the condensed phase to the analyte, generating a gas mixture in which the matrix carries the analyte. Ionization occurs in the gas phase between the matrix and the analyte, where bimolecular proton transfer, due to the acidic nature of the matrix, may occur by a mechanism that is not well described to transform peptides into detectable MH^+ ions. ESI, on the other hand, involves the transport of ions from solution to the gas phase rather than ionization. Typically ESI is interfaced with HPLC, in which the sample moves through the capillary inlet into a vacuum and the MS. This requires the application of a large potential difference applied between the capillary and the MS instrument inlet. The high voltage applied to the capillary overcomes surface tension and results in the formation of a Taylor cone, a hallmark of the ESI process, due to a charged pair deconvolution, in which cations get pushed away and anions are held back within the capillary. This process generates droplets with an electrical double layer and a net positive charge. In this state the solvent continues to evaporate from the droplet until the droplet reaches the Rayleigh limit, at which point the coulombic repulsion exceeds the surface tension of the droplet. This situation results in droplet fission and, ultimately, one ion per droplet. This process requires low salt concentration and can often generate multiply charged ions.

Additional information can be obtained about a particular peptide by the use of tandem MS/MS, which requires the use of ESI technology. Tandem MS/MS allows the isolation and fragmentation of a specific ion. The fragments undergo further MS analysis to generate information about the sequence of the peptide. The isolation of a single ion is accomplished by scanning all of the ions that were generated from a sample, followed by the application of a wide range of frequencies, except for the resonating frequency of the ion of interest. This allows for the ion of interest to be retained in the trap. The ion is then fragmented and analyzed to generate information about the sequence of the peptide aiding in identification and, possibly, information about modifications of the specific amino acids in the peptide (de Hoffmann, 1996; March, 1997).

2. SELDI-TOF

Surface-enhanced laser desorption ionization time-of-flight (SELDI-TOF) is a novel approach to proteomics that couples the classical methods of chromatographic sample preparation with MS analysis. The SELDI technique consists of a chip, which has been modified on the surface, either chemically or biochemically, in such a way as to optimize the isolation of a particular group of proteins. Chemical modifications include making the surface hydrophobic, hydrophilic, anionic, cationic, or metallic, while biochemical modifications take advantage of antibody-antigen, receptor-ligand, and DNA-protein interactions (Merchant and Weinberger, 2000). Advantages of SELDI-TOF technology include the potential to screen biomarkers from a variety of complex samples, including blood, urine, serum, plasma, etc., which are typically difficult to work with under 2D-PAGE conditions because of the high abundance of albumin and immunoglobulins. Additionally, SELDI has detection limits at the attomolar level and thus requires a small sample volume. SELDI can also be used to detect posttranslational modifications such as glycosylation and phosphorylation by screening for particular mass shifts in the protein peaks; however, the technology depends on a change in the expression profiles between samples and is limited because the technique cannot be used to specifically identify a protein that is differentially expressed. Consequently, isolation of the protein itself is required (Issaq *et al.*, 2002). Moreover, SELDI is limited to detection of proteins of relatively low molecular mass (Issaq *et al.*, 2002).

D. DATABASE SEARCHING

Informatics is the final, and perhaps, most critical stage of the protein identification process. Once the list of peptide masses has been generated by MS analysis, it is necessary to utilize various search algorithms of various available databases to compare and match the peptide masses with those of proteins in the database (Butterfield *et al.*, 2003). The search engines provide a theoretical digestion of the proteins contained within the database with which the peptide masses generated by MS can be compared. The search also takes into account a variety of factors, including protein size and the probability of a single peptide to occur within the database. The search engine provides a probability score for each entry based on the mathematical algorithms that are specific to the individual search engine used. The score corresponds to the probability the peptides match those of the theoretical digest of a particular protein contained in the database, and therefore the

TABLE I

TABLE OF MASS SPECTROMETRY DATABASES AND SEARCH ENGINES

Name	Address
MassSearch	http://cbrg.inf.ethz.ch
PeptideSearch	www.mann.embl-heidelberg.de
ExPASy	www.expasy.ch/tools
Mascot	www.matrixscience.com
MOWSE	www.hgmp.mrc.ac.uk/Bioinformatics/Webapp/mowse
SEQUEST	http://thompson.mbt.washington.edu/sequest
ProFound	www.prowl.rockefeller.edu/sgi-bin/profound
MS-Fit	http://prospector.ucsf.edu/ucsfhtml4.0/msfit.htm

correct identification of the protein. Any hit with a probability score corresponding to p<0.05, which can be set by the database, is generally considered to have a legitimate chance of being the protein cut from the gel, thereby allowing for the unambiguous identification of the protein of interest. Table I outlines some of the databases and search engines available online.

III. Proteomic Studies in AD

A. PROTEIN EXPRESSION ALTERATIONS

Proteomics is an invaluable resource for the investigation of neurodegenerative disease and offers the potential to identify protein and modifications of proteins involved in disease processes. As a result, proteomics offers the capabilities to identify biomarkers of disease and potential therapeutic targets. Expression proteomics, in particular, has enabled researchers to compare and contrast various conditions due to its ability to quickly and reproducibly map, screen, quantitate, and identify a vast number of proteins at once. Such principles have been used to detect specific alterations in the protein expression levels of various regions of the AD brain compared to control brain, which may in turn facilitate an explanation of the mechanisms by which the disease progresses.

Extensive protein expression analysis has been reported by Lubec and co-workers. Table II summarizes the results. This group and others have contributed to the identification of a number of protein expression alterations in the AD brain, which offer substantial speculation into the possible mechanisms underlying the pathogenesis of the disease.

In addition to the presence of neurofibrillary tangles and senile plaques, AD is associated with synapse loss, oxidative stress, altered glucose metabolism,

TABLE II
Protein Expression in AD Brain

Protein	Tissue	Expression alteration	Reference
Proapoptotic proteins			
ZIPK	Frontal cortex	Increase	Engidawork *et al.*, 2001c
BIM/BOD	Frontal cortex	Increase	
RICK	Frontal cortex	Increase	Engidawork *et al.*, 2001b
FLIP	Frontal cortex	Decrease	
	Cerebellum	Decrease	
Procaspase-3	Frontal cortex	Decrease	
	Cerebellum	Decrease	
Procaspase-8	Frontal cortex	Decrease	
	Cerebellum	Decrease	
Procaspase-9	Frontal cortex	Decrease	
GFAP	Frontal cortex	Increase	Greber *et al.*, 1999
	Temporal cortex	Increase	
	Parietal cortex	Increase	
	Occipital cortex	Increase	
Antiapoptotic proteins			
p21	Frontal cortex	Increase	Engidawork *et al.*, 2001c
Bcl-2	Cerebellum	Increase	
ARC	Frontal cortex	Increase	Engidawork *et al.*, 2001b
DFF45	Frontal cortex	Decrease	
	Cerebellum	Decrease	
Metabolic proteins			
VDAC *pI* 10.0	Frontal cortex	Decrease	Yoo *et al.*, 2001a
	Temporal cortex	Decrease	
	Occipital cortex	Decrease	
VDAC *pI* 7.5	Occipital cortex	Increase	
VDAC *pI* 7.5, 8.5, 10.0	Frontal cortex	Decrease	
	Thalamus	Decrease	
VDAC-2	Temporal cortex	Increase	
Complex I 24-kDa subunit	Temporal cortex	Decrease	Kim *et al.*, 2001d
	Occipital cortex	Decrease	
Complex I 75-kDa subunit	Parietal cortex	Decrease	
Antioxidant proteins			
CBR	Temporal cortex	Increase	Balcz *et al.*, 2001
	Parietal cortex	Increase	
	Caudate nucleus	Increase	
	Thalamus	Increase	
	Cerebellum	Increase	
ADH	Temporal cortex	Increase	
	Occipital cortex	Increase	
	Cerebellum	Increase	

(Continued)

TABLE II   (*Continued*)

Protein	Tissue	Expression alteration	Reference
Prx-I	Temporal cortex	Increase	Kim *et al.*, 2001b
	Occipital cortex	Increase	
	Thalamus	Increase	
Prx-II	Thalamus	Increase	
Prx-III	Occipital cortex	Decrease	
	Thalamus	Decrease	Kim *et al.*, 2001b
Synaptic proteins			
NDPK-A	Frontal cortex	Decrease	Kim *et al.*, 2002
	Parietal cortex	Decrease	
	Occipital cortex	Decrease	
CNPase	Frontal cortex	Decrease	Vlkolinský *et al.*, 2001
SNAP-25	Frontal cortex	Decrease	Greber *et al.*, 1999
	Temporal cortex	Decrease	
	Parietal cortex	Decrease	
	Occipital cortex	Decrease	
	Cerebellum	Decrease	
TCP-1	Frontal cortex	Decrease	Schuller *et al.*, 2001
	Temporal cortex	Decrease	
	Parietal cortex	Decrease	
	Thalamus	Decrease	
NF-L	Occipital cortex	Decrease	
DRP-2	Frontal cortex	Decrease	Lubec *et al.*, 1999
Drebrin	Frontal cortex	Decrease	Shim and Lubec, 2002
	Temporal cortex	Decrease	
Stathmin	Frontal cortex	Decrease	Cheon *et al.*, 2001
	Temporal cortex	Decrease	
α-Endosulfine	Frontal cortex	Decrease	Kim and Lubec, 2001
	Cerebellum	Decrease	
Neurotransmitter functions			
HRF			
	Temporal cortex	Decrease	Kim *et al.*, 2001a
	Caudate nucleus	Decrease	
45-kDa subunit nAChR	Thalamus	Decrease	
26-kDa subunit nACHR	Frontal cortex	Increase	Engidawork *et al.*, 2001a
α7 Subunit nACHR	Frontal cortex	Decrease	
PKA	Frontal cortex	Decrease	
	Temporal cortex	Decrease	Kim *et al.*, 2001c
Chaperone proteins			
HSP60	Parietal cortex	Decrease	Yoo *et al.*, 2001b
HSC71	Temporal cortex	Decrease	
GRP75	Temporal cortex	Decrease	
	Parietal cortex	Decrease	
Alpha crystalline B	Temporal cortex	Increase	
HSP70 RY	Caudate nucleus	Increase	
GRP94	Parietal cortex	Increase	

mitochondrial deficit, increased protein misfolding, and decreased protein turnover (Butterfield and Lauderback, 2002). The expression alterations observed in many proteins involved in a number of pathways help to develop testable hypotheses of neurodegenerative mechanisms in AD brain, as discussed in the following sections of this chapter.

1. *Altered Energy Metabolism*

The accumulation of glycolytic enzymes such as α- and γ-enolase and glyceraldehyde 3-phosphate dehydrogenase confirms the indication that glucose metabolism is affected in AD (Schonberger *et al.*, 2001). Additionally, the decrease in the expression of voltage-dependent anion-selective channel protein-1 (VDAC-1), which is responsible for the regulation of mitochondrial metabolism by manipulating the ion flux of metabolites such as adenosine triphosphate (ATP), supports this hypothesis (Yoo *et al.*, 2001a). Decreased expression of β-enolase, one of the subunits that compose the enzyme enolase, which catalyzes the reversible conversion of 2-phosphoglycerate to phosphoenolpyruvate in glycolysis, has also been reported. Moreover, a decrease in the precursor α- and β-subunits of mitochondrial ATP synthase has been reported (Tsuji *et al.*, 2002).

Decreased glucose metabolism is also associated with the decrease in expression of the 24- and 75-kDa subunits of the multiprotein enzyme complex NADH:ubiquinone oxidoreductase, more commonly known as complex I of the mitochondrial electron transport chain. This complex is located on the mitochondrial membrane and is responsible for the flow of electrons from NADH to ubiquinone in the initiating steps of oxidative phosphorylation to produce ATP (Kim *et al.*, 2001d). A decrease in complex I expression, consistent with altered message (Aksenov *et al.*, 1999), may result in impaired ATP production, as well as a decrease in the activity of the entire electron transport chain. This in turn may result in the departure of electrons from their carrier molecules to generate reactive oxygen species (ROS). ROS production caused by the decreased expression of complex I suggests an alternative rationalization for the well-documented existence of oxidative stress in AD (Butterfield and Lauderback, 2002; Kim *et al.*, 2001d). Additionally, a decrease in core protein 1 of ubiquinol-cyctochrome c oxidoreductase (complex III) has been reported. Complex III consists of nine polypeptides and catalyzes the transfer of electrons from ubiquinol to cytochrome c. A decrease in core protein 1 of complex III supports the proposed model of oxidative stress and, consequently, altered energy metabolism in AD (Kim *et al.*, 2000).

2. *Altered Antioxidant Expression*

An increase in the expression of several antioxidant proteins was also observed in AD brain, which agrees with the premise of oxidative stress in the pathogenesis of the disorder (Butterfield, 2002; Butterfield and Lauderback,

2002; Butterfield *et al.*, 2001, 2002). An increase in carbonyl reductase (CBR), alcohol dehydrogenase (ADH), peroxiredoxin-I (Prx-I), peroxiredoxin-II (Prx-II), antioxidant protein 2, and Cu/Zn superoxide dismutase was detected (Balcz *et al.*, 2001; Kim *et al.*, 2001b; Krapfenbauer *et al.*, 2003; Schonberger *et al.*, 2001). Moreover, a decrease in peroxiredoxin-III (Prx-III), metallothionein-1 (MT-1), and metallothionein-3 (MT-3) expression was found (Kim *et al.*, 2001b; Prange *et al.*, 2001). CBR and ADH are cytosolic enzymes that catalyze the reduction of carbonyls to their corresponding alcohols. Carbonyls are generally toxic metabolic intermediates that serve as a marker of oxidative stress (Butterfield and Stadtman, 1997). An elevation in the expression of the enzymes involved in the removal of these cytotoxic intermediates suggests an adaptive mechanism of up-regulation to counteract the accumulation of these species (Balcz *et al.*, 2001). Prx-I and Prx-II play an important antioxidant role in the protection of neurons from damage induced by hydrogen peroxide. The up-regulation of these enzymes is consistent with the role of oxidative stress in AD. However, Prx-III, found only in mitochondria, was decreased in AD brain. This could be a result of damage to the enzyme caused by ROS produced within the mitochondria (Kim *et al.*, 2001b). MT-1 and MT-3 are proteins with antioxidant function, with respect to the clearing of heavy metals. The reduced expression of these proteins is consistent with the notion that metals in AD brain may play a role in this disorder (Bush, 2003; Lovell *et al.*, 1998; Prange *et al.*, 2001).

3. *Altered Synaptic Function*

Synaptic dysfunction and alterations in neuronal growth in AD can be related to the decrease in nucleoside diphosphate kinase-A (NDPK-A), $2',3'$-cyclic nucleotide-$3'$-phosphodiesterase (CNPase), synaptosomal associated protein 25-kDa (SNAP-25), vesicular-fusion protein N-ethylmaleimide-sensitive factor (NSF), t-complex polypeptide 1 (TCP-1), stathmin, neurofilament protein-L (NF-L), drebrin, dihydropyrimidinase related protein-2 (DRP-2), and α-endosulfine. NDPK-A has been reported to be colocalized with microtubules and is believed to be involved in neuronal cell proliferation and neurite outgrowth (Kim *et al.*, 2002). CNPase is associated with oligodendrocytes and therefore myelination (Vlkolinský *et al.*, 2001). SNAP-25 is believed to play a role in neurotransmission via the exocytosis and docking of synaptic vesicles (Greber *et al.*, 1999). Vesicular-fusion protein NSF is associated with synaptic transmission and neuronal outgrowth (Schonberger *et al.*, 2001). TCP-1 is a protein complex involved in the folding of actin and various isoforms of tubulin (Schuller *et al.*, 2001), whereas stathmin is responsible for the integration of multiple signal-transduction cascades and the destabilization of microtubules (Cheon *et al.*, 2001). NF-L is a protein implicated in maintaining the integrity of the neuronal cytoskeleton (Bajo *et al.*, 2001). Drebrin is a dendritic spine protein that modulates synaptic plasticity (Kim and Lubec, 2001). DRP-2 is a pathfinding protein associated with axonal outgrowth and guidance (Castegna *et al.*, 2002b; Lubec *et al.*, 1999; Schonberger *et al.*, 2001; Tsuji *et al.*, 2002). α-Endosulfine is an endogenous regulator of ATP-sensitive potassium channels (Kim and Lubec, 2001). All of the aforementioned differences in expression alterations reported in AD could result in the loss of synaptic function and neuronal communication, cognitive decline, and neuronal death.

4. *Neurotransmitter and Receptor Dysfunction*

Cognitive decline is associated with neurotransmitter imbalance and neuronal death, both of which can be conceivably explained by changes in protein expression levels. Histamine-releasing factor (HRF), which regulates the release of the neurotransmitter histamine, is expressed ubiquitously throughout the brain. The decrease in HRF expression may be associated with cognitive decline, indicating that histamine plays a role in whole-brain function (Kim *et al.*, 2001a). The α7 and 26-kDa truncated isoform of the α3 subunit of nicotinic acetylcholine receptors (nAchRs) were significantly reduced in AD brain, suggesting the decreased expression may influence the function of cholinergic neurons, which are the most affected neurons in AD (Engidawork *et al.*, 2001a). Interaction of Aβ(1-42) with the α7 nAchR, which regulates acetylcholine release and calcium homeostasis, is reported. Aβ(1-42) binds to the α7 nAchR with high affinity, and the complex is endocytosed, resulting in intraneuronal accumulation of Aβ (Nagele *et al.*, 2002). Consequently, Aβ exhibits an inhibitory effect on α7 nAchR, resulting in altered release of acetylcholine and therefore memory and learning deficits (Tozaki *et al.*, 2002). Alternatively, the 45-kDa α3 subunit was increased. The expression of the α3 nAchR subunit is normally down-regulated by cyclic adenosine monophosphate (cAMP) via protein kinase A (PKA). The decreased basal level of cAMP and PKA (Kim *et al.*, 2001c) in AD brain likely results in dysregulation in which the expression of the α3 subunit goes unchecked and therefore increases (Engidawork *et al.*, 2001a).

5. *Apoptotic and Antiapoptotic Regulation*

Apoptosis may play a role in the neuronal loss exhibited in AD. The pro-apoptotic proteins zipper-interacting protein kinase (ZIPK), Bcl-2-interacting mediator of cell death/Bcl-2 related ovarian death gene (Bim/BOD), and the receptor interacting protein (RIP)-like interacting CLARP kinase (RICK) were found to be increased in AD brain, whereas the antiapoptotic protein p21 is up-regulated in response to oxidative stress (Engidawork *et al.*, 2001c). Protein p21 is believed to involve the inhibition of the MAPK/JNK pathway, which has been shown to be activated in AD brain and by Aβ peptide *in vitro* (Morishima *et al.*, 2001). The antiapoptotic protein Bcl-2 is up-regulated only in the cerebellum of AD brain, suggesting a possible mechanism by which this area of the brain is less affected in AD (Engidawork *et al.*, 2001c; Hensley *et al.*, 1995). Likewise the apoptosis repressor with caspase recruitment domain (ARC) was also up-regulated as an antiapoptotic mechanism in response to apoptotic signals such as Aβ-peptide (Engidawork *et al.*, 2001b). Conversely, the Fas-associated death domain (FADD)-like interleukin-1β-converting enzyme inhibitory protein (FLIP) was decreased because it is a substrate for caspases and forms an inactivating complex with caspase-8. Additionally, the antiapoptotic protein DNA fragmentation factor 45 is decreased due to degradation by caspase-3. The down-regulation of FLIP and DFF45 also provides supporting evidence for the activation of caspases as well as the down-regulation of procaspase-3, procaspase-8, and procaspase-9 (Engidawork *et al.*, 2001b). Additionally, the activation of capspase-3 in the limbic cortex has been shown to be an early event in the pathogenesis of AD (Gastard *et al.*, 2003). Finally, glial fibrillary acidic protein (GFAP), a marker of glia, was elevated in AD brain, supporting the hypothesis of neuronal cell death (Greber *et al.*, 1999; Tsuji *et al.*, 1999, 2002).

6. Chaperone Proteins

AD is associated with protein misfolding and decreased protein turnover. Stress or chaperone proteins are thought to play an important role in protecting cells by accelerating protein degradation and preventing the binding of aggregated proteins to hydrophobic surfaces (Anthony *et al.*, 2003). The protein misfolding and decreased protein turnover associated with AD can be related to the dysregulation, and possibly dysfunction, of these molecular chaperone, or stress, proteins in AD brain. Heat shock protein 60 (HSP60), heat shock conjugate 71 (HSC71), glucose-regulated protein 75 (GRP75), and alpha crystalline B have all been reported to be down-regulated in AD. Conversely, heat shock protein 70 RY (HSP70 RY) and glucose regulated protein 94 (GRP94) are up-regulated (Yoo *et al.*, 2001b). Down-regulation of HSP60 (resident in mitochondria) conceivably could be related to elevated oxidative stress, as already noted.

7. Plasma and CSF Studies

For AD reseach using proteomics, brain is not the only tissue that has been examined to elicit protein expression changes. Blood plasma samples have been examined for apolipoprotein E (ApoE), tau, and presenillin-2 in order to develop a less invasive screening process for AD using immunodetection (Ueno *et al.*, 2000). Cerebrospinal fluid (CSF) has also been used to determine differences between control and AD patients (Davidsson *et al.*, 2002). Several significant protein expression changes were determined in this study, including a decrease in the isoforms of ApoE and proapolipoprotein, suggesting that there may be a decrease in these levels in the brain as well (Davidsson *et al.*, 2002). An additional study detected nine proteins that were differentially expressed in AD CSF versus control, although these biomarkers have yet to be identified (Choe *et al.*, 2002).

8. SELDI and AD Studies

SELDI has been used as a nontraditional method of proteomics study in AD. For example, SELDI has been used to demonstrate that PS1 plays a role, either directly or indirectly, in the production of Aβ as either γ-secretase itself or in the function of γ-secretase, respectively (Chen et al., 2000). Also, SELDI studies have shown that BACE1 is the primary neuronal β-secretase (Cai et al., 2001), and that an increase in intracellular cholesterol in cells transfected with APP increased the production of Aβ(1-42) (Austen et al., 2000). Likewise, SELDI technology has shown that in the presence of γ-secretase inhibitors, truncated amyloid β-peptides are not produced for the C99 fragment that results from the cleavage of APP by β-secretase. Additionally, increased cleavage of the membrane-bound C99 fragment by α-secretase was detected (Beher et al., 2002). Additionally, it has been shown that Aβ(1-40) and Aβ(1-42) are deposited in the lens in AD, resulting in increased protein aggregation and supranuclear cataract formation (Goldstein et al., 2003). A SELDI analysis of CSF detected five proteins that were differentially expressed in AD, including cystatin c, two β-2-microglobulin isoforms, a nerve growth factor (VGF polypeptide), and a 7.69 kDa polypeptide, which was not identified (Carrette et al., 2003). SELDI has also been used to study the variants of Aβ-peptide present in CSF and brain homogenates of AD versus control. A peptide with a molecular mass corresponding to Aβ(1-45) or Aβ(2-46) was observed only in AD CSF. Additionally, in the AD CSF the ratio of Aβ(1-38) to total Aβ was increased. Several variants of Aβ peptide were present in AD brain but not in control, including Aβ(1-29), Aβ(2-33), Aβ(1-40), Aβ(1-42), Aβ(2-46) or Aβ(1-45), Aβ(8-42), Aβ(7-42), Aβ(6-42), Aβ(5-42), Aβ(4-42), and Aβ(2-42). The molecular mass of Aβ(3-42) is very similar to that of Aβ(1-40) and therefore could not be differentiated (Lewczuk et al., 2003).

It is important to note that the expression changes detected in AD do not provide information regarding the integrity of the function of the proteins themselves, and that these changes are not global but correspond to specific brain regions. Consequently, protein expression changes provide only a clue as to the altered state of the protein that the disease causes. More research is required to determine if these proteins are modified in some way, which would result in loss of function (i.e., oxidation). For example, up-regulation of antioxidant proteins such as CBR, ADH, Prx-I, Prx-II, antioxidant protein 2, and Cu/Zn superoxide dismutase, may be a compensatory action; however, if the proteins do not function properly, the up-regulation is all for naught. Additionally, increased expression may be caused by decreased protein turnover, which has been implicated in AD. Nevertheless, this proteomics work has validated the association of altered energy metabolism, decreased synaptic function, and oxidative stress in AD; however, this work has provided only the beginning from which researchers can, in future studies, determine how these individual alterations affect the brain and lead to cognitive decline in AD.

B. OXIDATIVELY MODIFIED PROTEINS IN AD

Extensive protein oxidation is evident in AD, as indexed by protein carbonyls and 3-nitroyrosine (Butterfield and Lauderback, 2002; Butterfield et al., 2001, 2002; Castegna et al., 2003; Good et al., 1996; Smith et al., 1997). However, the detection of markers of oxidative stress offers little insight into the proteins that are specifically oxidatively modified and, subsequently, the cellular mechanisms and pathways that are affected. Identification of proteins specifically oxidized in AD brain allows for the determination of proteins that are more susceptible to oxidation and, consequently, more prone to inactivation and loss of function (Table III). Our initial attempts along this area of research identified creatine kinase BB and β-actin as oxidized proteins in AD by coupling immunochemical quantitation of carbonyl reactivity with immunochemical detection on the protein on 2D gels (Aksenov et al., 2000, 2001). This process is time-consuming, laborious, and requires a good educated guess as to the identity of the protein based on pI and molecular weight. This method also ultimately depends on the availability of specific antibodies. Consequently, our laboratory has turned to the techniques of proteomics to provide a method of screening oxidized proteins in AD brain (Butterfield, 2004; Butterfield and Castegna, 2003a,b,c; Butterfield et al., 2003; Castegna et al., 2002a,b, 2003).

The first proteomics analysis to detect specifically oxidized proteins in AD brain (short PMI of <4 hr) led to the identification of five proteins, including: creatine kinase BB (CK), glutamine synthase (GS), ubiquitin carboxy-terminal hydrolyze L-1 (UCH L-1), α-enolase, and DRP-2 (Castegna et al., 2002a,b). These techniques have recently been modified to detect proteins that are

TABLE III
OXIDATIVELY MODIFIED PROTEINS IN AD BRAIN

Biochemical alteration in AD	Protein
Energy metabolism	Creatine kinase BB
	α-Enolase
	Triosephospate isomerase
Glutamate uptake and excitotoxicity	Glutamine synthetase
Proteasomal dysfunction	Ubiquitin carboxy-terminal hydrolyze L-1
Membrane structure/cholinergic function	Neuropolypeptide H3
Neuritic abnormalities	Dihydropyrimidinase-related protein-2

specifically modified by 3-NT. Three proteins were found to be specifically nitrated in AD—neuropolypeptide H3, triosephosphate isomerase, and α-enolase (Castegna et al., 2003). These oxidatively modified proteins vary across a wide range of classes of proteins, including those dealing with energy metabolism, excitotoxicity, proteosomal function, membrane structure, apoptosis, and neuronal communication (Butterfield, 2004; Butterfield et al., 2003). Based on the principle that oxidative modification affects protein function, as has been demonstrated with respect to the glutamate transporter EAAT2 (Lauderback et al., 2001), CK, and GS (Hensley et al., 1995), a number of plausible mechanisms of neurodegeneration can be proposed based on each of the oxidized proteins.

1. Energy Metabolism

Either directly or indirectly, creatine kinase BB, α-enolase, and triosephosphate isomerase are all involved in the synthesis of ATP. CK activity is severely compromised in AD brain (Hensley et al., 1995). Thus oxidation of CK leads to loss of its function, which would suggest that ATP synthesis is severely affected in AD. Such alterations in energy metabolism and ATP production are consistent with positron-emission tomographic (PET) scanning studies of AD patients (Blass and Gibson, 1991; Scheltens and Korf, 2000) and with the altered accumulation of glycolytic enzymes in AD, such as α-enolase, γ-enolase, and glyceraldehyde 3-phosphate dehydrogenase (Schonberger et al., 2001). Likewise, the expression of CK was also found to be altered in AD brain (Schonberger et al., 2001). Lack of ATP would consequently lead to dysfunction in ion pumps, electrochemical gradients, voltage-gated ion channels, and cell potential.

2. Glutamate Uptake and Excitotoxicity

It has been previously reported that $A\beta(1\text{-}42)$ leads to the production of the lipid peroxidation product, 4-hydroxy-2-nonenal (HNE) (Mark et al., 1997). Additionally, $A\beta(1\text{-}42)$ has been shown to induce oxidative modification of the glutamate transporter EAAT2 by HNE in synaptosomal preparations (Lauderback et al., 2001). Likewise, EAAT2 is oxidatively modified by HNE in AD brain (Lauderback et al., 2001). HNE has been shown to induce protein conformational changes that could lead to loss of protein function (Subramaniam et al., 1997). Therefore it has been proposed that the loss of activity of EAAT2 in AD (Masliah et al., 1995) is due to oxidative modification by HNE (Lauderback et al., 2001). Likewise, it is likely that oxidative modification of GS explains the loss of activity of GS reported in AD (Hensley et al., 1995). Loss of function of these proteins would result in a decreased conversion or uptake of glutamate, resulting in accumulation of extracellular glutamate. The excess glutamate would stimulate N-methyl-D-aspartate (NMDA) receptors, leading to an increase in Ca^{2+} influx. Altered calcium homeostasis would lead to alteration in long-term potentiation (LTP) and, consequently, learning and memory, mitochondrial swelling with consequent ROS leakage and release of proapoptotic cytochrome c, stress in the endoplasmic reticulum, as well as activation of calcium-sensitive proteases such as calpain. Clearly such changes would lead to neuronal death and may be important in AD.

3. Proteasomal Dysfunction

Proteasomal dysfunction has been reported in AD (Keller *et al.*, 2000) and leads to a buildup of damaged, misfolded, and aggregated proteins (Shringarpure *et al.*, 2001). Protein oxidation typically results in protein cross-linking and aggregation (Butterfield and Stadtman, 1997). Such aggregated proteins could "clog" the pore of the proteasome, leading to a compromise in proteasomal function. Loss of activity of UCH L-1, which was found to be oxidized in AD (Castegna *et al.*, 2002a), would lead to excess protein ubiquitination, loss of activity of the proteasome, and accumulation of damaged or aggregated proteins, all of which are found in AD.

4. Membrane Structure and Cholinergic Dysfunction

Neuropolypeptide h3 has been identified as specifically nitrated in AD (Castegna *et al.*, 2003). Neuropolypeptide h3 has a variety of names and functions, two of which are phosphatidylethanolamine-binding protein (PEBP) and hippocampal cholinergic neurostimulating peptide (HCNP). It is possible that loss of function of PEBP could lead to loss of phospholipid asymmetry, resulting in the exposure of phosphatidylserine on the outer leaflet of the lipid bilayer, a signal of apoptosis. Among the functions of HCNP is *in vitro* up-regulation of the production of choline acetyltransferase in cholinergic neurons following NMDA receptor activation (Ojika *et al.*, 1998). Choline acetyltransferase activity is known to be decreased in AD (Rossor *et al.*, 1982), and cholinergic deficits are prominent in AD brain (Giacobini, 2003; Katzman and Saitoh, 1991). Nitration of neuropolypeptide h3 may help to explain the decline in cognitive function caused by lack of neurotrophic action on cholinergic neurons of the hippocampus and basal forebrain.

5. Neuritic Abnormalities

DRP-2 has been shown to be decreased (Lubec *et al.*, 1999; Schonberger *et al.*, 2001; Tsuji *et al.*, 2002) and is oxidatively modified in AD brain (Castegna *et al.*, 2002b). DRP-2 is a pathfinding and guidance protein for axonal outgrowth. Additionally, DRP-2 interacts with and modulates collapsin, a protein responsible for the elongation and guidance of dendrites. Consequently, DRP-2 plays an important role in forming neuronal connections and maintaining neuronal communication. The oxidation and impaired activity of DRP-2 could result in the known shortened dendritic lengths in AD brain (Coleman and Flood, 1987). Neurons with shortened neurites would not be expected to communicate well with adjacent neurons, a process that could conceivably contribute to memory and cognitive loss in AD.

6. Oxidized Proteins in AD Plasma

Recently, similar proteomics techniques have been applied to identify specifically oxidized proteins in AD plasma. Isoforms of γ-chain precursor protein and α-1-antitrypsin precursor were identified, both of which have previously been implicated in the disease process (Choi et al., 2003).

IV. Proteomics Analysis of Transgenic Models of AD

Application of proteomics to transgenic models of AD is an increasing field of research in AD. Such approaches allow methods of testing the effects of genetic mutations associated with AD on specific proteins at both the expression and post-translational modification levels. Additionally, transgenic knock-in and knock-out mice allow for the study of the effect of inactivation of specific proteins, which have been found to be oxidized in AD brain. For example, the gracile axonal dystrophy (GAD) mouse model allows for the study of the consequences of the inactivation of UCH L-1 in the brain, which was found to be oxidized in AD brain (Castegna et al., 2002a, 2004). Loss of function of UCH L-1 led to specifically oxidized proteins in brain as identified by proteomics (Castegna et al., 2004).

MudPIT techniques were combined with a hydrazide biotin-streptavidin isolation of carbonylated proteins to identify oxidized proteins in aged mice (Soreghan et al., 2003a). These techniques have recently been applied to the study of the PS1/APP transgenic mouse model, which develops both the amyloid and tau pathologies of AD (Soreghan et al., 2003b). Several membrane proteins were identified in both models; however, this technique is not quantitative. Therefore no information was generated with regard to the extent of carbonylation of the individual proteins.

Studies by Tilleman et al. (2002a,b) have led to the identification of 51 proteins differentially expressed in glycogen synthase-3β (GSK-3β) mutant mice compared to control. GSK-3β is believed to play a role as a tau kinase, resulting in hyperphoshorylation of tau and, consequently, the formation of paired helical filaments and, ultimately, neurofibrillary tangles. Cytoskeletal proteins were identified as well as those involved in energy metabolism, vesicle transport, protein folding, signal transduction, amino acid synthesis, and detoxification (Tilleman, 2002a). Likewise, studies of a mutant mouse model expressing human tau have resulted in the identification of 34 differentially expressed proteins (Tilleman, 2002b). The proteins implicated were involved in similar processes as those described in the GSK-3β study. Taken together, four proteins were differentially regulated between the two models. These include α-enolase, D-3-phosphoglycerate dehydrogenase, NADH:ubiquinone oxidoreductase, and nucleoside diphosphate kinase, almost all of which have been described as having altered expression in AD (Kim *et al.*, 2001d, 2002; Schonberger *et al.*, 2001).

V. Future of Proteomics in AD

In summary, a number of proteins are oxidatively modified in AD brain. Likewise, the expression of many proteins is altered in the AD brain, resulting in a cascade of potential alterations of multiple pathways within the brain. Perhaps it is the relationship between these pathways that maintains the careful balance between neuronal survival and neuronal death. To date, proteomics has shed light on only a small portion of the puzzle; however, with improved techniques that allow for increased solubilization and loading of membrane-bound proteins and very basic proteins, along with better detection limits, more information will become available on the pathogenesis of AD.

Acknowledgments

This work was supported in part by grants from the National Institutes of Health (AG-05119; AG-10836).

References

Aebersold, R., and Goodlett, D. R. (2001). Mass spectrometry in proteomics. *Chem. Rev.* **101,** 269–295.

Aksenov, M. Y., Aksenova, M. V., Butterfield, D. A., and Markesbery, W. R. (2000). Oxidative modification of creatine kinase BB in Alzheimer's disease brain. *J. Neurochem.* **74,** 2520–2527.

Aksenov, M. Y., Aksenova, M. V., Butterfield, D. A., Geddes, J. W., and Markesbery, W. R. (2001). Protein oxidation in the brain in Alzheimer's disease. *Neuroscience* **103,** 373–383.

Aksenov, M. Y., Tucker, H. M., Nair, P., Askenova, M. V., Butterfield, D. A., Estus, S., and Markesbery, W. R. (1999). The expression of several mitochondrial and nuclear genes encoding the subunits of electron transport chain enzyme complexes, cytochrome c oxidase, and NADH dehydrogenase in different brain regions in Alzheimer's disease brain. *Neurochem. Res.* **24,** 767–774.

Anthony, S. G., Schipper, H. M., Tavares, R., Hovanesian, V., Cortez, S. C., Stopa, E. G., and Johanson, C. E. (2003). Stress protein expression in the Alzheimer-diseased choroid plexus. *J. Alzheimer's Dis.* **5,** 171–177.

Austen, B. M., Frears, E. R., and Davies, H. (2000). The use of Seldi ProteinChip arrays to monitor production of Alzheimer's β-amyloid in transfected cells. *J. Peptide Sci.* **6,** 459–469.

Bajo, M., Yoo, B. C., Cairns, N., Gratzer, M., and Lubec, G. (2001). Neurofilament proteins NF-L, NF-M, and NF-H in brain of patients with Down syndrome and Alzheimer's disease. *Amino Acids* **21,** 293–301.

Balcz, B., Kirchner, L., Cairns, N., Fountoulakis, M., and Lubec, G. (2001). Increased brain protein levels of carbonyl reductase and alcohol dehydrogenase in Down syndrome and Alzheimer's disease. *J. Neural. Transm.* **61**(Suppl.), 193–201.

Beher, D., Wrigley, J. D., Owens, A. P., and Shearman, M. S. (2002). Generation of C-terminally truncated amyloid β-peptides is dependent on γ-secretase activity. *J. Neurochem.* **82,** 563–575.

Berggren, K. N., Schulenberg, B., Lopez, M. F., Steinberg, T. H., Bogdanova, A., Smejkal, G., Wang, A., and Patton, W. F. (2002). An improved formulation of SYPRO ruby protein gel stain: Comparison with the original formulation and with a ruthenium II tris (bathophenanthroline disulfonate) formulation. *Proteomics* **2,** 486–498.

Blass, J. P., and Gibson, G. E. (1991). The role of oxidative abnormalities in the pathophysiology of Alzheimer's disease. *Rev. Neurol.* **147,** 513–525.

Bush, A. I. (2003). The metallobiology of Alzheimer's disease. *Trends Neurosci.* **26,** 207–214.

Butterfield, D. A. (2002). Amyloid beta-peptide (1-42)-induced oxidative stress and neurotoxicity: Implications for neurodegeneration in Alzheimer's disease brain. *Free Radic. Res.* **36,** 1307–1313.

Butterfield, D. A. (2003). Amyloid beta-peptide [1-42]-associated free radical-induced oxidative stress and neurodegeneration in Alzheimer's disease brain: Mechanisms and consequences. *Curr. Med. Chem.* **10,** 2651–2659.

Butterfield, D. A. (2004). Proteomics: A new approach to investigate oxidative stress in Alzheimer's disease brain. *Brain Research* **1000,** 1–7.

Butterfield, D. A., and Castegna, A. (2003a). Proteomic analysis of oxidatively modified proteins in Alzheimer's disease brain: Insights into neurodegeneration. *Cell Mol. Biol.* **49,** 747–751.

Butterfield, D. A., and Castegna, A. (2003b). Proteomics for the identification of specifically oxidized proteins in brain: Technology and application to the study of neurodegenerative disorders. *Amino Acids* **25,** 419–425.

Butterfield, D. A., and Castegna, A. (2003c). Energy metabolism in Alzheimer's disease brain: Insights from proteomics. *Appl. Proteomics Genomics* **2,** 67–70.

Butterfield, D. A., and Lauderback, C. M. (2002). Lipid peroxidation and protein oxidation in Alzheimer's disease brain: Potential causes and consequences involving amyloid beta-peptide-associated free radical oxidative stress. *Free Rad. Biol. Med.* **32,** 1050–1060.

Butterfield, D. A., and Stadtman, E. R. (1997). Protein oxidation processes in aging brain. *Adv. Cell. Aging Gerontol.* **2,** 161–191.

Butterfield, D. A., Castegna, A., Lauderback, C. M., and Drake, J. (2002). Evidence that amyloid beta-peptide-induced lipid peroxidation and its sequelae in Alzheimer's disease brain contribute to neuronal death. *Neurobiol. Aging* **23,** 655–664.

Butterfield, D. A., Drake, J., Porcernich, C., and Castegna, A. (2001). Evidence of oxidative damage in Alzheimer's disease brain: Central role for amyloid beta-peptide. *Trends Mol. Med.* **7,** 548–554.

Butterfield, D. A., Boyd-Kimball, D., and Castegna, A. (2003). Proteomics in Alzheimer's disease: Insights into potential mechanisms of neurodegeneration. *J. Neurochem.* **86,** 1313–1327.

Cai, H., Wang, Y., McCarthy, D., Wen, H., Borchett, D. R., Price, D. L., and Wong, P. C. (2001). BACE1 is the major β-secretase for generation of Aβ peptides by neurons. *Nat. Neurosci.* **4,** 233–234.

Carrette, O., Demalte, I., Scherl, A., Yalkinoglu, O., Corthals, G., Burkhard, P., Hochstrasser, D. F., and Sanchez, J. C. (2003). A panel of cerebrospinal fluid potential biomarkers for the diagnosis of Alzeimer's disease. *Proteomics* **3,** 1486–1494.

Castegna, A., Aksenov, M., Aksenova, M., Thongboonkerd, V., Klein, J. B., Pierce, W. M., Booze, R., Markesbery, W. R., and Butterfield, D. A. (2002a). Proteomic identification of oxidatively modified proteins in Alzheimer's disease brain. I. Creatine kinase BB, glutamine synthetase, and ubiquitin carboxy-terminal hydrolase L-1. *Free Rad. Biol. Med.* **33,** 562–571.

Castegna, A., Aksenov, M., Thongboonkerd, V., Klein, J. B., Pierce, W. M., Booze, R., Markesbery, W. R., and Butterfield, D. A. (2002b). Proteomics identification of oxidatively modified proteins in Alzheimer's disease brain. II. Dihydropyrimidinase related protein II, α-enolase, and heat schock cagnate 71. *J. Neurochem.* **82,** 1524–1532.

Castegna, A., Thongboonkerd, V., Klein, J. B., Lynn, B., Markesbery, W. R., and Butterfield, D. A. (2003). Proteomic identification of nitrated proteins in Alzheimer's disease brain. *J. Neurochem.* **85,** 1394–1401.

Castegna, A., Thongboonkerd, V., Klein, J., Lynn, B. C., Wang, Y. L., Osaka, H., Wada, K., and Butterfield, D. A. (2004). Proteomic analysis of brain proteins in the gracile axonal dystrophy (gad) mouse, a syndrome that emanates from dysfunctional ubiquitin carboxyl terminal hydrolase L-1, reveals oxidation of key proteins. *J. Neurochem.* **88,** 1540–1546.

Chen, F., Yang, D. S., Petanceska, S., Yang, A., Tandon, A., Yu, G., Rozmahel, R., Ghiso, J., Nishimura, M., Zhang, D. M., Kawarai, T., Leveeque, G., Mills, J., Levesque, L., Song, Y. Q., Rogaeva, E., Wastaway, D., Mount, H., Gandy, S., St. George-Hyslop, P., and Fraser, P. E. (2000). Carboxy-terminal fragments of Alzheimer's β-amyloid precursor protein accumulate in restricted and unpredicted intracellular compartments in presenillin 1-deficient cells. *J. Biol. Chem.* **275,** 36794–36802.

Cheon, M. S., Fountoulakis, M., Cairns, N., Dierssen, M., Herkner, K., and Lubec, G. (2001). Decreased protein levels of stathmin in adult brains with Down syndrome and Alzheimer's disease. *J. Neural. Transm.* **61**(Suppl.), 281–288.

Choe, L. H., Dutt, M. J., Relkin, N., and Lee, K. H. (2002). Studies of potential cerebrospinal fluid molecular markers for Alzheimer's disease. *Electrophoresis* **23,** 2247–2251.

Choi, J., Malakowsky, C. A., Talent, J. M, Conrad, C. C., Carrll, C. A., Weintraub, S. T., and Gracy, R. W. (2003). Antiapoptotic proteins are oxidized by Aβγ5–35 in Alzheimer's fibroblasts. *Biochim. Biophys. Acta* **1637,** 135–141.

Coleman, P. D., and Flood, D. G. (1987). Neuron numbers and dendritic extent in normal aging and Alzheimer's disease. *Neurobiol. Aging* **8,** 521–545.

Davidsson, P., Westman-Brinkmalm, A., Nilsson, C. L., Lindbjer, M., Paulson, L., Andreasen, N., Sjogren, M., and Blennow, K. (2002). Proteome analysis of cerebrospinal fluid proteins in Alzheimer patients. *Clin. Neurosci. Neuropathol.* **13,** 611–615.

De Hoffmann, E. (1996). Tandem mass spectrometry: A primer. *J. Mass Spectrom.* **31,** 129–137.

Engidawork, E., Gulesserian, T., Balic, N., Cairns, N., and Lubec, G. (2001a). Changes in nicotinic acetylcholine receptor subunits expression in brain of patients with Down syndrome and Alzheimer's disease. *J. Neural. Transm.* **61**(Suppl.), 211–222.

Engidawork, E., Gulesserian, T., Yoo, B. C., Cairns, N., and Lubec, G. (2001b). Alteration of caspases and apoptosis-related proteins in brains of patients with Alzheimer's disease. *Biochem. Biophys. Res. Commun.* **281,** 84–93.

Engidawork, E., Gulesserian, T., Seidl, R., Cairns, N., and Lubec, G. (2001c). Expression of apoptosis-related proteins in brains of patients with Alzheimer's disease. *Neurosci. Lett.* **303,** 79–82.

Ferguson, P. L., and Smith, R. D. (2003). Proteome analysis by mass spectrometry. *Annu. Rev. Biophys. Biomol. Struct.* **32,** 399–424.

Friso, G., and Wikstrom, L. (1999). Analysis of proteins from membrane-enriched cerebellar preparations by two-dimensional gel electrophoresis and mass spectrometry. *Electrophoresis* **20,** 917–927.

Gastard, M. C., Troncoso, J. C., and Koliasos, V. E. (2003). Caspase activation in the limbic cortex of subjects with early Alzheimer's disease. *Ann Neurol.* **54,** 393–398.

Gauss, C., Kalkum, M., Lowe, M., Lehrach, H., and Klose, J. (1999). Analysis of the mouse proteome. I. Brain proteins: Separation by two-dimensional electrophoresis and identification by mass spectrometry and genetic varation. *Electrophoresis* **20,** 575–600.

Giacobini, E. (2003). Cholinergic function and Alzheimer's disease. *Int. J. Geriatr. Psychiatr.* **18,** S1–S5.

Goldstein, L. E., Muffat, J. A., Chemy, R. A., Moir, R. D., Ericsson, M. H., Huang, X., Mavros, C., Coccia, J. A., Faget, K. Y., Fitch, K. A., Masters, C. L., Tanzi, R. E., Chylack, L. T., Jr., and Bush, A. I. (2003). Cytosolic β-amyloid deposition and supranuclear cataracts in lenses from people with Alzheimer's disease. *Lancet* **361,** 1258–1265.

Good, P. F., Werner, P., Hsu, A., Olanow, C., and Perl, D. P. (1996). Evidence for neuronal oxidative damage in Alzheimer's disease. *Am. J. Pathol.* **149,** 21–27.

Goshe, M. B., Conrads, T. P., Panisko, E. A., Angell, N. H., Veenstra, T. D., and Smith, R. D. (2001). Phosphoprotein isotope-coded affinity tag approach for isolating and quantitating phosphopeptides in proteome-wide analyses. *Anal. Chem.* **73,** 2578–2586.

Greber, S., Lubec, G., Cairns, N., and Fountoulakis, M. (1999). Decreased levels of synaptosomal associated protein 25 in the brain of patients with Down syndrome and Alzheimer's disease. *Electrophoresis* **20,** 928–934.

Gygi, S. P., Rist, B., Gerber, S. A., Tureck, F., Gelb, M. H., and Aebersold, R. (1999). Quantitative analysis of complex protein mixtures using isotope-coded affinity tags. *Nat. Biotechnol.* **17,** 994–999.

Hensley, K., Hall, N., Subramaniam, R., Cole, P., Harris, M., Aksenov, M., Aksenova, M., Gabbita, P., Wu, J. F., Carney, J. M., Lovell, M., Markesbery, W. R., and Butterfield, D. A. (1995). Brain regional correspondence between Alzheimer's disease histopathology and biomarkers of protein oxidation. *J. Neurochem.* **65,** 2146–2156.

Herbert, B. (1999). Advances in protein solubilization for two-dimensional gel electrophoresis. *Electrophoresis* **20,** 660–663.

Herbert, B. R., Molloy, M. P., Gooley, A. A., Walsh, B. J., Bryson, W. G., and Williams, K. L. (1998). Improved protein solubility in two-dimensional electrophoresis using tributyl phosphine as reducing agent. *Electrophoresis* **19,** 845–851.

Hoving, S., Gerrits, B., Voshol, H., Muller, D., Roberts, R. C., and Oostrum, J. V. (2002). Preparative two-dimensional gel electrophoresis at alkaline pH using narrow range immobilized pH gradients. *Proteomics* **2,** 127–134.

Issaq, H. J., Conrads, T. P., Janini, G. M., and Veenstra, T. D. (2002a). Methods for fractionation, separation, and profiling of proteins and peptides. *Electrophoresis* **23,** 3048–3061.

Issaq, H. J., Veenstra, T. D., Conrads, T. P., and Felschow, D. (2002b). The SELDI-TOF MS approach to proteomics: Protein profiling and biomarker identification. *Biochem. Biophys. Res. Commun.* **292,** 587–592.

Katzman, R., and Saitoh, T. (1991). Advances in Alzheimer's disease. *FASEB J.* **5,** 278–286.

Keller, J. N., Hanni, K. B., and Markesbery, W. M. (2000). Impaired proteasome function in Alzheimer's disease. *J. Neurochem.* **75,** 436–439.

Kim, S. H., and Lubec, G. (2001). Brain α-endosulfine is manifold decreased in brains from patients with Alzheimer's disease: A tentative marker and drug target? *Neurosci. Lett.* **310,** 77–80.

Kim, S. H., Cairns, N., Fountoulakis, M., and Lubec, G. (2001a). Decreased brain histamine-releasing factor protein in patients with Down syndrome and Alzheimer's disease. *Neurosci. Lett.* **300,** 41–44.

Kim, S. H., Fountoulakis, M., Cairns, N., and Lubec, G. (2001b). Protein levels of human peroxiredoxin subtypes in brains of Alzheimer's disease and Down syndrome. *J. Neural. Transm. Suppl.* **61,** 223–235.

Kim, S. H., Fountoulakis, M., Cairns, N. J., and Lubec, G. (2002). Human brain nucleoside diphosphate kinase activity is decreased in Alzheimer's disease and Down syndrome. *Biochem. Biophys. Res. Commun.* **296,** 970–975.

Kim, S. H., Nairn, A. C., Cairns, N., and Lubec, G. (2001c). Decreased levels of ARPP-19 and PKA in brains of Down syndrome and Alzheimer's disease. *J. Neural. Transm.* **61**(Suppl.), 263–272.

Kim, S. H., Vlkolinsky, R., Cairns, N., Fountoulakis, M., and Lubec, G. (2001d). The reduction of NADH ubiquinone oxidoreducatase 24- and 75-kDa subunits in brains of patients with Down syndrome and Alzheimer's disease. *Life Sci.* **68**, 2741–2750.

Kim, S. H., Vlkolinský, R., Cairns, N., and Lubec, G. (2000). Decreased levels of complex III core protein 1 and complex V beta chain in brains from patients with Alzheimer's disease and Down syndrome. *Cell Mol. Life Sci.* **57**, 1810–1816.

Knight, Z. A., Schilling, B., Row, R. H., Kenski, D. M., Gibson, B. W., and Shokat, K. M. (2003). Phosphospecific proteolysis for mapping sites of protein phosphorylation. *Nat. Biotechnol.* **21**, 1047–1054.

Krapfenbauer, K., Engidawork, E., Cairns, N., Fountoulakis, M., and Lubec, G. (2003). Aberrant expression of peroxiredoxin subtypes in neurodegenerative disorders. *Brain Res.* **967**, 152–160.

Larsen, M. R., Sorensen, G. L., Fey, S. J., Larsen, P. M., and Poepstorff, P. (2001). Phospho-proteomics: Evaluation of the use of enzymatic de-phosphorylation and differential mass spectrometric peptide mass mapping for site specific phosphorylation assignment in proteins separated by gel electrophoresis. *Proteomics* **1**, 223–238.

Lauderback, C. M., Hackett, J. M., Huang, F. F., Keller, J. N., Szweda, L. I., Markesbery, W. R., and Butterfield, D. A. (2001). The glial glutamate transporter, GLT-1, is oxidatively modified by 4-hydroxy-2-nonenal in the Alzheimer's disease brain: The role of Abeta 1-42. *J. Neurochem.* **78**, 413–416.

Lewczuk, P., Esselmann, H., Meyer, M., Wollscheid, V., Neumann, M., Otto, M., Maler, J. M., Ruther, E., Kornhuber, J., and Wiltfang, J. (2003). The amyloid-β (Aβ) peptide pattern in cerebrospinal fluid in Alzheimer's disease: Evidence of a novel carboxyterminally elongated Aβ peptide. *Rapid Comm. Mass Spectrom.* **17**, 1291–1296.

Lovell, M. A., and Markesbery, W. R. (2001). Ratio of 8-hydroxyguanine in intact DNA to free 8-hydroxyguanine is increased in Alzheimer disease ventricular cerebrospinal fluid. *Arch. Neurol.* **58**, 392–396.

Lovell, M. A., Robertson, J. D., Teesdale, W. J., Campbell, J. L., and Markesbery, W. R. (1998). Copper, iron, and zinc in Alzheimer's disease senile plaques. *J. Neurol. Sci.* **158**, 47–52.

Lubec, G., Nonaka, M., Krapfenbauer, K., Gratzer, M., Cairns, N., and Fountoulakis, M. (1999). Expression of the dihydropyrimidinase related protein 2 (DRP-2) in Down syndrome and Alzheimer's disease brain is downregulated at the mRNA and dysregulated at the protein level. *J. Neural. Transm.* **57**(Suppl.), 161–177.

March, R. E. (1997). An introduction to quadrupole ion trap mass spectrometry. *J. Mass Spectrom.* **32**, 351–369.

Mark, R. J., Lovell, M. A., Markesbery, W. R., Uchida, K., and Mattson, M. P. (1997). A role for 4-hydroxynonenal, an aldehydic product of lipid peroxidation, in disruption of ion homeostasis and neuronal death induced by amyloid beta-peptide. *J. Neurochem.* **68**, 255–264.

Markesbery, W. R. (1997). Oxidative stress hypothesis in Alzheimer's disease. *Free Radic. Biol. Med.* **23**, 134–147.

Masliah, E., Alford, M., De Teresa, R., Mallory, M., and Hansen, L. (1995). Deficient glutamate transport is associated with neurodegeneration in Alzheimer's disease. *Ann. Neurol.* **40**, 759–766.

Merchant, M., and Weinberger, S. R. (2000). Recent advancements in surface-enhanced laser desorption/ionization-time of flight-mass spectrometry. *Electrophoresis* **21**, 1164–1167.

Molloy, M. P., Herbert, B. R., Walsh, B. J., Tyler, M. I., Traini, M., Sanchez, J. C., Hochstrasser, D. F., Williams, K. L., and Gooley, A. A. (1998). Extraction of membrane proteins by differential solubilization for separation using two-dimensional gel electrophoresis. *Electrophoresis* **19**, 837–844.

Molloy, M. P. (2000). Two-dimensional electrophoresis of membrane proteins using immobilized pH gradients. *Anal. Biochem.* **280,** 1–10.

Morishima, Y., Gotoh, Y., Zeig, J., Barrett, T., Takano, H., Flavell, R., Davis, R. J., Shirasaki, Y., and Greenberg, M. E. (2001). Beta-amyloid induces neuronal apoptosis via a mechanism that involves the c-Jun-N-terminal kinase pathway and the induction of Fas ligand. *J. Neurosci.* **21,** 7551–7560.

Moseley, M. A. (2001). Current trends in differential expression proteomics: Isotopically coded tags. *Trends Biotechnol.* **19,** S10–S16.

Nagele, R. G., D'Andrea, M. R., Anderson, W. J., and Wang, H. Y. (2002). Intracellular accumulation of β-amyloid (1-42) in neurons is facilitated by the α7 nicotinic receptor in Alzheimer's disease. *Neuroscience* **110,** 199–211.

Oda, Y., Nagasu, T., and Chait, B. T. (2001). Enrichment analysis of phosphorylated proteins as a tool for probing the phosphoproteome. *Nat. Biotechnol.* **19,** 379–382.

Ojika, K., Tsugu, Y., Mitake, S., Otsuka, Y., and Takada, E. (1998). NMDA receptor activation enhances the release of a cholinergic differentiation peptide (HCNP) from hippocampal neurons in vitro. *Neuroscience* **101,** 341–352.

Pasquali, C., Fialka, I., and Huber, L. A. (1997). Preparative two-dimensional gel electrophoresis of membrane proteins. *Electrophoresis* **18,** 2573–2581.

Prange, A., Schaumlöffel, D., Brätter, P., Richarx, A., and Wolf, C. (2001). Species analysis of metallothionein isoforms in human brain cytosols by use of capillary electrophoresis hyphenated to inductively coupled plasma-sector field mass spectrometry. *J. Anal. Chem.* **371,** 764–774.

Qian, W. J., Goshe, M. B., Camp, D. G., III, Yu, L. R., Tang, K., and Smith, R. D. (2003). Phosphoprotein isotope-coded solid-phase tag approach for enrichment and quantitative analysis of phosphopeptides from complex mixtures. *Anal. Chem.* **75,** 5441–5450.

Rabilloud, T. (1998). Use of thiourea to increase the solubility of membrane proteins in two-dimensional electrophoresis. *Electrophoresis* **19,** 758–760.

Rossor, M. N., Svendsen, C., Hunt, S. P., Mountjoy, C. Q., Roth, M., and Iversen, L. L. (1982). The substantia innominata in Alzheimer's disease: A histochemical and biochemical study of cholinergic marker enzymes. *Neurosci. Lett.* **28,** 217–222.

Santoni, V., Molloy, M., and Rabilloud, T. (2000). Membrane proteins and proteomics: Un amour impossible? *Electrophoresis* **21,** 1054–1070.

Scheltens, P., and Korf, E. S. C. (2000). Contribution of neuroimaging in the diagnosis of Alzheimer's disease and other dementias. *Curr. Opin. Neurol.* **13,** 391–396.

Schonberger, S. J., Edgar, P. F., Kydd, R., Faull, R. L. M., and Cooper, G. J. S. (2001). Proteomic analysis of the brain in Alzheimer's disease: Molecular phenotype of a complex disease process. *Proteomics* **1,** 1519–1528.

Schuller, E., Gulesserian, T., Seidl, R., Cairns, N., and Lubec, G. (2001). Brain t-complex polypeptide 1 (TCP-1) related to its natural substrate β1 tubulin is decreased in Alzheimer's disease. *Life Sci.* **69,** 263–270.

Selkoe, D. J., and Podlisny, M. B. (2002). Deciphering the genetic basis of Alzheimer's disease. *Annu. Rev. Genomics Hum. Genet.* **3,** 67–99.

Selkoe, D. J. (2001a). Alzheimer's disease results from the cerebral accumulation and cytotoxicity of amyloid beta-protein. *J. Alzheimers Dis.* **3,** 75–80.

Selkoe, D. J. (2001b). Presenilin, Notch, and the genesis and treatment of Alzheimer's disease. *Proc. Natl. Acad. Sci. USA* **98,** 11039–11041.

Shim, K. S., and Lubec, G. (2002). Drebrin, a dendritic protein, is manifold decreased in brains of patients with Alzheimer's disease and Down syndrome. *Neurosci. Lett.* **324,** 209–212.

Shringarpure, R., Grune, T., and Davies, K. J. (2001). Protein oxidation and 20S proteasome-dependent proteolysis in mammalian cells. *Cell Mol. Life Sci.* **58,** 1442–1450.

Smith, M. A., Richey Harris, P. L., Sayre, L. M., Beckman, J. S., and Perry, G. (1997). Widespread peroxynitrite-mediated damage in Alzheimer's disease. *J. Neurosci.* **17,** 2653–2657.

Soreghan, B. A., Yang, F., Thomas, S. N., Hsu, J., and Yang, A. J. (2003a). High-throughput proteomic-based identification of oxidatively induced protein carbonylation in mouse brain. *Pharm. Res.* **20**, 1713–1720.

Soreghan, B. A., Thomas, S. N., Duff, K. E., and Yang, A. J. (2003b). Identification of oxidatively induced protein carbonylation in an APP/PS1 mouse model of Alzheimer's disease by a shotgun proteomics approach. *Soc. Neurosci. Abs.* 629.22.

Steinberg, T. H., Agnew, B. J., Gee, K. R., Laung, W. Y., Goodman, T., Schulenberg, B., Hendrickson, J., Beechem, J. M., Haugland, R. P., and Patton, W. F. (2003). Global quantitative phosphorylation analysis using multiplexed proteomics technology. *Proteomics* **3**, 1128–1144.

Stevens, S. M., Jr., Zharikova, A. D., and Prokai, L. (2003). Proteomic analysis of the synaptic plasma membrane fraction isolated from rate forebrain. *Mol. Brain Res.* **117**, 116–128.

Subramaniam, R., Roediger, F., Jordan, B., Mattson, M. P., Keller, J. N., Waeg, G., and Butterfield, D. A. (1997). The lipid peroxidation product, 4-hydroxy-2-trans-nonenal, alters the conformation of cortical synaptosomal membrane proteins. *J. Neurochem.* **69**, 1161–1169.

Tilleman, K., Stevens, I., Spittaels, K., Van der Haute, C., Clerens, S., Van den Bergh, G., Geerts, H., Van Lauven, F., Vandesande, F., and Moens, L. (2002a). Differential expression of brain proteins in glycogen synthase kinase-3β transgenic mice: A proteomics point of view. *Proteomics* **2**, 94–104.

Tilleman, K., Van den Haute, C., Geerts, H., van Leuven, G., Esmans, E. L., and Moens, L. (2002b). Proteomics analysis of the neurodegeneration in the brain of tau transgenic mice. *Proteomics* **2**, 656–665.

Tsuji, T., Shimohama, S., Kamiya, S., Sazuka, T., and Ohara, O. (1999). Analysis of brain proteins in Alzheimer's disease using high-resolution two-dimensional gel electrophoresis. *J. Neurol. Sci.* **166**, 100–106.

Tozaki, H., Matsumoto, A., Kanno, T., Nagai, K., Nagata, T., Yamamoto, S., and Nishizaki, T. (2002). The inhibitory and facilitatory actions of amyloid-beta peptide on nicotinic ACh receptors and AMPA receptors. *Biochem. Biophys. Res. Commun.* **294**, 42–45.

Tsuji, T., Shiozaki, A., Kohno, R., Yoshizato, K., and Shimohama, S. (2002). Proteomic profiling and neurodegeneration in Alzheimer's disease. *Neurochem. Res.* **27**, 1245–1253.

Ueno, I., Sakai, T., Yamaoka, M., Yoshida, R., and Tsugita, A. (2000). Analysis of blood plasma proteins in patients with Alzheimer's disease by two-dimensional electrophoresis, sequence homology and immunodetection. *Electrophoresis* **21**, 1832–1845.

Vlkolinský, R., Cairns, N., Fountoulakis, M., and Lubec, G. (2001). Decreased brain levels of 2',3-cyclic nucleotide-3'-phosphodiesterase in Down syndrome and Alzheimer's disease. *Neurobiol. Aging* **22**, 547–553.

Wagner, Y., Sickmann, A., Meyer, H. E., and Daum, G. (2003). Multidimensional nano-HPLC for analysis of protein complexes. *J. Am. Soc. Mass Spectrom.* **14**, 1003–1011.

Wang, H., and Hanash, S. (2003). Multi-dimensional liquid phase separations in proteomics. *J. Chromatogr. B.* **787**, 11–18.

Washburn, M. P., Wolters, D., and Yates, J. R. (2001). Large-scale analysis of the yeast proteome by multidimensional protein identification technology. *Nat. Biotechnol.* **19**, 242–247.

Wu, C. C., MacCoss, M. J., Howell, K. E., and Yates, J. R., III (2003). A method for the comprehensive proteomic analysis of membrane proteins. *Nat. Biotechnol.* **21**, 532–538.

Yatin, S. M., Varadarajan, S., and Butterfield, D. A. (2000). Vitamin E prevents Alzheimer's amyloid beta-peptide (1-42)-induced neuronal protein oxidation and reactive oxygen species production. *J. Alzheimers Dis.* **2**, 123–131.

Yoo, B. C., Fountoulakis, M., Cairns, N., and Lubec, G. (2001a). Changes of voltage-dependent anion-selective channel proteins VDAC1 and VDAC2 brain levels in patients with Alzheimer's disease and Down syndrome. *Electrophoresis* **22**, 172–179.

Yoo, B. C., Kim, S. H., Cairns, N., Fountoulakis, M., and Lubec, G. (2001b). Deranged expression of molecular chaperones in brains of patients with Alzheimer's disease. *Biochem. Biophys. Res. Commun.* **280**, 249–258.

PROTEOMICS AND ALCOHOLISM

Frank A. Witzmann* and Wendy N. Strother[†]

*Department of Cellular and Integrative Physiology
Indiana University School of Medicine
Indianapolis, Indiana 46202
[†]Department of Psychiatry
Institute of Psychiatric Research
Indiana University School of Medicine
Indianapolis, Indiana 46202

I. Introduction

Approximately 66% of the U.S. population will consume alcohol at some point in their lifetimes, with roughly 13% developing alcohol dependence (Grant, 1997). The risk factors that lead some individuals to develop alcohol dependency are many, from genetic factors to psychosocial and environmental influences. The unique pharmacological properties of alcohol that promote dependency and alcohol-seeking behaviors occur in multiple neurochemical systems located in anatomically distinct, but functionally connected, brain regions. Challenges in the alcohol research community continue to focus on how alcohol modifies brain structure and function differently in individuals at risk for developing alcohol dependence versus those individuals at low or no risk. The use of animal models of alcoholism has been of paramount importance for providing insight into the neurochemical and cellular changes associated with alcohol use and abuse.

INTERNATIONAL REVIEW OF
NEUROBIOLOGY, VOL. 61

189

A. Animal Models of Alcoholism

There are currently several rodent models of alcoholism, which were recently reviewed by Spanagel (2000). Of them, the alcohol-preferring (P) line of rats meets all the criteria proposed by Cicero (1979) for a suitable animal model of alcoholism (reviewed in McBride and Li, 1998; Murphy *et al.*, 2002). The alcohol-preferring and alcohol-nonpreferring (NP) lines of rats were originally obtained through a selective breeding program from an outbred, closed colony of Wistar rats (Lumeng *et al.*, 1977). Selection criteria include ethanol intakes by the P rat with free-choice access to 10% ethanol and water at least 5 g/kg per day, with a preference of ethanol to water of at least 2:1, whereas the NP rat line displays ethanol intake of less than 1 g/kg per day and a preference ratio of less than 0.5:1 (Lumeng *et al.*, 1977). The production of these selectively bred rat lines provides convincing data that genetics can significantly impact alcohol-drinking behaviors. Studies aimed at identifying neurochemical and behavioral differences between the NP and P rat lines have helped to distinguish potential phenotypic traits associated with alcohol preference and nonpreference.

B. Brain Regions of Interest

The extended amygdala and associated Central nervous system (CNS) regions (e.g., nucleus accumbens, prefrontal cortex, amygdala) have been implicated in mediating alcohol-reward and alcohol-seeking behaviors (Koob *et al.*, 1998; McBride, 2002; McBride and Li, 1998). Other brain structures have been shown to be involved in mediating the motor-impairing effects of ethanol (e.g., caudate-putamen) and in the development of tolerance to ethanol (e.g., hippocampus). Innate differences have been found in several neurotransmitters and receptors between the P and NP rat lines within several brain regions, including such key limbic structures as the nucleus accumbens, amygdala, and hippocampus (reviewed in McBride and Li, 1998; Murphy *et al.*, 2002). In the P rat line, serotonin (5-HT) content is lower in several brain regions compared to the NP rat, (Murphy *et al.*, 1982, 1987), and the number of serotonin immunopositive fibers is also decreased in numerous brain regions of the P rat (Zhou *et al.*, 1991, 1994). Further, higher densities of 5-HT_{1A} receptors (McBride *et al.*, 1994) and lower densities of 5-HT_2 receptors (McBride *et al.*, 1993) have been also been demonstrated in the P line compared to the NP line. Innate differences in dopamine (DA) content (Murphy *et al.*, 1987), DA D_2 receptor densities (McBride *et al.*, 1993), and dopaminergic innervation (Zhou *et al.*, 1995) have also been reported in several key limbic regions between the P and NP lines. Additionally, innate differences in the opioid and other neuropeptide systems have been found between the two rat lines (reviewed in McBride and Li, 1998; Murphy *et al.*, 2002).

The sum of these studies is that the predisposition for high alcohol-drinking behavior is likely a complex interaction between numerous neurotransmitter systems and neuroanatomical locations.

How ethanol alters neuronal function also has been an area of intense investigation. Early theories focused on nonselective changes in membrane fluidity (reviewed in Goldstein, 1986), but researchers have come to realize that ethanol acts directly on certain proteins and can, in fact, occupy specific regions of select proteins (reviewed in Peoples *et al.*, 1996; Yamakura *et al.*, 2001). Protein-protein interactions are necessary for almost every physiological process, drug addiction included. Linkage and association studies in humans and animal models have provided several key candidate genes for alcoholism (reviewed in Dick and Foroud, 2003), but investigations of the proteome and alcoholism remain to be done. This chapter will review the findings from recent proteomic investigations using the P and NP rat lines.

C. 2DE Gel-Based Proteomics Technology

We have begun to analyze regional brain proteomes to determine basal protein expression differences between these lines as a foundation for developing a brain protein expression profile database similar to other two-dimensional gel electrophoretic (2DE) knowledge databases under development, such as brain (Comings, 1982), serum (Anderson and Anderson, 1991), heart (Arnott *et al.*, 1998; Corbett *et al.*, 1995), colon (Ji *et al.*, 1997), liver (Anderson *et al.*, 1995), and a database of drug and chemical effects (the Molecular Effects of Drugs, or MED, database) (Anderson and Anderson, 1998). It is our belief that by comparing innate differences in protein expression in the brains of rats with varying preference for alcohol, we will gain insights into those protein factors that may contribute to vulnerability to alcohol addiction in human beings.

In 2DE, complex protein mixtures are solubilized, denatured, and subjected to orthogonal separation methods—first by protein charge via isoelectric focusing (IEF), then by mass in sodium dodecyl sulfate polyacrylamide gel electrophoresis (SDS-PAGE). The final product of 2DE separation is essentially an in-gel array of proteins, each assuming a coordinate position corresponding to the unique combination of isoelectric point (pI) and mass (MW). Resultant 2D protein patterns are visualized by any of a number of methods, such as visible and/or fluorescent dyes, silver stains, and autoradiography. Typically, scanned gel images are analyzed by variety of ever-improving 2D gel analysis software packages. It is at this point that both the strengths and weaknesses of this approach become evident. Protein abundance comparisons (e.g., differential expression) are easily made, because differences in protein spot density are readily detectable, can be quantified robustly, and compared statistically.

However, because the dynamic range of protein expression in most whole cell or tissue lysates is vast, only the most abundant proteins from 2D gels can be analyzed, and many proteins are overlooked. Furthermore, proteins with pIs at extreme pH and significant hydrophobicity are typically absent from 2D gel patterns. Typically only 2000 or so of the most abundant proteins in a particular cell or tissue can be reliably separated and identified.

Despite its shortcomings, 2D gel-based experimentation remains an exceptional approach for assessing differential protein expression. It not only enables one to separate, detect, and quantify the proteins, but it is also a preparative technique. Proteins separated on a 2D gel are isolated at their unique pI and MW coordinates and therefore can be physically excised, identified, and characterized using a variety of mass spectrometric techniques. This approach enables one to: (1) determine relative expression levels of cellular proteins, (2) identify the resolved proteins, (3) characterize modifications such as phosphorylation, glycosylation, and proteolytic cleavage, and (4) discover unpredicted gene products.

II. Proteomics of the Hippocampus and Nucleus Accumbens

A. Two-Dimensional Electrophoresis-Based Proteomics

1. *Electrophoresis and Image Analysis*

Because of the innate differences previously observed between the NP and P rat lines, and the involvement of the nucleus accumbens and hippocampus in mediating ethanol drinking and the development of tolerance, respectively, these structures were selected as regions to examine using proteomics technology. Relative abundances of proteins were determined to test the hypothesis that innate differences in the expression of proteins associated with synaptic function and cellular signaling pathways would be found in the nucleus accumbens and hippocampus of the inbred NP and P rats (Witzmann *et al.*, 2003).

Samples of NP and P rat brain tissue from the hippocampal and nucleus accumbens regions were solubilized and separated by 2DE using a 20-gel platform, as described previously (Anderson, 1981). The resulting slab gels were stained using a colloidal Coomassie Blue G-250 procedure, and were scanned and analyzed using PDQuest software. Statistical comparisons between individual protein abundances were conducted by calculation of Student t after data export to Excel. Typical hippocampus and nucleus accumbens 2D gel patterns are shown in Fig. 1.

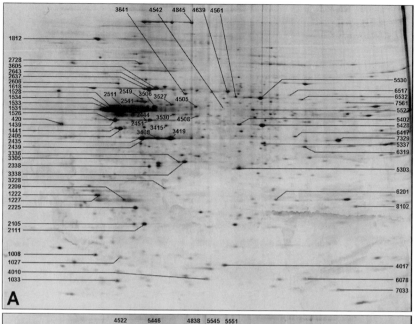

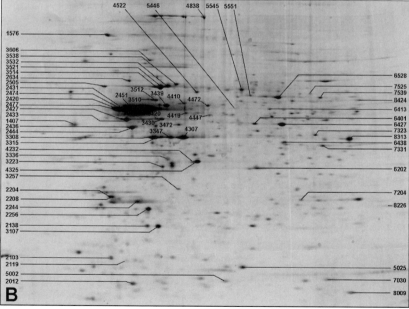

2. *Protein Indentification Using MALDI-TOF MS*

Protein spots that differed in abundance between NP and P groups were cut from the *stained* gels and processed for tryptic digestion, peptide recovery, and mass analysis (Witzmann *et al.*, 2003). After acquisition of the peptide mass spectra, proteins were identified by manual ProFound (Proteometrics, LLC NY, NY) database searches. Proteins common to gel patterns of both regions were selected for identification using matrix-assisted laser desorption ionization time-of-flight mass spectometry (MALDI-TOF MS), and these are presented in Table I.

B. PROTEOMIC DIFFERENCES IN THE NP AND P RAT

1. *Brain Region Similarities*

The 2DE protein patterns obtained from hippocampus and nucleus accumbens are shown in Figs. 1A and B. Visual inspection demonstrates their striking similarity. This resemblance is to be expected given the predominance of glial cells in the brain samples studied. If one assumes that 90–95% of cells in the brain are glial (Williams and Herrup, 1988), and the majority of these are protoplasmic astrocytes (Hansson and Rönnbäck, 2003), then the bulk of the approximately 1500 proteins resolved in the 2D gel patterns are presumably of glial origin. For instance, a dominant group of proteins was identified as glial fibrillary acidic protein (GFAP), an intermediate filament protein (MW 51,000) found only in glial cells or cells of glial origin. These proteins are completely absent from neuron-specific subcellular fraction patterns such as synaptosomes (Fig. 2). Consequently, functional inferences made regarding neuronal hippocampus and nucleus accumbens protein expression differences with respect to alcohol preference must be made cautiously when using heterogeneous brain tissues, because glial-specific proteins will dominate the detectable proteome.

2. *Hippocampal Protein Expression*

Of the more than 1500 neuronal/glial protein spots analyzed in the hippocampus, the abundance of only eight proteins was significantly different ($p < 0.05$) between the NP and P rats, representing 0.5% of the proteins analyzed.

FIG. 1. Colloidal Coomassie blue stained 2DE gel image of rat hippocampus (A) and nucleus accumbens (B). Proteins from whole sections of these brain regions were solubilized by standard methods and separated on 23.5-cm IEF tube gels and 20-by 25-by 0.15-cm slab gels. By convention, the horizontal dimension represents a pH gradient of approximately 4–7.5 and the vertical dimension a polyacrylamide gradient of 11–17%. The protein spots were cut from the gel and analyzed by peptide mass fingerprinting using MALDI-TOF MS. Those proteins successfully identified are designated by their spot number, corresponding protein names, and the expression information listed in Table I.

TABLE I

MEAN ABUNDANCES AND FOLD DIFFERENCES BETWEEN NP and P RATS FOR HIPPOCAMPUS AND NUCLEUS ACCUMBENS PROTEINS IDENTIFIED BY PEPTIDE MASS FINGERPRINTING

GENBANK accession	Protein name	Hippocampus abundance				Nucleus accumbens abundance			
		Spot number[a]	NP	P	FOLD[b]	Spot number	NP	P	FOLD
AAF22214	syndapin llbb	420	1881	1467	1.3	1407	2754	1532	1.8
AAK64519	BM259 (stroke prone associated)	1008	1804	1164	1.5	2103	2950	1787	1.7
P02695	retinoic acid-binding protein	1027	405	34	11.8	2119	575	104	5.5
NP_074055	complexin I	1033	2006	1646	1.2	2012	3858	2824	1.4
AAC53002	calpain small subunit (charge variant)	1222	1992	1333	1.5	2204	2621	1552	1.7
AAC53002	calpain small subunit	1227	1360	988	1.4	2208	1754	1368	1.3
AAB02288	ATP synthase beta	1439	8794	7582	1.2	2433	15662	12978	1.2
AAF27283	yotiao protein	1441	1219	1752	0.7	2436	2048	2103	1.0
A28701	ATP synthase beta	1526	1685	1753	1.0	2427	2530	3015	0.8
NP_073169	RP58 protein	1528	1042	1273	0.8	2431	1811	2003	0.9
AAB70013	ryanodine receptor type	1531	2513	2248	1.1	2477	1435	1739	0.8
O35568	fibulin-3	1533	3164	2977	1.1	2420	5865	5181	1.1
NP_058890	acetylcholine receptor epsilon	1534	2680	1721	1.6	2474	3262	2641	1.2
P15385	voltage-gated potassium channel protein KV1.4	1618	3776	2895	1.3	2505	2968	2209	1.3
NP_037177	tenascin-R	1812	3090	2514	1.2	1576	5675	5191	1.1
NP_058865	thioredoxin peroxidase	2105	1359	1125	1.2	2138	2830	1940	1.5
NP_058932	hippocampal cholinergic neurostimulating peptide	2111	4882	3981	1.2	3107	7264	5249	1.4

(Continued)

TABLE I (*Continued*)

GENBANK accession	Protein name	Hippocampus abundance				Nucleus accumbens abundance			
		Spot number[a]	NP	P	FOLD[b]	Spot number	NP	P	FOLD
JC2502	mitochondrial import stimulation factor S1 chain	2209	1977	1282	1.5	2244	3664	2773	1.3
AAC53002	calpain small subunit	2225	4354	3437	1.3	2256	8634	6208	1.4
P02650	Apo-E	2338	1682	1383	1.2	3223	2688	2202	1.2
P07323	enolase, gamma	2405	7548	7195	1.0	2444	12729	10714	1.2
NP_112406	actin, beta	2435	5914	4470	1.3	3308	11029	9095	1.2
P02571	actin, gamma	2439	2829	2743	1.0	3315	5015	4862	1.0
AAD01873	glial fibrillary acidic protein alpha	2444	995	1339	0.7	3420	711	591	1.2
AAD01873	glial fibrillary acidic protein alpha	2451	4916	3539	1.4	3430	6136	5648	1.1
NP_073169	RP58 protein	2511	749	1473	0.5	2451	1686	2728	0.6
AAD26207	unknown (specific to rat suprachiasmatic nucleus)	2541	994	1093	0.9	3510	1627	1738	0.9
NP_062001	intermexin, alpha	2549	3176	2604	1.2	3512	5115	4684	1.1
P06761	GRP78	2606	1147	854	1.3	2634	2009	1599	1.3
S31716	HSc70 (charge variant)	2637	2184	2620	0.8	3514	3143	3421	0.9
NP_077327	HSc70	2643	11424	8960	1.3	3521	19308	15062	1.3
NP_077377	Pervin	2728	801	672	1.2	3606	1335	1361	1.0
NP_114039	Prohibitin	3228	846	638	1.3	3257	1407	1047	1.3
1A06	calmodulin-dependent protein kinase	3305	528	177	3.0	3336	1231	520	2.4
NP_036727	lactate dehydrogenase B	3336	713	823	0.9	4232	1086	890	1.2

NP_036727	lactate dehydrogenase B	3338	5426	4621	1.2	4325	10887	9240	1.2
ATRTC	actin, beta	3408	3060	2443	1.3	3347	4747	3739	1.3
AAK54603	protein kinase C-binding protein	3415	1051	932	1.1	3472	2471	1462	1.7
AAA40933	creatine kinase B	3419	11169	9523	1.2	4307	17912	15260	1.2
NP_071565	HSP60	3506	4289	3672	1.2	3439	7433	5537	1.3
NP_036697	Glucokinase	3527	1059	930	1.1	4410	1797	1354	1.3
P50517	vacuolar ATP synthase subunit B, brain	3530	1041	856	1.2	4419	1466	1394	1.1
NP_067466	neutral sphingomyelinase II	3605	5621	3899	1.4	3532	7260	4308	1.7
S31716	GRP75	3614	1920	1353	1.4	3538	3540	2081	1.7
AAB61241	integrin beta-7 subunit	3641	1748	1442	1.2	4522	2441	2226	1.1
AAB32800	protein tyrosine phosphatase (frag)	4010	1217	914	1.3	5002	1703	1278	1.3
CAA29121	dismutase	4017	1503	1827	0.8	5025	3199	2654	1.2
P11598	HIP-70	4505	1536	1144	1.3	4472	2502	2055	1.2
AAA41239	glucokinase	4508	905	724	1.3	4447	495	404	1.2
NP_064670	serotonin receptor 3B	4542	110	101	1.1	5546	92	89	1.0
P11516	lamins C and C2	4561	718	936	0.8	5551	1629	1377	1.2
P02770	serum albumin	4639	1672	2216	0.8	5545	3122	3934	0.8
P97924	kalirin	4815	844	735	1.1	4838	1556	1869	0.8
P53812	phosphatidylinositol transfer protein beta	5303	2082	1899	1.1	6202	3635	4517	0.8
NP_058748	sorbitol dehydrogenase	5337	1196	770	1.6	6348	1459	1082	1.3
P56932	protein phosphatase 2A	5402	1911	2264	0.8	6401	3590	3172	1.1
AAF68666	parkin	5428	14233	10859	1.3	6427	21982	17066	1.3
P49187	c-Jun N-terminal kinase 3	5522	1062	1202	0.9	6413	1404	1256	1.1
NP_0622345	pyruvate dehydrogenase phosphatase isoenzyme 1	5530	5916	5127	1.2	6528	9606	8593	1.1
S42723	matricin	5546	828	617	1.3	6444	1252	1218	1.0
2207299A	insulin-like growth factor-binding protein	6078	785	714	1.1	7030	813	810	1.0

(*Continued*)

TABLE I (*Continued*)

GENBANK accession	Protein name	Hippocampus abundance				Nucleus accumbens abundance			
		Spot number[a]	NP	P	FOLD[b]	Spot number	NP	P	FOLD
NP_445742	phosphoglycerate mutase 1	6201	760	732	1.0	7204	1090	1020	1.1
NP_037022	zinc transporter 2	6319	1251	1196	1.0	7331	2005	1934	1.0
P38918	aflatoxin B1 aldehyde reductase	6417	1159	1006	1.2	7323	1417	1800	0.8
NP_036878	proprotein convertase subtilisin/ kexin type 2	6517	418	275	1.5	7525	463	419	1.1
AAC21449	TIC.	6532	1234	982	1.3	7539	1773	1752	1.0
NP_445853	p75NTR-associated cell death executor	7033	974	849	1.1	8009	1580	1412	1.1
1717354A	glutamine synthetase	7329	5163	4896	1.1	8313	8216	7807	1.1
CAA75351	p60 protein	7561	857	717	1.2	8424	1019	793	1.3
P49897	type 3 5deiodinase	8102	853	722	1.2	8226	1140	1381	0.8

[a]Protein spot number in Figs. 1A and B;
[b]NP protein abundance/P protein abundance; adapted from Witzmann *et al.* (2003).

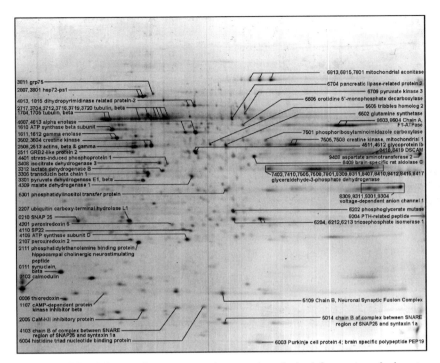

FIG. 2. 2DE gel image of a synaptosomal preparation obtained from rat cerebral cortex. Synaptosomes were isolated by discontinuous sucrose gradient centrifugation, solubilized by standard methods, separated on 24-cm, pH 3–10 linear IPG strips and 20-by-25-by 0.15-cm slab gels, and stained using colloidal Coomassie Blue. The protein spots were cut from the gel and analyzed by peptide mass fingerprinting using MALDI-TOF MS. A list of these proteins is presented in Table II.

Based on mean integrated densities determined by image analysis, the expression of all eight proteins was higher in the NP group than in the P group. Because of their very low abundance and other analytical peculiarities, six of these proteins eluded identification. Only cellular retinoic acid-binding protein 1 and a calmodulin-dependent protein (CAM) kinase were identified. The expression of cellular retinoic acid-binding protein was nearly 12-fold higher in the hippocampus of the NP rat. In comparison to other proteins in the 2D pattern this protein was present in relatively low abundance (see Table I). CAM kinase expression was found to be threefold higher in the hippocampus of the NP rats.

Although fold differences of 1.3 and higher were found in another 27 identified proteins in the hippocampus, these differences were statistically insignificant. Even so, the expression of nearly all was greater in the NP rats compared to the P rats, including syndapin IIbb, BM259, two forms of the calpain small subunit, acetylcholine-receptor epsilon, voltage-gated K channel protein KV1.4, mitochondrial import stimulation factor S1 chain, beta actin, GFAP alpha (spot #2451), glucose regulated protein 78 (GRP78), heat shock cognate protein 70 (HSC70), prohibitin, neutral sphingomyelinase II, GRP75, protein tyrosine phosphatase (fragment), protein disulfide isomerase er-60 precursor (HIP-70), hexokinase, sorbitol dehydrogenase, parkin, matricin, R8f DNA-binding protein, and arylhydrocarbon receptor nuclear translocator-like protein 1. Three proteins—yotiao protein, GFAP alpha (spot #2444, the more acidic charge variant of spot #2451), and repressor protein 58 (RP58), tended to be higher in the hippocampus of the P rat. The contradictory differences in the two GFAP charge forms (2451 versus 2444) probably relates to variable chemical modification (e.g., post-translational) of GFAP and, consequently, the variable appearance of this unknown modification in NP and P hippocampi. The nature of this modification remains to be characterized.

3. Nucleus Accumbens Protein Expression

In the nucleus accumbens the expression of 32 proteins differed significantly (P < 0.05). Similar to the hippocampus, nearly all of these were more abundant in the NP group, and 21 of them were identified by peptide mass fingerprinting. They included syndapin IIbb, BM259, cellular retinoic acid-binding protein 1, complexin 1, thioredoxin peroxidase, hippocampal cholinergic neurostimulating peptide (HCNP), calpain small subunit 1, apolipoprotein E (Apo-E), gamma enolase, GRP78, HSC70, prohibitin, CAM kinase, beta actin, protein kinase C-binding protein, heat shock protein 60 (HSP60), glucokinase, GRP75, sorbitol dehydrogenase, and parkin. The abundance of only one protein, an HSC70 charge variant (a post-translationally modified form, with lower pI), was statistically higher in the P rats.

Consistent with the hippocampal observations, the largest-fold differences in nucleus accumbens protein expression between the NP and P rats were found in cellular retinoic acid-binding protein 1 (5.5-fold) and a CAM kinase (2.4-fold). Other abundant proteins that differed to a lesser degree were gamma enolase, HSC70, parkin, syndapin IIbb, BM259, protein kinase C-binding protein, and GRP75 (see Table I).

The observations previously described support the hypothesis that innate differences exist in protein expression in two key limbic structures of rat lines selectively bred for disparate alcohol-drinking behaviors. The greatest dissimilarity between these lines appears in the nucleus accumbens, a key structure in the regulation of alcohol consumption (Koob *et al.*, 1998; McBride and Li, 1998). Despite the quantitative preponderance of glial proteins in the data sets, differential expression of proteins with known neuronal functions suggests some basic differences in the mechanisms underlying synaptic transmission in the nucleus accumbens between the P and NP rats. For instance, differences in the abundances of the following proteins were found: complexin 1, which plays a key role in Ca^{++}-dependent transmitter release (Chen *et al.*, 2002); gamma enolase, which plays a role in the fusion of the synaptic vesicle with the synaptic plasma membrane (Bulliard *et al.*, 1997); HSC70, which is part of a protein complex isolated from purified synaptic plasma membranes and synaptic vesicles and may be involved in endocytosis (Bulliard *et al.*, 1997); syndapin IIbb, a member of a family of cytoplasmic phosphoproteins that appears to be involved in synaptic vesicle recycling (endocytosis) and actin cytoskeletal organization (Qualmann and Kelly, 2000); and GRP78, which has a role in calcium homeostasis (Rao *et al.*, 2002). Higher abundance of these five proteins in the nucleus accumbens of the NP rat suggests that the mechanisms mediating exocytoxic transmitter release and vesicle recycling may be operating at a lower capacity in the P rat nucleus accumbens. Alternatively, the lower abundances of these five proteins in the P rat nucleus accumbens may reflect lower *serotonin* (5-HT) and DA innervation (Zhou *et al.*, 1991, 1994, 1995) and therefore fewer nerve terminals and synaptic vesicles in the P rat nucleus accumbens.

Other protein differences suggest different cellular signaling systems in the P rat; for example, protein kinase C-binding protein, which affects the interaction of protein kinase C with its substrates, as well as its cellular location (Jaken and Parker, 2000); CAM kinase, which can phosphorylate several proteins involved in synaptic function (Kitamura *et al.*, 1993; Risinger and Bennett, 1999; Yokoyama *et al.*, 1997); and cellular retinoic acid-binding protein 1, which can negatively regulate protein kinase C activity (Cope *et al.*, 1986) in the nucleus accumbens of P compared to NP rats. On the other hand, the lower abundances of these three proteins may reflect the reduced 5-HT and DA innervation noted earlier.

Several proteins involved in anterograde axonal transport of proteins had lower abundances in the P rat. These proteins ensure that transported proteins are properly incorporated into the functional elements of the synaptic terminal and include beta actin; the endoplasmic reticular molecular chaperones GRP78, HSC70 and HSC60 (Gupta, 1990; Rao *et al.*, 2002), and GRP75; and prohibitin, a membrane-bound mitochondrial chaperone (Massa *et al.*, 1995; Nijtmans *et al.*, 2000). Lower expression of these proteins may also reflect reduced 5-HT and DA innervation to the nucleus accumbens.

Another relatively abundant protein detected in the nucleus accumbens, HCNP, had a 1.4-fold higher expression in the NP rat. HCNP is an undecapeptide involved in differentiation of presynaptic cholinergic neurons in the medial septum and can enhance the production of choline acetyl transferase (Ojika *et al.*, 2000). The lower abundance of HCNP in the nucleus accumbens of the P rat may suggest that the cholinergic system within the nucleus accumbens is less developed than in NP rats.

Several proteins involved in various aspects of cellular metabolism (e.g., protein degradation, glucose metabolism, and peroxide degradation) were expressed differently in the nucleus accumbens of P and NP rats. Calpain (small subunit 1), a Ca^{++}-activated neutral protease that has been implicated in playing a role in neuronal injury and excitotoxicity (Hajimohammadreza et al., 1997), and parkin, a ubiquitin protein ligase that tags proteins for degradation (Hyun et al., 2002), were less abundant in the P rat, suggesting lower protein degradation capacity in the nucleus accumbens. Glucokinase, a modulator of adenosine triphosphate (ATP)-sensitive K^+ channel activity that can alter the rate of cell firing in specialized cells using glucose as a regulator of cell activity (Dunn-Meynell et al., 2002), and sorbitol dehydrogenase, a critical component of the polyol pathway (an alternate route of glucose metabolism) (Maekawa et al., 2001), are both less abundant in the P rat, which suggests strain-differences in glucose utilization, a condition that could result in differences in basal firing rates of glucose sensitive cells in the nucleus accumbens. In fact, basal local cerebral glucose utilization rates have been found to be significantly different in many brain regions, including the nucleus accumbens, between the P and NP rat lines (Smith et al., 2001). Finally, thioredoxin peroxidase is an antioxidant that eliminate peroxides (Rabilloud et al., 2002), thereby combatting oxidative stress. Lower levels of thioredoxin peroxidase in the nucleus accumbens of P rats suggest that P rats may be more vulnerable to oxidative stress. Accordingly, the CNS of the P line of rats may be more vulnerable to the chronic effects of high-dose ethanol through its oxidation to acetaldehyde by hydrogen peroxide via a catalase-mediated reaction.

As mentioned earlier in this chapter, the nucleus accumbens has been implicated in regulating alcohol-drinking behavior, whereas the hippocampus appears to be involved in the development of tolerance (Kalant, 1993). The P and NP rats differ in alcohol-drinking behavior, as well as in the development and persistence of tolerance (Gatto et al., 1987; Waller et al., 1983). If decreased expression of proteins in the nucleus accumbens and, to a lesser extent, in the hippocampus of the aforementioned P rat reflects reduced monoamine innervation, then it is highly likely that the innately lower DA and 5-HT innervation of these regions in the P rats may be major factors that contribute to high alcohol-drinking behavior and more rapid development of acute and persistent ethanol tolerance.

Based on the preliminary study described in this chapter, proteins associated with receptor function (e.g., 5-HT_{1A}, delta and mu-opioid receptors in the hippocampus, and D2 and 5-HT2 receptors in the nucleus accumbens) or DA and 5-HT innervation (e.g., DA or 5-HT transporters) have not been identified on the 2DE gels. Given the huge number of glial cells contributing to the sample, these relatively low abundance neuronal proteins may have fallen below the level of detection in this gel analysis system. Additionally, 2DE is notoriously ill-suited for resolving highly hydrophobic proteins, as are most other proteomic techniques (Patton et al., 2002). Consequently, the combination of low abundance and poor extraction may have prevented the detection and analysis of these relevant membrane-associated proteins.

III. Future Directions

The results of this preliminary proteomics investigation of the heritable molecular mechanisms underlying alcoholism are encouraging. The protein expression differences observed, although subtle, lend some support to current understanding of this phenomenon and reinforce the legitimacy of our approach. At the same time it is clear that our analysis is by no means global, and improvements in the approach are required. In this respect the problems we have identified are common to differential expression proteomics analysis of any whole (or regional) tissue. In the present case we are faced with too many glial cells and not enough neurons, when it is the neuron proteome in which we are currently most interested. That our approach has detected only a fraction of the cellular proteome raises the question, "How can we detect and quantify the expression of those proteins present at relatively low copy number; for example, 5-HT_{1A}, delta and mu-opioid receptors in the hippocampus, and D2 and 5-HT_2 receptors?" In response to the analytical issues and questions raised, we have developed a strategy to continue to take advantage of the unique utility of 2DE as a differential expression proteomics platform.

A. ANALYZING NEURONAL PROTEINS INDEPENDENT OF THE GLIAL PROTEOME

If one is interested in analyzing the purely neuronal proteome, primary dissociated neuronal cell culture systems seem to be the only solution (Potter and DeMarse, 2001). Like many *in vitro* systems, this artificial paradigm eliminates the considerable influences of surrounding cells (e.g., glia), making extrapolation to intact systems problematic. Nevertheless, it is an option that should be explored for comparing protein expressions in the genetically different NP and P rats.

A more practical and relevant approach involves the isolation of synaptosomes from NP and P rats. For instance, when hippocampal synaptosomes are prepared by discontinuous sucrose gradient centrifugation (Simon and Martin, 1973) and subjected to 2DE, as described earlier in this chapter, the protein pattern shown in Fig. 2 results (Witzmann *et al.*, unpublished). Mass spectrometric identification of some of the prominent constituents of this pattern (Table II) reveals a portion of the proteome devoid of GFAP, suggesting that this is a neuron specific preparation. This pattern also includes a number of proteins generally considered to be neuron-specific, such as neuron-specific enolase (NSE; gamma enolase), beta synuclein (phosphoneuroprotein 14), SNAP-25 (synaptosomal-associated protein), hippocampal cholinergic neurostimulating peptide, brain specific polypeptide PEP19, chain B, and neuronal synaptic fusion complex.

TABLE II

SYNAPTOSOMAL (CEREBRAL CORTEX) PROTEINS SEPARATED BY 2DE AND IDENTIFIED BY PEPTIDE MASS FINGERPRINTING (SEE GEL IMAGE IN FIG. 2)

Spot number[a]	Accession #	Protein name	Z score[b]	%C[c]	pI[d]	MW[d] (kDa)
6	NP_035790.1	thioredoxin 1; thioredoxin [Mus musculus]	1.43	40	4.8	12.00
103	AAB22151.1	calmodulin Ca(2+)-dependent ganglioside-binding protein	1.34	47	4.1	5.65
111	NP_542955.1	synuclein beta [Rattus norvegicus]	1.51	26	4.5	14.49
210	NP_112253.1	SNAP-25 synaptosomal-associated protein 25 kDa [Rattus norvegicus]	2.43	33	4.7	23.53
1107	NP_032889.2	cAMP-dependent protein kinase inhibitor beta [Mus musculus]	2.43	53	4.7	9.65
1610	AAB02288.1	ATP synthase beta subunit	2.43	28	4.9	51.18
1611	NP_647541.1	neuron specific enolase (NSE) enolase gamma [Rattus norvegicus]	2.43	25	5.0	47.52
1612	NP_647541.1	neuron specific enolase (NSE) enolase gamma [Rattus norvegicus]	2.43	25	5.0	47.52
1704	A25113	tubulin beta chain 15 - rat	2.43	31	4.8	50.38
1705	NP_775125.1	tubulin beta 5 [Rattus norvegicus]	2.39	31	4.8	50.11
2005	NP_067710.1	CAM-KII inhibitory protein [Rattus norvegicus]	2.43	38	5.3	8.67
2107	NP_058865.1	peroxiredoxin 2; thioredoxin peroxidase 1 [Rattus norvegicus]	2.43	34	5.3	21.94
2111	NP_058932.1	hippocampal cholinergic neurostimulating peptide [Rattus norvegicus]	2.40	60	5.5	20.9
2207	NP_058933.1	ubiquitin carboxy-terminal hydrolase L1 [Rattus norvegicus]	2.43	51	5.1	25.11
2508	NP_112406.1	cytoplasmic beta-actin [Rattus norvegicus]	2.43	28	5.3	42.06
2511	NP_003017.1	SH3-domain GRB2-like protein 2 [Homo sapiens]	2.43	37	5.3	40.12
2513	ATRTC	actin beta - rat	2.43	32	5.3	42.08
2604	IMAB	rat liver F1-ATPase chain B	2.43	19	4.9	51.33
2717	NP_775125.1	tubulin beta 5 [Rattus norvegicus]	2.43	23	4.8	50.11
2807	S31716	dnaK-type molecular chaperone HSP72-PS1 - rat	2.43	34	5.4	71.14

3204	XP_214724.1	prohibitin [Rattus norvegicus]	2.43	30	5.4	27.76
3301	P49432	pyruvate dehydrogenase E1 component beta subunit	2.43	34	5.9	39.34
3306	P54311	transducin beta (Guanine nucleotide-binding protein beta subunit 1)	2.43	24	5.5	38.17
3312	NP_036727.1	lactate dehydrogenase B; lactate dehydrogenase B [Rattus norvegicus]	2.29	25	5.7	36.88
3408	NP_446090.1	isocitrate dehydrogenase 3 (NAD+) alpha [Rattus norvegicus]	2.43	33	6.5	40.05
3502	AAA40933.1	creatine kinase-B	2.43	29	5.3	40.89
3504	NP_036661.2	creatine kinase brain [Rattus norvegicus]	2.43	48	5.3	42.98
3704	NP_775125.1	tubulin beta chain 15 - rat	2.43	27	4.8	50.11
3705	NP_775125.1	tubulin beta chain 15 - rat	2.43	27	4.8	50.11
3712	A25113	tubulin beta chain 15 - rat	2.43	36	4.8	50.38
3716	A25113	tubulin beta chain 15 - rat	2.43	36	4.8	50.38
3719	A25113	tubulin beta chain 15 - rat	2.43	36	4.8	50.38
3720	A25113	tubulin beta chain 15 - rat	2.43	36	4.8	50.38
3801	S31716	dnaK-type molecular chaperone HSP72-ps1 - rat	2.43	38	5.4	71.14
3811	156581	dnaK-type molecular chaperone GRP75 precursor - rat	2.43	35	5.9	74.01
4103	1JTH	chain B, complex between N-terminal region of SNAP-25 and Snare region of Syntaxin 1a	2.38	19	5.9	9.07
4109	NP_062256.1	ATP synthase subunit d [Rattus norvegicus]	2.3	42	6.2	18.8
4110	NP_476484.1	fertility protein; SP22 [Rattus norvegicus]	2.43	39	6.3	20.18
4201	NP_446028.1	peroxiredoxin 6 [Rattus norvegicus]	2.43	23	5.6	24.86
4309	NP_150238.1	malate dehydrogenase 1 [Rattus norvegicus]	2.21	28	6.2	36.64
4401	XP_218684.1	similar to stress-induced phosphoprotein 1 [Rattus norvegicus]	1.56	31	6.1	40.73
4511	NP_446383.1	glycoprotein Ib (platelet) beta polypeptide [Rattus norvegicus]	2.43	40	6.3	44.36
4512	NP_446383.1	glycoprotein Ib (platelet) beta polypeptide [Rattus norvegicus]	2.43	15	6.3	44.36
4607	P04764	Alpha enolase (Nonneural enolase) (NNE)	2.43	23	5.8	47.53
4613	NP_036686.1	enolase 1 alpha	2.43	50	6.2	47.44

(Continued)

TABLE II (Continued)

Spot number[a]	Accession #	Protein name	Z score[b]	%C[c]	pI[d]	MW[d] (kDa)
4813	P47942	dihydropyrimidinase related protein-2	2.30	20	6.0	62.66
4815	P47942	dihydropyrimidinase related protein-2	2.37	24	6.0	62.66
5004	XP_220432.1	similar to histidine triad nucleotide binding protein [Rattus norvegicus]	2.43	28	6.2	11.6
5014	1JTH	chain B, complex between N-terminal region of SNAP-25 and Snare region of Syntaxin 1a	2.43	30	5.9	9.07
5109	1SFC	Chain B neuronal synaptic fusion complex	2.43	35	5.1	9.57
5505	NP_653134.2	tribbles homolog 2 [Mus musculus]	2.43	11	5.8	39.38
6003	NP_006189.1	Purkinje cell protein 4; brain specific polypeptide PEP19 [Homo sapiens]	1.81	44	6.2	6.8
6202	JC1132	JC1132 phosphoglycerate mutase (EC 5.4.2.1) B chain-rat	2.43	65	6.7	28.93
6204	NP_075211.1	triosephosphate isomerase 1 [Rattus norvegicus]	2.43	62	6.5	27.42
6212	NP_075211.1	triosephosphate isomerase 1 [Rattus norvegicus]	2.43	39	6.5	27.42
6213	NP_075211.1	triosephosphate isomerase 1 [Rattus norvegicus]	2.43	43	6.5	27.42
6301	NP_058927.1	phosphatidylinositol transfer protein	2.43	22	6.0	32.15
6409	CAA30044.1	unnamed protein product [Rattus norvegicus] brain-specific rat aldolase C	2.43	23	6.8	39.6
6502	1717354A	Gln synthetase	2.43	19	6.4	41.16
6605	AAA61256.1	orotidine 5-monophosphate decarboxylase (EC 4.1.1.23)	2.43	15	6.6	51.48
6704	NP_476554.1	pancreatic lipase-related protein 2 [Rattus norvegicus]	2.43	10	6.0	54.84
6709	NP_445749.1	pyruvate kinase 3 [Rattus norvegicus]	2.39	20	6.6	58.31
6813	NP_077374.1	mitochondrial aconitase (nuclear aco2 gene) [Rattus norvegicus]	1.07	13	8.2	86.2
6815	NP_077374.1	mitochondrial aconitase (nuclear aco2 gene) [Rattus norvegicus]	2.40	20	8.2	86.2

ID	Accession	Description				
7403	NP_058704.1	glyceraldehyde-3-phosphate dehydrogenase [Rattus norvegicus]	1.45	20	8.4	36.1
7409	NP_034342.1	four and a half LIM domains 2 [Rattus norvegicus]	2.43	40	7.8	34.05
7410	XP_214333.1	similar to glyceraldehyde-3-phosphate dehydrogenase [Rattus norvegicus]	2.43	29	7.8	36.09
7501	NP_080215.1	phosphoribosylaminoimidazole carboxylase [Mus musculus]	2.43	17	7.0	47.73
7505	XP_215806.1	creatine kinase, mitochondrial 1 ubiquitous [Rattus norvegicus]	2.38	28	8.9	47.34
7508	XP_215806.1	creatine kinase, mitochondrial 1 ubiquitous [Rattus norvegicus]	2.26	29	8.9	47.34
7801	NP_077374.1	mitochondrial aconitase (nuclear aco2 gene) [Rattus norvegicus]	2.39	23	8.2	86.2
8309	NP_112643.1	voltage-dependent anion channel 1 [Rattus norvegicus]	2.43	24	8.8	30.85
8311	NP_112643.1	voltage-dependent anion channel 1 [Rattus norvegicus]	2.43	24	8.8	30.85
8407	NP_058704.1	glyceraldehyde-3-phosphate dehydrogenase [Rattus norvegicus]	2.40	44	8.4	36.1
8410	NP_058704.1	glyceraldehyde-3-phosphate dehydrogenase [Rattus norvegicus]	2.40	44	8.4	36.1
8412	NP_058704.1	glyceraldehyde-3-phosphate dehydrogenase [Rattus norvegicus]	2.40	44	8.4	36.1
8415	NP_058704.1	glyceraldehyde-3-phosphate dehydrogenase [Rattus norvegicus]	2.40	44	8.4	36.1
8417	NP_058704.1	glyceraldehyde-3-phosphate dehydrogenase [Rattus norvegicus]	2.40	44	8.4	36.1
8418	AAL99984.1	Down syndrome cell adhesion molecule-like protein [Mus musculus]	2.08	22	9.6	40.69
8419	AAL99984.1	Down syndrome cell adhesion molecule-like protein [Mus musculus]	2.08	22	9.6	40.69
8603	1MAB	rat liver F1-ATPase chain A	2.23	22	8.4	55.38
8604	1MAB	rat liver F1-ATPase chain A	2.23	22	8.4	55.38

(Continued)

TABLE II (*Continued*)

Spot number[a]	Accession #	Protein name	Z score[b]	%C[c]	pI[d]	MW[d] (kDa)
9204	NP_032996.1	parathyroid hormone-related protein; PTH-related peptide [Mus musculus]		61	10.7	20.08
9301	NP_112643.1	voltage-dependent anion channel 1 [Rattus norvegicus]	2.43	43	8.8	30.85
9304	NP_112643.1	voltage-dependent anion channel 1 [Rattus norvegicus]	2.43	43	8.8	30.85
9408	NP_037309.1	glutamate oxaloacetate transaminase 2 [Rattus norvegicus]	2.43	33	9.4	47.7

[a]Spot number from PDQuest imaging software; image shown in Fig. 2.
[b]Z-score from ProFound peptide mass database.
[c]% = sequence coverage.
[d]pI and MW estimates from ProFound peptide mass database.

208

These data suggest sample homogeny, but the limited brain proteomic literature is not clear as to which proteins uniquely reside in neurons or glial cells. In fact, a number of proteins appear in both Table 1 (predominantly glial) and Table II. Accordingly, studies of differential expression proteomics in the CNS might well be advised to first determine the basal proteomes of various neural cell types and establish their heterogeneity and homogeneity, which is no small undertaking. Currently, only few investigations of this type that use a proteomic approach have been undertaken (Lubec *et al.*, 2003). Even well-established markers such as GFAP may not be so specific. Although GFAP is considered a specific marker for astrocytes, Bicknese *et al.* (2002) has shown that GFAP is also found in umbilical cord multipotent stem cells.

B. Reducing Sample Complexity and Increasing Analytical 'Depth of Field'

It has been estimated that from the 30,000 or so human genes available, hundreds of thousands of individual protein forms may exist, and with large differences in copy number, their abundance may span seven to eight orders of magnitude (Anderson and Anderson, 1998). No current proteomics technique can hope to detect and quantify them all in a single tissue sample. Hence the 1500+ proteins in rat hippocampus and nucleus accumbens discussed in this chapter (see Fig. 1) represent a mere fraction of the actual rat brain proteome, hardly a "global" assessment. Despite the valuable and relevant information provided by these results, it is clear that a greater percentage of the proteome must be rendered analyzable.

To address the issues of dynamic range and detection sensitivity, researchers using proteomics approaches have begun to incorporate various methods of sample fractionation to reduce sample complexity and dig deeper into the broad dynamic range of protein expression. The simplest of these methods is subcellular fractionation by differential centrifugation, yielding cytosol, mitochondria, microsomes, and nuclei/membranes, whose proteomes are subsequently separated on individual 2D gels. For example, this approach has significantly improved the utility of 2D gel-based proteomics in brain analysis (Krapfenbauer, 2003) and should become standard operating procedure when analyzing tissues or organs electrophoretically in general.

We propose an additional level of sample complexity reduction, accompanied by an increased analytical depth of field, through the serial fractionation of subcellular components into more manageable compartments. This is similar to a strategy proposed by Cordwell *et al.* (2000), in which tissue samples were fractionated on the basis of subcellular location *and* their relative solubilities. Although this approach increased the resolution of a microbial proteome by

30%, it necessitated up to 40 2D gels per sample to do so. We are using a strategy that similarly fractionates tissues by differential centrifugation but adds a further reduction in complexity achieved by solution isoelectric focusing (Weber and Bocek, 1996, 1998). A number of previous investigations support the use of this approach in concept (Zuo and Speicher, 2000, 2002; Zuo *et al.*, 2001, 2002). In effect, the subcellular protein fractions are subdivided into approximately two pH unit fractions by free-flow electrophoresis (FFE) (Burggraf *et al.*, 1995; Ros *et al.*, 2002; Zischka *et al.*, 2003) that can then be resolved on large-format 2D gels whose horizontal dimension (pI) is defined by a linear 2 pH unit gradient. The overall approach is illustrated in Fig. 3. Our initial experiments using liver cell fractions (Witzmann, unpublished) suggest that from a single tissue sample fractionated into four subcellular fractions and five solution IEF fractions will yield 2DE differential expression data for approximately 20,000 protein spots (i.e., 1000 on 20 individual gels). Referring to the synaptosomal fraction mentioned earlier and illustrated in Fig. 2 (a 2D pattern containing approximately 1000 protein spots), implementation of FFE-IEF to this fraction, as described previously, will specifically address the issue of dynamic range and significantly improve our proteomic comparisons of NP and P rat brain regions.

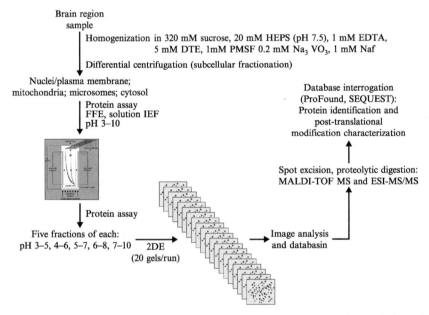

FIG. 3. This diagram illustrates a strategy for reducing brain protein sample complexity and increasing analytical depth of field for 2DE gel-based proteomics. This approach is designed to increase the number of proteins that can be detected, comparatively quantified, and identified by at least one order of magnitude over current methods. (See Color Insert.)

IV. Conclusion

Proteomic analysis using 2DE separation and relative quantitation, followed by MALDI-TOF MS-identification of relevant protein spots in alcohol-preferring (P) and alcohol-nonpreferring (NP) lines of rat hippocampus and nucleus accumbens demonstrates subtle but significant between-line differences in basal protein expression. However, the more substantive, anticipated differences between them may be masked by limitations of the current proteomics approach. As described in other chapters of this book, a number of alternative proteomic techniques and approaches are available (e.g., multidimensional protein identification technology [MudPIT], isotope-code affinity tags [ICAT], stable-isotope labeling, surface-enhanced laser desorption ionization [SELDI]) and their application to alcoholism should be explored. Then again, by combining a sample complexity reduction strategy with 2DE and mass spectrometric identification and characterization of the resolved proteins, the genetic differences between P and NP rats, as manifest in their unique proteomes, may be determined and the molecular underpinnings of alcoholism explained.

References

Anderson, N. G., and Anderson, N. L. (1998). Proteome and proteomics: New technologies, new concepts, and new words. *Electrophoresis* **19,** 1853–1861.

Anderson, N. L. (1981). "Two-Dimensional Electrophoresis: Operation of the ISO-DALT System." Large Scale Biology Press, Washington.

Anderson, N. L., and Anderson, N. G. (1991). A two-dimensional gel database of human plasma proteins. *Electrophoresis* **12,** 883–906.

Anderson, N. G., Esquer-Blasco, R., Hofmann, J.-P., Meheus, L., Raymackers, J., Steiner, S., Witzman, F. A., and Anderson, N. G. (1995). An updated two-dimensional gel database of rat liver proteins useful in gene regulation and drug effects studies. *Electrophoresis* **16,** 1977–1981.

Arnott, D., O'Connell, K. L., King, K. L., and Stults, J. T. (1998). An integrated approach to proteome analysis: Identification of proteins associated with cardiac hypertrophy. *Anal. Biochem.* **258,** 1–18.

Bicknese, A. R., Goodwin, H. S., Quinn, C. O., Henderson, V. C., Chien, S. N., and Wall, D. A. (2002). Human umbilical cord blood cells can be induced to express markers for neurons and glia. *Cell Transplant.* **11,** 261–264.

Bulliard, C., Zurbriggen, R., Tornare, J., Faty, M., Dastoor, Z., and Dreyer, J. L. (1997). Purification of a dichlorophenol-indophenol oxidoreductase from rat and bovine synaptic membranes: Tight complex association of a glyceraldehyde-3-phosphate dehydrogenase isoform, TOAD64, enolase-gamma and aldolase C. *Biochem. J.* **324,** 555–563.

Burggraf, D., Weber, G., and Lottspeich, F. (1995). Free flow-isoelectric focusing of human cellular lysates as sample preparation for protein analysis. *Electrophoresis* **16,** 1010–1015.

Chen, X., Tomchick, D. R., Kovrigin, E., Arac, D., Machius, M., Sudhof, T. C., and Rizom, J. (2002). Three-dimensional structure of the complexin/SNARE complex. *Neuron* **33,** 397–409.

Cicero, T. J. (1979). A critique of animal analogs of alcoholism. In "Biochemistry and Pharmacology of Ethanol" (E. Majchrowich and E. P. Noble, Eds.), vol. 2, pp. 533–560. Plenum Press, New York.

Comings, D. E. (1982). Two-dimensional gel electrophoresis of human brain proteins. III. Genetic and non-genetic variations in 146 brains. *Clin. Chem.* **28**, 798–804.

Cope, F. O., Howard, B. D., and Boutwell, R. K. (1986). The *in vitro* characterization of the inhibition of mouse brain protein kinase-C by retinoids and their receptors. *Experientia* **42**, 1023–1027.

Corbett, J. M., Wheeler, C. H., and Dunn, M. J. (1995). Coelectrophoresis of cardiac tissue from human, dog, rat and mouse: Toward the establishment of an integrated two-dimensional protein database. *Electrophoresis* **16**, 1524–1529.

Cordwell, S. J., Nouwens, A. S., Verrills, N. M., Basseal, D. J., and Walsh, B. J. (2000). Subproteomics based upon protein cellular location and relative solubilities in conjunction with composite two-dimensional electrophoresis gels. *Electrophoresis* **21**, 1094–1103.

Dick, D. M., and Foroud, T. (2003). Candidate genes for alcohol dependence: A review of genetic evidence from human studies. *Alcohol Clin. Exp. Res.* **27**, 868–879.

Dunn-Meynell, A. A., Routh, V. H., Kang, L., Gaspers, L., and Levin, B. E. (2002). Glucokinase is the likely mediator of glucosensing in both glucose-excited and glucose-inhibited central neurons. *Diabetes* **51**, 2056–2065.

Gatto, G. J., Murphy, J. M., Waller, M. B., McBride, W. J., Lumeng, L., and Li, T.-K. (1987). Persistence of tolerance to a single dose of ethanol in the selectively-bred alcohol-preferring P rat. *Pharmacol. Biochem. Behav.* **28**, 105–110.

Goldstein, D. B. (1986). Effect of alcohol on cellular membranes. *Ann. Emerg. Med.* **15**, 1013–1008.

Grant, B. F. (1997). Convergent validity of DSM-III-R and DSM-IV alcohol dependence: Results from the National Longitudinal Alcohol Epidemiologic Survey. *J. Subst. Abuse* **9**, 89–102.

Gupta, R. S. (1990). Microtubules, mitochondria, and molecular chaperones: A new hypothesis for *in vivo* assembly of microtubules. *Biochem. Cell. Biol.* **68**, 1352–1363.

Hajimohammadreza, I., Raser, K. J., Nath, R., Nadimpalli, R., Scott, M., and Wang, K. K. (1997). Neuronal nitric oxide synthase and calmodulin-dependent protein kinase IIalpha undergo neurotoxin-induced proteolysis. *J. Neurochem.* **69**, 1006–1013.

Hansson, E., and Rönnbäck, L. (2003). Glial neuronal signaling in the central nervous system. *FASEB J.* **17**, 341–348.

Hyun, D. H., Lee, M., Hattori, N., Kubo, S., Mizuno, Y., Halliwell, B., and Jenner, P. (2002). Effect of wild-type or mutant Parkin on oxidative damage, nitric oxide, antioxidant defenses, and the proteasome. *J. Biol. Chem.* **227**, 28572–28577.

Jaken, S., and Parker, P. J. (2000). Protein kinase C binding partners. *Bioassays* **22**, 245–254.

Ji, H., Reid, G. E., Moritz, R. L., Eddes, J. S., Burgess, A. W., and Simpson, R. J. (1997). A two-dimensional gel database of human colon carcinoma proteins. *Electrophoresis* **18**, 605–613.

Kalant, H. (1993). Problems in the search for mechanisms of tolerance. *Alcohol Alcohol. Suppl.* **2**, 1–8.

Kitamura, Y., Miyazaki, A., Yamanaka, Y., and Nomura, Y. J. (1993). Stimulatory effects of protein kinase C and calmodulin kinase II on N-methyl-D-aspartate receptor/channels in the postsynaptic density of rat brain. *Neurochem.* **61**, 100–109.

Koob, G. F., Roberts, A. J., Schulteis, G., Parsons, L. H., Heyser, C. J., Hyytia, P., Merlo-Pich, E., and Weiss, F. (1998). Neurocircuitry targets in ethanol reward and dependence. *Alcohol Clin. Exp. Res.* **22**, 3–9.

Krapfenbauer, K., Fountoulakis, M., and Lubec, G. (2003). A rat brain protein expression map including cytosolic and enriched mitochondrial and microsomal fractions. *Electrophoresis* **24**, 1847–1870.

Lubec, G., Krapfenbauer, K., and Fountoulakis, M. (2003). Proteomics in brain research: Potentials and limitations. *Prog. Neurobiol.* **69**, 193–211.

Lumeng, L., Hawkins, T. D., and Li, T.-K. (1977). New strains of rats with alcohol preference and nonpreference. In "Alcohol and Aldehyde Metabolizing Systems." (R. G. Thurman, J. R. Williamson, H. Drott, and B. Chance, Eds.), pp. 537–544. Academic Press, New York.

Maekawa, K., Tanimoto, T., Okada, S., Suzuki, T., Suzuki, T., and Yabe-Nishimura, C. (2001). Analysis of gene expression of aldose reductase and sorbitol dehydrogenase in rat Schwann cells by competitive RT-PCR method using non-homologous DNA standards. Brain Res. Brain Res. Protoc. **8,** 219–227.

Massa, S. M., Longo, F. M., Zuo, J., Wang, S., Chen, J., and Sharp, F. R. (1995). Cloning of rat grp75, an hsp70-family member, and its expression in normal and ischemic brain. J. Neurosci. Res. **40,** 807–819.

McBride, W. J. (2002). Central nucleus of the amygdala and the effects of alcohol and alcohol-drinking behavior in rodents. Pharmacol. Biochem. Behav. **71,** 509–515.

McBride, W. J., Chernet, E., Dyr, W., Lumeng, L., and Li, T.-K. (1993). Densities of dopamine D_2 receptors are reduced in CNS regions of alcohol-preferring P rats. Alcohol **10,** 387–390.

McBride, W. J., Chernet, E., Rabold, J. A., Lumeng, L., and Li, T.-K. (1993). Serotonin-2 receptors in the CNS of alcohol-preferring and–nonpreferring rats. Pharmacol. Biochem. Behav. **46,** 631–636.

McBride, W. J., Guan, X. M., Chernet, E., Lumeng, L., and Li, T.-K. (1994). Regional serotonin$_{1A}$ receptors in the CNS of alcohol-preferring and–nonpreferring rats. Pharmacol. Biochem. Behav. **49,** 7–12.

McBride, W. J., and Li, T.-K. (1998). Animal models of alcoholism: Neurobiology of high alcohol-drinking behavior in rodents. Crit. Rev. Neurbiol. **12,** 339–369.

Murphy, J. M., Mcbride, W. J., Lumeng, L., and Li, T.-K. (1982). Regional brain levels of monoamines in alcohol-preferring and -nonpreferring lines of rats. Pharmacol. Biochem. Behav. **16,** 145–149.

Murphy, J. M., McBride, W. J., Lumeng, L., and Li, T.-K. (1987). Contents of monoamines in forebrain regions of aclohol-preferring (P) and -nonpreferring (NP) lines of rats. Pharmacol. Biochem. Behav. **26,** 389–392.

Murphy, J. M., Stewart, R. B., Bell, R. L., Badia-Elder, N. E., Carr, L. G., McBride, W. J., Lumeng, L., and Li, T.-K. (2002). Phenotypic and genotypic characterization of the Indiana University rat lines selectively bred for high and low alcohol preference. Behav. Genet. **32,** 363–388.

Nijtmans, L. G., de Jong, L., Artal-Sanz, M., Coates, P. J., Berden, J. A., Back, J. W., Muijsers, A. O., van der Spek, H., and Grivell, L. A. (2000). Prohibitins act as a membrane-bound chaperone for the stabilization of mitochondrial proteins. EMBO J. **19,** 2444–2451.

Ojika, K., Mitake, S., Tohdoh, N., Appel, S. H., Otsuka, Y., Katada, E., and Matsukawa, N. (2000). Hippocampal cholinergic neurostimulating peptides (HCNP). Prog. Neurobiol. **60,** 37–83.

Patton, W. F., Schulenberg, B., and Steinberg, T. H. (2002). Two-dimensional gel electrophoresis; better than a poke in the ICAT? Curr. Opin. Biotechnol. **13,** 321–328.

Peoples, R. W., Li, C., and Weight, F. F. (1996). Lipid vs protein theories of alcohol action in the nervous system. Annu. Rev. Pharmacol. Toxicol. **36,** 185–201.

Potter, S. M., and DeMarse, T. B. (2001). A new approach to neural cell culture for long-term studies. J. Neurosci. Methods **110,** 17–24.

Qualmann, B., and Kelly, R. B. (2000). Syndapin isoforms participate in receptor-mediated endocytosis and actin organization. J. Cell Biol. **148,** 1047–1062.

Rabilloud, T., Heller, M., Gasnier, F., Luche, S., Rey, C., Aebersold, R., Benahmed, M., Louisot, P., and Lunardi, J. (2002). Proteomics analysis of cellular response to oxidative stress. Evidence for in vivo overoxidation of peroxiredoxins at their active site. J. Biol. Chem. **277,** 19396–19401.

Rao, R. V., Peel, A., Logvinova, A., del Rio, G., Hermel, E., Yokota, T., Goldsmith, P. C., Ellerby, L. M., Ellerby, H. M., and Bredesen, D. E. (2002). Coupling endoplasmic reticulum stress to the cell death program: Role of the ER chaperone GRP78. FEBS Lett. **514,** 122–128.

Risinger, C., and Bennett, M. K. (1999). Differential phosphorylation of syntaxin and synaptosome-associated protein of 25 kDa (SNAP-25) isoforms. J. Neurochem. **72,** 614–624.

Ros, A., Faupel, M., Mees, H., Oostrum, J., Ferrigno, R., Reymond, F., Michel, P., Rossier, J. S., and Girault, H. H. (2002). Protein purification by Off-Gel electrophoresis. *Proteomics* **2**, 151–156.

Simon, J. R., and Martin, D. L. (1973). The effects of L 2,4 diaminobutyric acid on the uptake of gamma aminobutyric acid by a synaptosomal fraction from rat brain. *Arch. Biochem. Biophys.* **157**, 348–355.

Smith, D. G., Learn, J. E., McBride, W. J., Lumeng, L., Li, T.-K., and Murphy, J. M. (2001). Alcohol-naïve alcohol-preferring (P) rats exhibit higher local cerebral glucose utilization than alcohol-nonpreferring (NP) and Wistar rats. *Alcohol Clin. Exp. Res.* **25**, 1309–1316.

Spanagel, R. (2000). Recent animal models of alcoholism. *Alcohol Res. Health* **24**, 124–131.

Waller, M. B., McBride, W. J., Lumeng, L., and Li, T.-K. (1983). Initial sensitivity and acute tolerance to ethanol in the P and NP lines of rats. *Pharmacol. Biochem. Behav.* **19**, 683–686.

Weber, G., and Bocek, P. (1996). Optimized continuous flow electrophoresis. *Electrophoresis* **17**, 1906–1910.

Weber, G., and Bocek, P. (1998). Recent developments in preparative free flow isoelectric focusing. *Electrophoresis* **19**, 1649–1653.

Williams, R. W., and Herrup, K. (1988). The control of neuron number. *Annu. Rev. Neurosci.* **11**, 423–453.

Witzmann, F. A., Li, J., Strother, W. N., McBride, W. J., Hunter, L., Crabb, D. W., Lumeng, L., and Li, T.-K. (2003). Innate differences in protein expression in the nucleus accumbens and hippocampus of inbred alcohol-preferring and -nonpreferring rats. *Proteomics* **3**, 1335–1344.

Yamakura, T., Bertaccini, E., Trudell, J. R., and Harris, R. A. (2001). Anesthetics and ion channels: Molecular models and sites of action. *Annu. Rev. Pharmacol. Toxicol.* **41**, 23–51.

Yokoyama, C. T., Sheng, Z. H., and Catterall, W. A. (1997). Phosphorylation of the synaptic protein interaction site on N-type calcium channels inhibits interactions with SNARE proteins. *J. Neurosci.* **17**, 6929–6938.

Zhou, F. C., Bledsoe, S., Lumeng, L., and Li, T.-K. (1991). Immunostained serotonergic fibers are decreased in selected brain regions of alcohol-preferring rats. *Alcohol* **8**, 425–431.

Zhou, F. C., Pu, C. F., Murphy, J., Lumeng, L., and Li, T.-K. (1994). Serotonergic neurons in the alcohol-preferring rats. *Alcohol* **11**, 397–403.

Zhou, F. C., Bledsoe, S., Lumeng, L., and Li, T.-K. (1994). Reduced serotonergic immunoreactive fibers in the forebrain of alcohol-preferring rats. *Alcohol. Clin. Exp. Res.* **18**, 571–579.

Zhou, F. C., Zhang, J. K., Lumeng, L., and Li, T.-K. (1995). Mesolimbic dopaminergic system in alcohol-preferring rats. *Alcohol* **12**, 403–412.

Zischka, H., Weber, G., Weber, P. J., Posch, A., Braun, R. J., Buhringer, D., Schneider, U., Nissum, M., Meitinger, T., Ueffing, M., and Eckerskorn, C. (2003). Improved proteome analysis of Saccharomyces cerevisiae mitochondria by free-flow electrophoresis. *Proteomics* **3**, 906–916.

Zuo, X., and Speicher, D. (2000). A method for global analysis of complex proteomes using sample prefractionation by solution isoelectrofocusing prior to two-dimensional electrophoresis. *Anal. Biochem.* **284**, 266–278.

Zuo, X., Echan, L., Hembach, P., Tang, H. Y., Speicher, D. K., Santoli, D., and Speicher, D. (2001). Towards global analysis of mammalian proteomes using sample prefractionation prior to narrow pH range two-dimensional gels and using one-dimensional gels for insoluble and large proteins. *Electrophoresis* **22**, 1603–1615.

Zuo, X., Hembach, P., Echan, L., and Speicher, D. (2002). Enhanced analysis of human breast cancer proteomes using micro-scale solution isoelectrofocusing combined with high-resolution 1-D and 2-D Gels. *J. Chromatog.* **782**, 253–265.

Zuo, X., and Speicher, D. (2002). Comprehensive analysis of complex proteomes using microscale solution isoelectrofocusing prior to narrow pH range two-dimensional electrophoresis. *Proteomics* **2**, 58–68.

PROTEOMICS STUDIES OF TRAUMATIC BRAIN INJURY

Kevin K. W. Wang,*, †, ‡, § Andrew Ottens,*, †, § William Haskins,*, †, §
Ming Cheng Liu,*, †, § Firas Kobeissy,*, †, ‡, § Nancy Denslow,*, ‖
SuShing Chen,*, ¶ and Ronald L. Hayes†, ‡, §

*Center of Neuroproteomics and Biomarkers Research, University of Florida
Gainesville, Florida 32610
†Center for Traumatic Brain Injury Studies, University of Florida, Gainesville, Florida 32610
‡Department of Psychiatry, University of Florida, Gainesville, Florida 32610
§Department of Neuroscience, University of Florida, Gainesville, Florida 32610
‖Interdisciplinary Center of Biomedical Research, University of Florida
Gainesville, Florida 32610
¶Computing and Information Science Engineering, University of Florida
Gainesville, Florida 32610

I. Introduction

With the completion of human and rat genomes, the next major technological challenge facing the biomedical community is the deciphering of the human proteome. Study of the proteome has been aided by recent advances in protein separation, protein identification/quantification, and bioinformatics. Although the application of proteomics technologies in brain injury research is still in its infancy, enormous insights can be achieved from such endeavors. There are approximately 30,000–40,000 hypothetical protein products transcribable from the human genome (Aebersold and Watts, 2002; Grant and Blackstock, 2001; Grant and Husi, 2001; Hanash, 2003; Hochstrasser et al., 2002; Service, 2001; Smith, 2000). Yet, the proteome is extremely complex. Even in a single cell type the set of proteins that are expressed, as well as their steady state levels, depend on time and the specific state of the cells in response to environmental stimuli or challenges. In addition, cellular proteins are almost constantly subjected to various forms of post-translational modifications (PTMs), including phosphory-lation/dephosphorylation by different kinases and phosphatases, proteolysis, or processing by different protease families, acetylation, glycosylation, and cross-linking by transglutaminases or conjugation to small protein tags such as ubiquitin or SUMO (similar to ubiquitin modifier) (Janssen, 2003; Schäfer et al., 2003; Schwartz and Hochstrasser, 2003). Because of these challenges, one often has to focus on a specific subproteome. The case in point is neuroproteomics, or the study of nervous system proteomes. The importance of neuroproteomics studies is that they will help elucidate the poorly understood biochemical mechanisms or pathways that currently underlie various psychiatric, neurological, and neurode-generative diseases. The example we will focus on here is traumatic brain injury (TBI), a neurological disorder currently with no Food and Drug Administration (FDA) approved therapeutic treatment.

II. Traumatic Brain Injury

Traumatic brain injury or traumatic head injury is characterized as a direct, physical impact or trauma to the head, causing brain injury (Denslow et al., 2003; Hayes et al., 2001). Annually there are 2 million TBI cases in the United States alone. They result in 500,000 hospitalizations, 100,000 deaths, 70,000–90,000 people with long-term disabilities, and 2000 people who survive but live in a permanent, vegetative state. Medical costs of TBI are estimated to be more than $48 billion annually in the United States. The cause of TBI can be broken down into the following catalogories: Motor vehicle accidents (50%), falls (21%), assault and violence (12%), sports and recreation (10%), and all others (7%) (Fig. 1). Importantly, 30–40% of all battlefield injuries also have a head injury component.

Because of intensive research both in clinical settings and in employing experimental animal models of TBI, there is now a general understanding of the pathology of TBI. Typically there is mechanical, compression-induced direct tissue injury often associated with hemorrhage and contusion at the site of

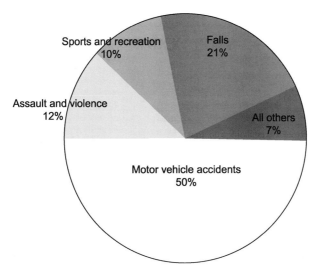

Fig. 1. Different causes of traumatic brain injury in humans.

impact. A significant amount of cell death will occur very rapidly in this zone. More distal to the injury zone, due to the impact of the force, long fiber tracts (axons) are especially at risk to this type of injury. Usually after the first phase of cell injury/death occurs, there is also the secondary injury, which is believed to be mediated by secondary biochemical events such as neurotoxic glutamate release (neurotoxicity) or oxidative damage. Other significant alterations include inflammation responses by microglia cells, astroglia activation, and proliferation. Over time, if the TBI patient survives, these events lead to long-lasting brain tissue remodeling, possibly including stem cells differentiation. Therefore the spatial and temporal levels of biochemical and proteomic changes of TBI can be investigated.

A. ANIMAL MODELS OF TBI

Over the past decades, basic science researchers have developed several animal models of TBI (Finnie, 2001; Raghupathi et al., 2000). There are several well-characterized models of TBI, including controlled cortical impact (CCI), which is controlled by compressed gas; a fluid percussion model that transduces a contusion force by the movement of fluid in the chamber, and vertical weight drop models in which a weight is dropped from a certain height within a hollow chamber for guidance. The weight drop model creates an acceleration force that

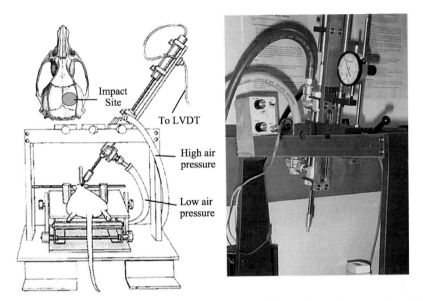

FIG. 2. Rat model of TBI: Controlled cortical impact (CCI). Left panel shows a schematic drawing of the CCI setup. Right panel is a photograph of the CCI device.

is directed to the top of the skull either unilaterally or bilaterally (reviewed by Finnie in 2001). In our work, we employ the rat CCI model of TBI (Dixon *et al.*, 1991; Fig. 2). We have argued that use of proteomics will greatly facilitate the biochemical mechanisms underlying the various phases of TBI pathology (Denslow *et al.*, 2003).

B. SOURCE OF BIOLOGICAL MATERIALS

Proteomics studies for TBI generally can be categorized into human studies, animal studies, and cell culture-based studies. For the purposes of this review, cell culture-based studies will not be discussed further. When comparing human versus. animal studies, there are pros and cons in each scenario (Table I). Regarding the sample types that can be exploited for proteomics analysis, they will include brain tissues, cerebrospinal fluid (CSF), and blood (serum and plasma). For human TBI studies, blood samples (which are further fractionated into plasma or serum) are the easiest to obtain. Interestingly, there is increasing interest now focused on using CSF because its status will reflect that status of the central nervous system itself. After severe traumatic brain injury, spinal shunt or spinal tap are routinely performed, thus obtaining CSF is not an issue. One of the major challenges of

Table I
COMPARING HUMAN VERSUS ANIMAL TBI PROTEOMIC STUDIES

	Human studies	Animal studies
Sample heterogeneity	High	Low
Environmental variables	High	Low
Brain tissue samples	Difficult to obtain (postmortem only)	Routine
CSF samples	Routine (large volume available)	Routine (small volume only)
Blood samples	Routine (large volume available)	Routine (sufficient volume available)
Results relevance to human disease	Yes	Likely (confirmation needed)

using clinical, samples-based proteomic studies is that it is extremely difficult to control individual (biological) and environmental variables (see Table I).

1. *Brain Samples*

Brain tissue from human TBI studies would inevitably come from deceased TBI patients. These brain samples could be subjected to postmortem artifacts, compounded by various and significant time delay before samples can be obtained. The biggest advantage of animal neuroproteomics studies over human counterparts is the ability to obtain brain tissues in a controlled laboratory environment. Furthermore, it is possible to harvest samples from defined anatomical regions. For example, for our TBI studies we often focus on cortical and hippocampal samples. This is important because different brain regions might be selectively more vulnerable to traumatic or ischemic insults.

2. *CSF*

CSF can be collected from the cisterna magna from lab animals such as rats and mice. CSF may contain rich brain proteome information that is relevant to disease diagnosis (Davidsson *et al.*, 2002). However, only approximate 50–100 μl can be withdrawn from rats and 25–30 μl from mice. Care must also be taken not to contaminate samples with blood as a result of puncture. Although more than one CSF draw might be possible, in our laboratory we generally withdraw only one CSF sample, followed by sacrifice. In the case of human TBI, CSF can also be collected routinely from ventriculotomy or from spinal tap. Importantly, a relatively large amount (2–5 ml) of CSF can be routinely obtained from human TBI patients from each CSF sampling time point, and repeating samples can often be achieved.

3. Blood Samples (Serum and Plasma)

In both human and animal TBI studies, blood can be routinely collected and usually further processed into either serum or plasma fractions before subjecting to proteomics analysis. Like CSF, most proteomics researchers believe there is significant proteomic information in the blood that would reflect the status of the brain, particularly after TBI caused by possible blood-brain barrier compromise (Raabe *et al.*, 1999; Romner, 2000).

C. Sample Collection and Processing Consistency

It needs to be emphasized that for proteomics results to be consistent and reproducible, one needs to use extra caution to ensure the variables can be kept to a minimum. All sample collection procedures should be discussed and finalized and the operators made familiar with the procedures. Some practice runs are highly desirable. For human studies, detailed record keeping is extremely important for future analysis or trouble-shooting purposes. For example, for human studies, CSF or blood samples should be taken at consistent intervals and before food consumption, because it might significantly affect the blood proteomics profile. For animal studies that are conducted in controlled environments, it should be possible to keep brains and biofluid sample collection time and routine as standardized as possible. Also, the animal subjects should be tagged and observed carefully and regularly, with any out-of-the-norm observations recorded. They might become very helpful in enhancing proteomics analysis. Tissue and biofluid samples, once obtained and processed, should be snap frozen and stored at $-85\ ^{\circ}C$ until use.

D. Sample Pooling Considerations

There is also an important decision to be made before the proteomics analysis (i.e., whether to pool samples for analysis or to analyze individual samples). Pooling samples significantly reduces minor individual variability and the amount of workload. Yet, at the same time its disadvantage is that it might miss certain proteomics changes that are present in only a subset of samples. On the other hand, analysis of individual samples has the advantage of being an exhaustive analysis of individual proteomics profiles but can be highly time consuming and cost-prohibitive. Another consideration is that it would be useful to pool samples when protein amount is a limiting factor.

A known biochemical marker that correlates with TBI, such as alphaII-spectrin breakdown products, can be used as positive control for quality assurance, and might even be used to guide inclusion criteria for sample pooling (Pike

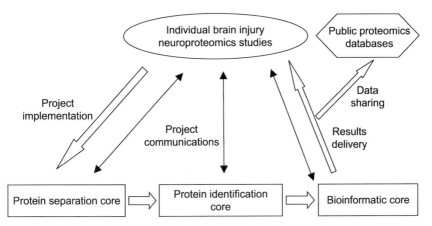

FIG. 3. Flowchart and organization of traumatic brain injury neuroproteomics studies. See text for details.

et al., 2001, 2004). It is also possible to incorporate both pooling and individual proteomics analysis in the same studies. For example, pilot studies or initial proteomics profiling of TBI can be performed with pooled samples while final detailed analysis can be done with individual samples.

III. Proteomics Analysis Overview

Regardless of whether we are dealing with human or animal samples, or whether they are tissue lysate or biofluid (CSF, serum, or plasma), the strategy we developed can be organized into three interacting, scientific disciplines or phases: protein separation, protein identification followed by quantification, and bioinformatics analysis (Fig. 3). By design, any proteomics center should spend two-thirds of its scientific and financial resources to establish a robust and readily usable proteomics platform. However, it is equally important for the center to develop new and improved neuroproteomics technologies on all fronts.

IV. Protein Separation Methods

In TBI neuroproteomics studies, we are less interested in descriptive and exhaustive characterization of the whole neuroproteome; rather we will focus on protein level or post-translational changes that occur in TBI. With this in mind, it is important to devise methods in comparing and contrasting the two proteomics data sets: control versus TBI. To productively identify all the proteins in a specific system of interest (subproteome) or a subset of proteins that are differentially expressed in TBI, it is essential that complex protein mixtures (e.g., brain samples or biofluids) be first subjected to multidimensional protein separation. Because proteins differ in size, hydrophobicity, surface charges, abundance, and other properties, there is no single protein separation method that can satisfactorily resolve all proteins in a proteome.

   To date there are two mainstream protein separation methods used for proteomic analysis: (1) two-dimensional gel isoelectrofocusing/electrophoresis and (2) multidimensional liquid chromatography.

A. Two-Dimensional Gel Electrophoresis Approach

   Two-dimensional gel electrophoresis (2DE) is the most established protein separation method for the analysis of a proteome or subproteome (Boguslavsky, 2003). It is achieved by subjecting protein mixtures to two protein separation methods under denaturing condition (in the presence of 6–8 M urea and cationic detergent such as sodium dodecylsulfate [SDS]). Traditionally proteins are first separated based on their isoelectric point (pI) value with a tube gel (polyacrylamide), by isoelectric focusing (IEF) with the aid of mobile ampholytes with different (pI) values. After IEF, the tube gel is placed atop a polyacrylamide gradient gel within which the SDS-bound proteins are separated by size. Because of poor gel consistency, the IEF step (the first dimension) is most variable. However, a recent breakthrough in IEF technology using immobilized pH gradient (IPG) strips, provides improved reproducibility (Bjellqvist *et al.*, 1982; Gorg *et al.*, 1988; Hanash, 2003; Jungblut *et al.*, 1996). Another disadvantage with 2D gels is the inevitable gel-to-gel variability in exact location and patterns of protein spots. This proves problematic when comparing two samples directly (e.g., control versus TBI brain samples).

   The recent advance of 2D-differential in-gel electrophoresis (2D-DIGE) has resolved this problem (Patton, 2002; Unlu *et al.*, 1997). The fluorescent cyanine dyes Cy3 and Cy5 are a match in molecular weight and charge but have distinct excitation and emission wavelengths (Yan, 2002). One dye is used to label control samples, and the other to label treated samples, which are then mixed and differentially compared in the same gel (Fig. 4). These advantages are incorporated into our approach, as outlined in Table I. They include in particular the high resolving power for complex mixtures of proteins and the capability of resolving post-translationally modified proteins, including acetylation, phosphorylation, glycosylation, and protein cross-linking (Janssen, 2003; Schäfer *et al.*, 2003). It is possible to annotate each protein of a proteome by pI and molecular

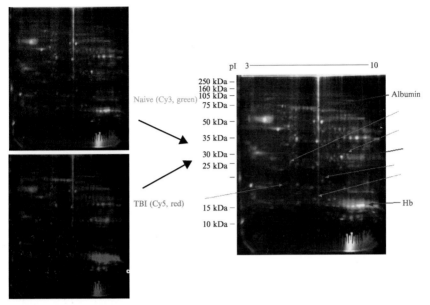

Fig. 4. Rat TBI protein separation by 2D differential in-gel electrophoresis *(DIGE)*. Pooled naïve and TBI rat cortex samples were labeled with Cy3 and Cy5 dyes, respectively (left panels) and co-run and resolved by 2DE. The fluorescence signals were merged, allowing the identification of differentially expressed proteins (right panel). Yellow spots represent proteins common to both samples. Green and orange-red spots are differentially expressed proteins in pooled naive and TBI sample, respectively. Blue arrows point to blood-borne protein contaminants found in TBI sample (e.g., albumin and hemoglobins [Hb]).

weight values in X-Y coordinates to form a 2D protein map, of which publicly accessible and searchable databases already exist (Appel *et al.*, 1999; Fountoulakis *et al.*, 1999, 2000; Lemkin, 1997; Lubec *et al.*, 2003). There are, however, several persistent weaknesses of 2D gels (See Table II). Proteins of extreme pI or minute quantity and proteins that are either very small or very large may be missed. Also, integral membrane proteins, of which many are central nervous system (CNS) disorder drug targets (membrane-bound receptors or neurotransmitter transporters), are lost because of their extreme hydrophobicity.

Regarding protein separation, there is also research in the direction of microfluidic 2D protein separation with miniaturized IEF and electrophoresis. This approach has the advantage of reducing sample usage with less waste and without compromising detection sensitivity (Derra, 2003; Reyes *et al.*, 2002).

B. Two-Dimensional Liquid Chromatography Approach

Alternative protein separation methods are needed to overcome some of the shortcoming of 2D gels. Recently there has been significant movement toward multidimensional liquid chromatography methods to resolve complex protein mixtures (Peng and Gygi, 2001). The general idea draws on classic chromatographic principles including size chromatography (gel filtration), ionic interaction (strong cation exchange [SCX] and strong anion exchange [SAX]), hydrophobic interaction (C4- or phenyl-agarose chromatography), and IEF chromatography. One can envision combining multiple chromatographic approaches in a series to achieve multidimensional separations. In our own work we have also combined the use of a size exclusion column (SEC) and a SAX column (Fig. 5) in series with some success. Challenging this method are: (1) incompatibilities of buffer components (e.g., salt concentration, organic components) and (2) the logistics of configuring fraction elution from one column with loading of a second column. Often, individual fractions are manually loaded onto the second column, but this is extremely labor intensive and may introduce run-to-run variability.

When selecting chromatographic separation methods, considerations must be given to take advantage of the size, pI, and hydrophobicity differences of the proteins of interest. In addition, when dealing with membrane-bound proteins, the chromatographic method must be compatible with the use of the proper

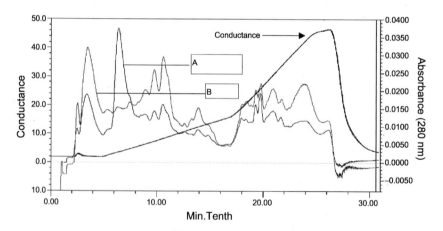

Fig. 5. Example of rat brain protein separation by strong ion exchange chromatography. Protein elution (30 min, 30 fractions) chromatograms (proteins are measured as absorbance at 280 nm). A = pooled rat cerebellum lysate and B = pooled rat cerebrum lysate. Chromatographic differences between A and B are detected readily throughout the elution. The third line is relative conductance measured over the NaCl gradient elution of the column.

neutral detergent (e.g., Triton X-100 or CHAPS). Importantly, minute proteins can be concentrated to enhance their detection. One weakness of this approach is that even with 2D liquid chromatographic (LC) separation, it is often not possible to separate all proteins individually. This problem will be addressed in the next section. In summary, when compared to 2DE, tandem LC is more compatible with membrane-bound proteins and can enrich proteins in minute quantity.

V. Protein Identification and Quantification Methods

The approach we are taking represents an effort to apply systematically the most contemporary proteomics approaches to identify and develop clinically useful biomarkers for brain injury from trauma, disease, or drugs. Classical methods of protein identification involving protein separation by gels or LC (see previous section), coupled with mass spectrometry, provide a potent and novel methodological array never before applied systematically to the detection of biomarkers of CNS injury, either alone or in combination. This integrated strategy makes possible both "targeted" analyses of known potential biomarker candidates as well as "untargeted" searches for novel proteins and protein fragments that could prove even more useful. Each of these technologies has advantages and disadvantages that together complement each other. Thus combining multiple proteomics strategies optimizes the opportunity for successful brain injury proteomics studies. Lastly, protein identification research also benefits from improved bioinformatics tools for protein database searching (Chakravarti et al., 2003). Thus, importantly, research designs must incorporate appropriate bioinformatics support (see next Section).

A. MASS SPECTROMETRY APPROACH

1. MALDI-TOF MS

The most classical method for protein identification in a given protein mixture is to perform 2DE, followed by in-gel digestion of the gel band(s) of interest with protein identification by mass spectrometry. The 2D-gel method has been improved by the use of IPG strips for the first dimension and the ability to label protein samples from control and experimental tissues with cyanine dyes (e.g., Cy3 and Cy5) that form co-migrating labeled samples that are compared in the same gel. Differentially expressed proteins are easily found, cut from the gel, digested in the gel spot with trypsin, and then identified by MALDI-TOF MS (matrix-assisted laser desorption ionization time-of-flight mass spectrometry) approach (Bienvenut et al., 2002). It is important to understand that

MALDI-TOF MS identifies peptides based on the accurate determination of peptide masses. Because each amino acid has a unique mass, any given peptide composed of a unique amino acid sequence will have a unique mass. However, this method of protein identification is not infallible. Peptides can have identical amino acid composition but with a different order, or more often peptides of similar length will have mass-to-charge values that are slightly, but indistinguishably, different from one another within the mass accuracy and resolution limits of the instrumentation. Thus it is common practice to use at least four to nine peptide fragments to positively identify a protein, which can be difficult with complex mixtures. In addition, any significant post-translational modifications that will change the mass-to-charge (m/z) value of multiple peptides will make protein identification extremely difficult (Table II).

By using 2D-gel separation, this method is useful for distinguishing proteins that are either up-regulated or down-regulated because of to injury, but it is suboptimal for finding very basic, very acidic, or hydrophobic proteins, and the identification of smaller peptides can be difficult because of chemical noise from matrix ions. Complementary to this method are direct MS procedures that capture the entire range of proteins and peptides but may not distinguish proteins that are post-translationally modified, and the maximal protein size is limited to approximately 25–30 kDa (kilodaltons). A modified MALDI approach, called surface-enhanced laser desorption ionization (SELDI) (invented by Ciphergen, Fremont, CA), combines an affinity matrix-based protein separation phase with the TOF MS-based protein mass determination (also called Protein Chips) (Wiesner, 2004).

2. LC-MS/MS Approach

Protein separations strategies including 1D- and 2D-LC techniques (Adkins *et al.*, 2002) and gel separations are commonly used to resolve complex protein mixtures. Subsequent LC fractions or gel bands are processed by in-solution or in-gel digestion (most often with trypsin) to form peptides small enough to be effectively measured by MS. Complex peptide mixtures of protein digests are typically separated by reverse-phase chromatography placed on-line with electrospray ionization mass spectrometry (ESI MS), which not only resolves peptides from one another but also concentrates them, providing greater sensitivity. LC-MS is most often performed on high-powered tandem mass spectrometers, including the quadrupole ion-traps (QIT), quadrupole time-of-flight (QTOF), and Fourier transform ion cyclotron resonance (FT-ICR) mass spectrometers. Tandem mass spectrometry (MS/MS) allows the advantage of providing peptide sequence information in addition to the parent peptide mass (Gygi *et al.*, 2000). (Figs. 6 and 7). In brief, ions of the peptide of interest are isolated (first stage of mass spectrometry) then fragment along the peptide backbone by colliding with neutrals. Pairs of b- and y-daughter ions, formed by fragmentation from the n- or c-terminal side of each residue, respectively, will predominantly be generated.

Table II

ATTRIBUTES OF VARIOUS PROTEIN IDENTIFICATION APPROACHES

Protein identification method	Strengths	Weaknesses
MALDI-TOF MS	-Can analyze both proteins and peptides	-Ion suppression with complex samples (no peptide separations)
	-High mass accuracy ± 0.01%	
	-Resolution 50 ppm	-Does not provide sequence information
	-Protein ID by mass mapping of peptides from tryptic digests	-Requires detection of multiple peptides for protein identification
	-Sensitive to 50 fmol routine	
	-Rapid analysis for high throughput	
	-Preserves sample for later analysis	
LC-MS/MS	-Provides peptide sequence for protein ID—less reliant on mass accuracy	-Slow sample analysis due to long chromatograms
	-Can reliably identify protein with 1 to 2 peptides	-Consumes entire sample loaded
	-Sensitive in the amol range	-Greater complexity of nano-LC requires dedicated operator
	-Provides precise/reproducible quantitation	
	-Routine analysis of multiprotein digests	
Antibody panels/arrays	-Easy protein ID decoding	-Non exhaustive
	-Easy confirmation	-Uneven sensitivity
	-Can potentially detect PTM	
	-Sensitive to high fmol range	

The b- and y-daughter ions are then mass analyzed to form a daughter ion spectrum (second stage of mass spectrometry). Using MS/MS information, the peptide sequence can be reconstructed, which can be performed rapidly with available bioinformatics software (see Table II). LC-MS/MS systems work extremely well for protein identification by coupling the generated mass and sequence information with database searches, and the technique is sensitive enough to identify pM levels of proteins present in complex mixtures such as tissue lysates.

B. PROTEIN AND PEPTIDE QUANTIFICATION BY MS

There are currently no less than half a dozen MS-based protein/peptide quantification methods, which were reviewed recently (Denslow, 2003). We will focus on two prominent quantification methods that are applicable to TBI proteomics.

1. *ICAT*

Isotope-coded affinity tags (ICAT) are a direct chromatographic approach to evaluate differential expression (Gygi *et al.*, 1999). ICAT reagent pairs are cysteine-binding tags that differ in molecular weight by use of hydrogen or carbon isotopes. These reagents are used to differentially label two protein samples, which are then mixed together and digested into peptides. Cysteine-containing fragments labeled with the tags can then be selectively isolated and analyzed by LC-MS/MS with differential expression determined from the peak height ratio of the tagged peptides. MS/MS data on the peptides is then searched against a protein database, providing the identity of the differentially expressed proteins (Peng *et al.*, 2003; Yates *et al.*, 1999).

2. *AQUA*

Another innovative method to quantify differential expression is through the use of *A*bsolute *qua*ntitation (AQUA) probes (Gerber *et al.*, 2003). Unlike ICAT, which can be used to tag any cysteine-containing protein, AQUA is applicable

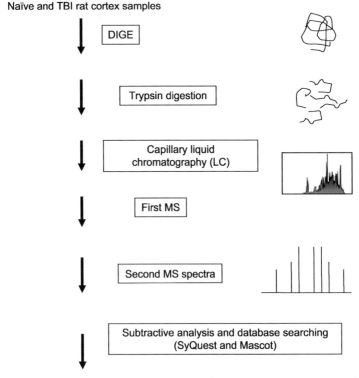

Fig. 6. Schematic sample flow of protein separation/protein identification by LC-MS/MS. See text for details.

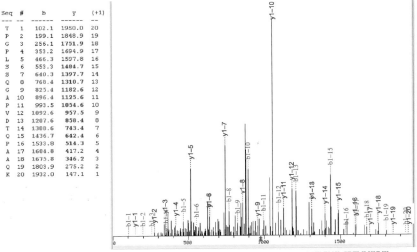

Seq	#	b	y	(+1)
T	1	102.1	1950.0	20
P	2	199.1	1848.9	19
G	3	256.1	1751.9	18
P	4	353.2	1694.9	17
L	5	466.3	1597.8	16
S	6	553.3	1484.7	15
S	7	640.3	1397.7	14
Q	8	768.4	1310.7	13
G	9	825.4	1182.6	12
A	10	896.4	1125.6	11
P	11	993.5	1054.6	10
V	12	1092.6	957.5	9
D	13	1207.6	858.4	8
T	14	1308.6	743.4	7
Q	15	1436.7	642.4	6
P	16	1533.8	514.3	5
A	17	1604.8	417.2	4
A	18	1675.8	346.2	3
Q	19	1803.9	275.2	2
K	20	1932.0	147.1	1

MAFSKGFRIY HKLDPPPFSL IVETRHKEEC LMFESGAVAV LSSAEKEAIK GTYAKVLDAY GLLGVLRLNL GDTMLHYLVL
VTGCMSVGKI QESEVFRVTS TEFISLRVDA SDEDRISEVR KVLNSGNFYF AWSASGVSLD LSLNAHRSMQ EHTTDNRFFW
NQSLHLHLKH YGVNCDDWLL RLMCGGVEIR TIYAAHKQAK ACLISRLSCE RAGTRFNVRG TNDDGHVANF VETEQVIYLD
DCVSSFIQIR GSVPLFWEQP GLQVGSHRVR MSRGFEANAP AFDRHFRTLK DLYGKQIVVN LLGSKEGEHM LSKAFQSHLK
ASEHASDIHM VSFDYHQMVK GGKAEKLHSV LKPQVQKFLD YGFFYFDGSA VQRCQSGTVR TNCLDCLDRT NSYQAFLGLE
MLAKQLEALG LAEKPQLVTR FQEVFRSMWS VNGDSISKIY AGTGALEGKA KLKDGARSVT RTIQNNFFDS SKQEAIDVLL
LGNTLNSDLA DKARALLTTG SLRVSEQTLQ SASSKVLKNM CENFYKYSKP KKIRVCVGTW NVNGGKQFRS IAFKNQTLTD
WLLDAPKLAG IQEFQDKRSK PTDIFAIDFE EMVELNAGNI VNASTTNQKL WAVELQKTIS RDNKYVLLAS EQLVGVCLFV
FIRPQHAFFI RDVAVDTVKT GMGGATGNKG AVAIRMLFHT TSLCFVCSHF AAGQSQVKER NEDFVEIARK LSFPMGRMLF
SHDYVFWCGD FNYRIDLPNE EVKELIRQQN WDSLIAGDQL INQKNAGQIF RGFLEGKVTF APTYKYDLFS EDYDTSEKCR
TPAWTDRVLW RRRKWPFDRS AEDLDLLNAS FQDESKILYT WTPGTLLHYG RAELKTSDHR PVVALIDIDI FEVEAEERQK
IYKEVIAVQG PPDGTVLVSI KSSAQENTFF DDALIDELLQ QFAHFGEVIL IRFVEDKMWV TFLEGSSALN VLSLNGKELL
NRTITITLKS PDWIKTLEEE MSLEKISVTL PSS~~TSTLLG EDAEVSADFD MEGDVIB~~DYSA EVEELLPQHL QPSSSGLGT
SPSSSPRTSP CQSPTAPEYS APSLPIRPSR APS⌈TPGPLS SQGAPVDTQP AAQK⌉SSQTI EPKRPPPPRP VAPPARPAPP
QRPPPPSGAR SPAPARKEFG APKSPGTARK DNIGRNQPSP QAGLAGPGPS GYGAARPTIP ARAGVISAPQ SQARVSAGRL
TPESQSKPLE TSKGPAVLPE PLKPQAAFPP QFSLFTPAQK LQDPLVPIAA PMPPSIPQSN LETPPLPPPR SRSSQSLPSD
SSPQLQQEQP TG

Mass (mono): 142869.8   **Identifier:** gi|1166575   **Database:** C:/Xcalibur/database/rat.fasta
Protein Coverage: 262/1292 = **20.3%** by amino acid count, 28224.7/142869.8 = **19.8%** by mass

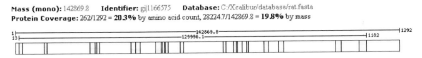

Tryptic peptide ID: TPGPLSSQGAPVDTQPAAQK

Fig. 7. Example of LC-coupled MS-MS identification of a protein differentially expressed in rat brain hippocampus after TBI. A protein band (in an SDS-PAGE gel) that is uniquely expressed in TBI-48 hr was cut out and digested with trypsin, and a distinct tryptic peptide was sequenced based on MS-MS data (top panel) and identified to be originated from a brain protein synaptojanin, based on proteomics database searching results (lower panel).

only to target proteins. A peptide of the selected protein is synthesized with an isotopically labeled amino acid. A known amount of the probe is then added to the digested sample, which is analyzed by LC-MS/MS. Because the probe exactly matches the endogenous peptide of interest except for a modest mass difference, the two will coelute with reverse-phase chromatography and have identical ionization properties, which minimizes variation in ion signal intensities. The tandem mass spectrometer then resolves the two peptides by the small m/z difference, allowing the ion signal of the two to be compared across the chromatographic peak. This method is very precise and can be applied to nearly any protein (with or without cysteine). By accurately measuring the amount of probe added, the absolute amount of a protein can also be determined, though relative protein amounts can also be determined without having to know the exact amount of probe added. In practice this method would follow a nontargeted differential method such as 2D-DIGE or ICAT, which produces a list of potential differentially expressed proteins. This method can then be used to quickly and precisely validate the differential expression of the targeted proteins across many samples. In comparison to the more traditional targeted quantitation of western analysis, AQUA is a much quicker way of validating differential expression than waiting for a specific antibody to be developed.

C. ANTIBODY PANEL/ARRAY APPROACH

Protein identification is also assisted by the availability of various platforms of antibody arrays or panels (e.g., Zyomyx protein biochips, BD Powerblot, and BD antibody arrays) (Graslund *et al.*, 2002; James 2002; Kusnezow and Hoheisel, 2002; Moody, 2001). These methods all rely on antibody-based capturing of the protein of interest. The quantitation of the captured protein can be performed by prelabeling (including differential labeling) of the protein with fluorescent dye(s) (dye-labeling detection) such as BD antibody arrays, which is similar to the gene chip mRNA quantification method. Alternatively, quantitative detection can be accomplished with a second primary antibody specific to the same protein antigen (sandwich detection), which is similar to the sandwich enzyme-linked immunoabsorbant assay (sandwich ELISA) method (e.g., Zyomyx protein Biochips). A third option is the BD Powerblot, which is a high-throughput Western blotting (immunoblotting) system with two distinct protein samples that are differentially subjected to a set of five blots. Each blot has 39 usable lanes with the use of a manifold system. Each lane is developed with five to six different fluorophore-linked monoclonal antibodies (toward antigen with nonoverlapping molecular weight). With this method samples are probed with a total of 1000 monoclonal antibodies. We have actually conducted several Powerblot experiments with animal TBI studies. Figure 8 gives examples of differential protein changes observed in the rat hippocampus after TBI.

The major advantage of the antibody panel or array approach is that proteins of interest can be readily identified, because all antibodies used have known antigens and their positional assignment on the antibody chip or panel is

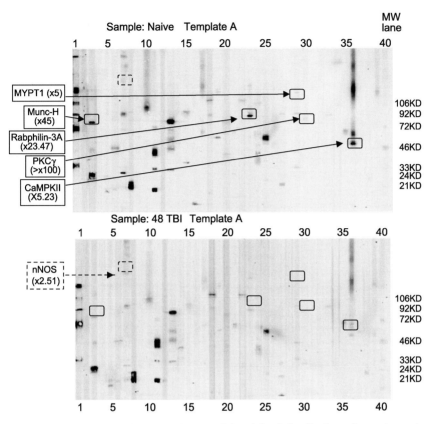

Fig. 8. Example of antibody panel approach-based by indentification of several protein differentially expressed in rat brain hippocampus after TBI. When comparing pooled naïve (top panel) and TBI-48 hr (bottom panel) hippocampal samples, five proteins (MYPT1, Munc-H, Rabphilin-3A, PKCdelta and CaMpKll; solid line) with reduced levels and one protein (nNOS; dotted line) with increased levels after TBI (average fold changes are shown in brackets) were identified.

known (See Table II). Also, quantification is already built into this antibody-based approach without any additional effort. On the other hand, the major disadvantage of this approach is that it is practically impossible to be exhaustive, because one would only have high fidelity antibodies to a subset of proteins. Furthermore, using antibodies collected from many different sources will likely result in uneven sensitivity. As in other immunoassay methods (e.g., Western blotting, immunostaining, or ELISA), it is a given that antibody array methods will likely detect nonspecifically bound proteins or other substances, affecting quantitation with high chemical noise and leading to false positive reactions. Despite its shortcoming, the antibody array-based protein identification approach is a useful complement to the MS-based approach discussed previously.

VI. TBI Proteomics Bioinformatics

The current advance in databases and web portals has a natural convergence for knowledge and data sharing among local and remote scientists in any National Institutes of Health (NIH) domain. Large databases will be networked, whereas web portals will "federate and access" large databases. Such efforts need to be developed for the neuroproteomics domain. Neuroscience has one of the most complex information structures—concepts, data types, and algorithms— among scientific disciplines. Its richness in organisms, species, cells, genes, and proteins and their signal-transduction pathways provides many challenging issues for biological sciences, computational sciences, and information technology. The advances in neuroscience urgently need developing portal services to access databases for analyzing and managing the following information: sequences, structures, and functions arising from genes, proteins, and peptides (e.g., protein segments and biomarkers) (Chakravarti *et al.*, 2003).

In the bioinformatic phase, two interlinked mandates are: (1) to build a local user-friendly proteomics database, and (2), to develop interoperable proteomics tools and architecture for multiple data integration and to integrate user and public domain-based databases (Fig. 9). Data analysis applications should interoperable with database operations and portal access. The TBI proteomics core technologies will provide an integrative approach to genomic and proteomics information by developing a common portal architecture—the TBI proteomics portal—at the University of Florida for data archiving and retrieval among core researchers and end users, and data linking and sharing to national and international neuroproteomics websites (e.g., Human Proteome Organization [HUPO, United States]) (Hanash, 2004) and Human Brain Proteome Project (HBPP, Germany) (Meyer *et al.*, 2003). Lastly, bioinformatic tools and software are also needed to enhance our ability to data mine as well as to study protein-protein interaction, protein pathways and networks, and complex post-translational modification such as protein phosphorylation, processing, cross-linking, and conjugation. This will help us develop knowledge bases about neuroproteomics functions and signal-transduction pathways in terms of dynamic objects and processes (Cattell, 1996; Mendes, 1993, 1997; Reddy, 1993; Somogyi, 1996). In addition, clinical information should be integrated with genomics and proteomics databases. The three major functions of the bioinformatic component of TBI proteomics studies can be further explained in the following section.

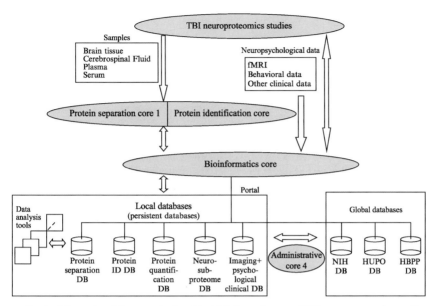

FIG. 9. Schematics of the central role of the bioinformatic core of TBI neuroproteomios studies. The bioinformatics core not only plays a key role in analyzing and archiving protein separation and identification data, but also plays a key role in integrating local TBI databases to global neuroproteome databases. See text for details.

A. PERMANENCE

Permanence is defined here as developing local databases for proteomics separation and identification and linking with national and international data sources. Local databases will include chromatograms, mass spectra, gel images, peptide and protein sequences, and functional magnetic resonance imaging (fMRI) images for control and TBI samples. Data modeling and semantics will be developed by proteomics and computer scientists together, so that semantic equivalence of search attributes and semantic associations can be established.

Our bioinformatics core is in the process of combining different data semantics and knowledge trees in separate genomics, proteomics, and clinical databases. A key requirement is the development of semantics (or ontology) of biological information, which is then captured in two components—semantic indexing and metainformation (i.e., "information about information")—of the intelligent search engines. A book by Chen (1998) has described these two important methods. Furthermore, semantic indexing and metainformation complement each other, reduce the complexity of neural taxonomy and classification, and correlate semantically the proteomics types and phenotypes (e.g., behavior in drug abuse) at various (e.g., subcellular, cellular, and tissue or fluid) levels of neural activities. Dissemination to national and international data sources (e.g., HUPO and HBPP) will be consistently maintained through our intelligent search engines.

B. INTEROPERABILITY

Interoperability is defined here as integrating existing data analysis tools with local databases. A proteomics problem-solving environment will be established to provide users with rapid access to TBI neuroproteome center databases and analysis tools. This will include existing tools for proteomics research and drug abuse research. The range of these tools is very broad, from peptide sequencing and protein identification to image processing for fMRI images and data analysis for neuropsychological tests and diagnosis.

A critical component of our bioinformatics core is to conduct research at widely distributed resources of data analysis and multiple levels of proteomic clinical and behavior information. The distributed collections of heterogeneous information resources will be large-scale. The intelligent search engines are beyond the capability of current web search engines and protocols. The TBI neuroproteome center distributed information retrieval component is a set of search engines that extend Emerge. Such an intelligent search engine should allow nomenclature, syntactic, and semantic differences in queries, data, and meta information. It should permit type, format, representation, and model differences as well in databases. In our TBI neuroproteome research, we have to compare information among proteomics and clinical data, such as chromatograms, mass spectra, gel images, peptide and protein sequences, and fMRI images. We will need a set of interoperable search engines to guide users finding information of various domains, formats, types, and levels of granularity (e.g., peptide, protein, cell, and system levels).

In addition, the interoperability of databases and analysis tools will establish a proteomics problem-solving environment. Thus users of the problem-solving environment will also be factored into the interoperability. Whatever users need—small versus large data sets, interactive versus batch computation—will require design and implementation of data and event services. For the current studies we intend to develop a neuroproteomics workbench to gather a collection of data analysis tools for neuroproteomics, as well as TBI neuroproteomics datasets:

1. Peptide sequencing and protein identification by MALDI-TOF MS and LC-MS/MS (Lu and Chen, 2003; Tabb et al., 2002).
2. Protein peak patterns and single protein retention time from 1D or 2D liquid chromatograms.

3. Protein database searching algorithms such as SEQUEST (Yates, 1998).

The integration of databases with proteomic computational algorithms will be based on the object-oriented data modeling and data semantics discussed earlier. The Object Data Management Group (ODMG)-compliant data analysis and databases are highly relevant to the Common Component Architecture. In high-throughput computing, in terms of parallel or multithreaded objects, components (data and algorithms alike) may be distributed over a wide area grid of resources and distributed services.

C. Data Mining

Our neuroproteomics initiative has placed significant effort in new data mining and analysis tools for differential protein expression, protein network and modification analysis, and validation. A unique data-mining workbench will be created to explore protein network and pathways underlying the pathobiology of TBI from a neuroproteomics perspective. Novel data-mining tools will include a differential analysis tool for research on proteins and protein fragments involved in TBI and construction of cognitive maps. Furthermore, the cognitive maps will be used for TBI-induced differential neuroproteome validation and possible brain injury diagnosis.

1. *Creating Cognitive Maps for TBI-Induced Differential Proteome*

New data mining tools for TBI-induced differential proteome analysis and validation are being developed at our center. There are three major zones of neuroproteomics information: (1) pathophysiological stasis (including TBI, other CNS injuries such as ischemic stroke, aging, environmental toxin or substance-abuse–induced brain injury, and neurodegenerative diseases such as Alzheimer's or Parkinson's), (2) neuroproteome stasis (pathology-mediated differential protein expression, protein synthesis and metabolism, alternative mRNA splicing and RNA editing, protein-protein interaction, enzymatic activity, or protein functions), post-translational modifications (e.g., protein cross-linking, acetylation, glycosylation protein proteolysis and processing, phosphorylation), and protein-protein interaction and networks and signal-transduction pathways, and (3) sources of neuroproteomics data (Fig. 10). These sources include brain tissue (from different areas or anatomical regions of the brain, such as hippocampus and cerebral cortex), biological fluids such as CSF, and blood samples (including plasma and serum) in which brain proteins stasis might be reflected upon via diffusion-based equilibrium or blood-brain barrier compromise (e.g., from brain to CSF to blood).

Collection of data from these three components will enable the construction of multiple cognitive maps (Axelrod, 1976; Kohn and Letzkus, 1983; Kosko,

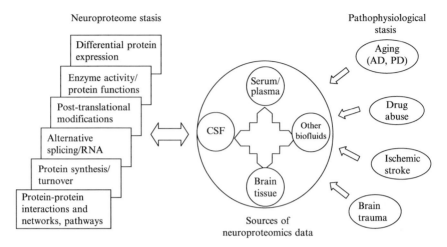

Fig. 10. Putative cognitive maps for the brain injury neuroproteome. The brain injury cognitive maps encompass three major areas (pathophysiological stasis, neuroproteome stasis, and sources of neuroproteomic data).

1986; Shi *et al.*, 2002; Zhang *et al.*, 1989). For instance, cognitive maps will be constructed for the TBI-induced differential proteome, such as the one shown in Fig. 9 for the brain injury neuroproteome. Automated reasoning and knowledge discovery algorithms (Chen, 1986, 1987; Chen and Markowitz, 1995, 1988, 2000a; Kitano, 2000) will distill the information and present the knowledge gained from a systems biology perspective. Thus cognitive maps will enable the brain trauma researchers to gain a greater understanding of the entire TBI-induced differential neuroproteome and hopefully the mechanistic protein-pathways of TBI.

2. Using Cognitive Maps for TBI-induced Differential Neuroproteome Validation

A statistical analysis tool is also being developed for TBI-induced differential neuroproteome validation and possible TBI protein-pathways elucidation. For example, up- or down-regulation of multiple proteins and protein fragments in control and injured samples will be quantified by ICAT, AQUA, or ELISA to validate differential TBI neuroproteome. Linear discriminant analysis (LDA) will be used to calculate the probability of a correct diagnosis given the number of injury-specific biomarkers measured the number of samples, etc. Thus statistical analysis tools are expected to provide an important component for all the TBI neuroproteomics research conducted at our neuroproteomics center.

VII. Prospective Utilities of TBI Proteomics Data

In summary, proteomics study of both human and rat traumatic brain injury, if approached systemically, is a very fruitful and powerful analytical technology. To obtain a comprehensive TBI neuroproteome dataset, it is important to integrate multiple protein separation and protein identification technologies. Equally important is the optimization of individual protein separation and identification methods. The bioinformatic platform then becomes the critical adhesive component by serving two purposes: (1) integrating all proteomics datasets and other relevant biological or clinical information, and (2) inferring and elucidating the protein-based pathways and biochemical mechanisms underlying the pathobiology of TBI and identifying and validating biomarkers for the diagnosis and monitoring of TBI (Goldknopf et al., 2003). Ultimately, if we are to be successful, the TBI proteomics approach outlined here must be further integrated with genomics, cytomics, as well as systems biology approaches (Kitano, 2002a,b).

References

Adkins, J. N., Varnum, S. M., Auberry, K. J., Moore, R. J., Angell, N. H., Smith, R. D., Springer, D. L., and Pounds, J. G. (2002). Toward a human blood serum proteome: Analysis by multidimensional separation coupled with mass spectrometry. *Mol. Cell Proteomics* **1,** 947–955.

Aebersold, R., and Watts, J. D. (2002). The need for national centers for proteomics. *Nature Biotech.* **20**(7), 651.

Appel, R. D., Bairoch, A., and Hochstrasser, D. F. (1999). 2-D databases on the World Wide Web in methods in molecular biology. *In* "2-D Proteome Analysis Protocols" (A. J. Link, Ed.), vol. 112, pp. 383–391. Humana Press, Totowa, N.J.

Axelrod, R. (1976). "Structure of Decision." Princeton University Press, Princeton, NJ.

Bienvenut, W. V., Deon, C., Pasquarello, C., Campbell, J. M., Sanchez, J. C., Vestal, M. L., and Hochstrasser, D. F. (2002). Matrix-assisted laser desorption/ionization-tandem mass spectrometry with high resolution and sensitivity for identification and characterization of proteins. *Proteomics* **2,** 868–876.

Bjellqvist, B., Ek, K., Righetti, P. G., Gianazza, E., Gorg, A., and Westermeier, R. (1982). Isoelectric focusing in immobilized pH gradients: Principle, methodology and some applications. *J. Biochem. Biophys. Methods* **6,** 317–339.

Boguslavsky, J. (2003). Resolving the proteome by relying on 2DE methods. *Drug Discovery Develop.* **6**(7), 57–60.

Cattell, R. G. G. (Ed.) (1996). "The Object Database Standard: ODMG-93." Morgan Kaufmann, San Mateo, CA.

Chakravarti, D. N., Chakrarti, B., and Moutsatsos, I. (2003). Informatic tools for proteome profiling. High throughput proteomics; protein arrays. *BioTechnoques* **3**(Suppl.), 4–15.

Chen, S. (1988). Knowledge acquisition on neural networks, uncertainty and intelligent systems. *In* "Lecture Notes in Computer Science" (B. Bouchon, L. Saitta, and R. R. Yager, Eds.), vol. 313, pp. 281–289. Springer-Verlag.

Chen, I. A., and Markowitz, V. M. (1995). An overview of the object protocol model (OPM) and the OPM data management tools. *Information Systems* **20**, 393–418.

Chen, S., (1986). Some extensions of probabilistic logic, Proc. AAAI Workshop on Uncertainty in Artificial Intelligence, Philadelphia, August 8–10, 1986, pp. 43–48, an extended version appeared in "Uncertainty in Artificial Intelligence," vol. 2, (L. N. Kanal, and J. F. Lemmer Eds.), North-Holland, Amsterdam, Holland.

Chen, S. (1987). Automated reasoning on neural networks: A probabilistic approach. IEEE First International Conference on Neural Networks, San Diego, June 21–24, 1987.

Chen, S. (2000a). Knowledge discovery of gene functions and metabolic pathways. IEEE BioInformatic and Biomedical Engineering Conference, Washington, November 2000.

Chen, S. (1998). "Digital Libraries: The Life Cycle of Information." BE Publisher, Columbus, OH.

Davidsson, P., Westman-Brinkmalm, A., Nilsson, C. L., Lindbjer, M., Paulson, L., Andreasen, N., Sjogren, M., and Blennow, K. (2002). Proteome analysis of cerebrospinal fluid proteins in Alzheimer patients. *Neuroreport* **13**(5), 611–615.

Denslow, N. D., Michel, M. E., Temple, M. D., Hsu, C., Saatman, K., and Hayes, R. L. (2003). Application of proteomics technology to the field of neurotrauma. *J. Neurotrauma* **20**, 401–407.

Derra, S. (2003). Lab-on-a-chip technologies emerging from infancy. *Drug Disc. Develop.* **6**(5), 40–45.

Dixon, C. E., Clifton, G. L., Lighthall, J. W., Yaghmai, A. A., and Hayes, R. L. (1991). A controlled cortical impact model of traumatic brain injury in the rat. *J. Neurosci. Methods* **39**(3), 253–262.

Fang, Z., Polacco, M., Chen, S., Schroeder, S., Hancock, D., Sanchez, H., and Coe, E. (2003). cMap: The comparative genetic map viewer. *Bioinformatics* **19**, 416–417.

Finnie, J. (2001). Animal models of traumatic brain injury: A review. *Aust. Vet. J.* **79**(9), 628–633.

Fountoulakis, M., Hardmaier, R., Schuller, E., and Lubec, G. (2000). Differences in protein level between neonatal and adult brain. *Electrophoresis* **21**(3), 673–678.

Fountoulakis, M., Schuller, E., Hardmeier, R., Berndt, P., and Lubec, G. (1999). Rat brain proteins: Two-dimensional protein database and variations in the expression level. *Electrophoresis* **20**(18), 3572–3579.

Gerber, S. A., Rush, J., Stemman, O., Kirschner, M. W., and Gygi, S. P. (2003). Absolute quantification of proteins and phosphoproteins from cell lysates by tandem MS. *Proc. Natl. Acad. Sci. USA* **100**, 6940–6945.

Goldknopf, I., Park, H. R., and Kuerer, H. M. (2003). Merging diagnostics with therapeutic proteomics. *IVD Technology* **9**(1), 1–6.

Gorg, A., Postel, W., and Gunther, S. (1988). The current state of two-dimensional electrophoresis with immobilized pH gradients. *Electrophoresis* **9**, 531–546.

Grant, S. G., and Blackstock, W. P. (2001). Proteomics in neuroscience: From protein to network. *J. Neurosci.* **21**(21), 8315–8318.

Grant, S. G. N., and Husi, H. (2001). Proteomics of multiprotein complexes: Answering fundamental questions in neuroscience. *Trends Biotechnol.* (Suppl. 10), S49–S54.

Graslund, S., Falk, R., Brundell, E., Hoog, C., and Stahl, S. (2002). A high-stringency proteomics concept aimed for generation of antibodies specific for cDNA-encoded proteins. *Biotechnol. Appl. Biochem.* **35**(Pt 2), 75–82.

Gygi, S. P., Rist, B., Gerber, S. A., Turecek, F., Gelb, M. H., and Aebersold, R. (1999). Quantitative analysis of complex protein mixtures using isotope-coded affinity tags. *Nat. Biotechnol.* **17**, 994–999.

Gygi, S. P., *et al.* (2000). Mass spectrometry and proteomics. *Analytical Techniques* **4**, 489–494.

Hanash, S. (2004). HUPO initiatives relevant to clinical proteomics. *Mol. Cell Proteomics.* 298–301.

Hanash, S. M. (2003). Disease proteomics. *Nature* **422**(6928), 226–232.

Hayes, R. L., Newcomb, J. K., Pike, B. R., and Deford, S. M. (2001). Contributions of calpains and caspases to cell death following traumatic brain injury. In "Head Trauma: Basic, Preclinical and Clinical Aspects" (L. P. Miller and R. L. Hayes, Eds.), vol. 10, pp. 219–237. Wiley & Sons, New York, NY.

Hochstrasser, D. F., Sanchez, J. C., and Appel, R. D. (2002). Proteomics and its trends facing nature's complexity. Proteomics 2(7), 807–812.

James, P. (2002). Chips for proteomics; a new tool or just hype? High throughput proteomics; protein arrays BioTechniques 12(Suppl.), 14–23.

Janssen, D. (2003). Major approaches to identifying key PTMs. Genomics and Proteomics 3(1), 38–41.

Jungblut, P., Thiede, B., Zimny-Arndt, U., Muller, E. C., Scheler, C., and Wittmann-Liebold, B. (1996). Resolution power of two-dimensional electrophoresis and identification of proteins from gels. Electrophoresis 17, 839–847.

Kitano, H. (2000). Perspectives on systems biology, "New Generation Computing," Vol. 18, No. 3. Ohm-sha, Springer-Verlag, New York Inc.

Kitano, H. (2002a). Systems biology: A brief overview. Science 295(5560), 1662–1664.

Kitano, H. (2002b). Computational systems biology. Nature 420(6912), 206–210 (review).

Kohn, M. C., and Letzkus, W. J. (1983). A graph theoretical analysis of metabolic regulation. J. Theoretical Biology 100, 293–304.

Kosko, B. (1986). Fuzzy cognitive maps. Int. J. Man-Machine Studies 24, 65–75.

Kusnezow, W., and Hoheisel, J. D. (2002). Antibody microarrays: Promises and problems. High throughput proteomics; protein arrays. Bio Tech. 12(Suppl.), 14–23.

Lemkin, P. F. (1997). Comparing two-dimensional electrophoretic gel images across the Internet. Electrophoresis 18, 2759–2773.

Lu, B., and Chen, T. (2003). A suffix tree approach to the interpretation of tandem mass spectra: Applications to peptides of non-specific digestion and post-translational modifications. Bioinformatics 19(Suppl. 2), II113–II121.

Lubec, G., Krapfenbauer, K., and Fountoulakis, M. (2003). Proteomics in brain research: Potentials and limitations. Prog. Neurobiol. 69(3), 193–211.

Mendes, P. (1993). GEPASI: A software package for modelling the dynamics, steady, states and control of biochemical and other systems. Comput. Appli. Biosci. 9, 563–571.

Mendes, P. (1997). Biochemistry by numbers: Simulation of biochemical pathways with Gepasi 3. Trends Biochem. Sci. 22, 361–363.

Meyer, H. E., Klose, J., and Hamacher, M. (2003). HBPP and the pursuit of standardisation. Lancet Neurol. 2(11), 657–658.

Moody, M. D. (2001). Array-based ELISAs for high-throughput analysis of human cytokines. Bio Tech. 31, 186–194.

Patton, W. F. (2002). Detection technologies in proteome analysis. J. Chromatogr. B. Analyt. Technol. Biomed. Life Sci. 771(1–2), 3–31.

Peng, J., Elias, J. E., Thoreen, C. C., Licklider, L. J., and Gygi, S. P. (2003). Evaluation of multidimensional chromatography coupled with tandem mass spectrometry (LC/LC-MS/MS) for large scale protein analysis: The yeast proteome. J. Proteome Res. 2, 43–50.

Peng, J., and Gygi, S. P. (2001). Proteomics: The move to mixtures. J. Mass. Spectrom. 36(10), 1083–1091.

Pike, B. R., Flint, J., Dave, J. R., Lu, X.-C. M., Wang, K. K. W., Tortella, F. C., and Hayes, R. L. (2004). Accumulation of calpain and caspase-3 proteolytic fragments of brain-derived all-spectrin in CSF after middle cerebral artery occlusion in rats. J. Cereb. Blood Flow Metab. 24(1), 98–106.

Pike, B. R., Flint, J., Dutta, S., Johnson, E., Wang, K. K. W., and Hayes, R. L. (2001). Accumulation of non-erythroid all-spectrin and calpain-cleaved all-spectrin breakdown products in cerebrospinal fluid after traumatic brain injury in rats. J. Neurochem. 78, 1297–1306.

Raabe, A., Grolms, C., and Seifert, V. (1999). Serum markers of brain damage and outcome prediction in patients after severe head injury. *Br. J. Neurosurg.* **13,** 56–59.

Raghupathi, R., Graham, D. I., and McIntosh, T. K. (2000). Apoptosis after traumatic brain injury. *J. Neurotrauma* **17**(10), 927–938.

Reddy, V. N., Mavrovouniotis, M. L., and Liebman, M. N. (1993). Petri net representations in metabolic pathways. *Proc. ISMB* **1,** 328–336.

Reyes, D. R., Iossifidis, D., Auroux, P. A., and Manz, A. (2002). Micro total analysis systems. I. Introduction, theory, and technology. *Anal. Chem.* **74**(12), 2623–2636.

Romner, B., Ingebrigtsen, T., Kongstad, P., and Borgesen, S. E. (2000). Traumatic brain damage: Serum S-100 protein measurements related to neuroradiological findings. *J. Neurotrauma* **17**(8), 641–647.

Schäfer, H., Marcus, K., Sickmann, A., Herrmann, M., Klose, J., and Meyer, H. E. (2003). Identification of phosphorylation and acetylation sites in alphaA-crystallin of the eye lens (mus musculus) after two-dimensional gel electrophoresis. *Anal. Bioanal. Chem.* **376**(7), 966–972.

Schwartz, D. C., and Hochstrasser, M. (2003). A superfamily of protein tags: Ubiquitin, SUMO and related modifiers. *Trends Biochem. Sci.* **28**(6), 321–328.

Service, R. F. (2001). Gold rush—High-speed biologists search for gold in proteins. *Science* **294**(5549), 2074–2077.

Shi, H., Rodriguez, O., Shang, Y., and Chen, S. (2002). Integrating adaptive and intelligent techniques into a web-based environment for active learning. *In* "Intelligent Systems: Technology and Applications" (C. T. Leondes, Ed.), vol. 4, pp. 229–260. CRC Press, Boca Raton, Fla.

Smith, R. D. (2000). Probing proteomes—seeing the whole picture? *Nat. BioTech.* **18,** 1041–1042.

Somogyi, R., and Sniegoski, C. A. (1996). Modeling the complexity of genetic networks: Understanding multigenic and pleiotropic regulation. *Complexity* **1,** 45–63.

Tabb, D. L., McDonald, W. H., and Yates, J. R. (2002). DTASelect and contrast: Tools for assembling and comparing protein identifications from shotgun proteomics. *J. Proteome Res.* **1,** 21–26.

Unlu, M., Morgan, M. E., and Minden, J. S. (1997). Difference gel electrophoresis: A single gel method for detecting changes in protein extracts. *Electrophoresis* **18**(11), 2071–2077.

Wiesner, A. (2004). Detection of tumor markers with ProteinChip technology. *Curr. Pharm. Biotechnol.* **5**(1), 45–67.

Yan, J. X., Devenish, A. T., Wait, R., Stone, T., Lewis, S., and Fowler, S. (2002). Fluorescence two-dimensional difference gel electrophoresis and mass spectrometry based proteomic analysis of *Escherichia coli. Proteomics* **2**(12), 1682–1698.

Yates, J. R., III, Carmack, E., Hays, L., Link, A. J., and Eng, J. K. (1999). Automated protein identification using microcolumn liquid chromatography-tandem mass spectrometry. *In* "Methods in Molecular Biology" (A. J. Link, Ed.), vol. 112, pp. 553–569. Human Press, Totowa, N. J.

Yates, J. R., Morgan, S. F., Gatlin, C. L., Griffin, P. R., and Eng, J. K. (1998). Method to compare collision-induced dissociation spectra of peptides: Potential for library searching and subtractive analysis. *Anal. Chem.* **70,** 3557–3565.

Zhang, W. R., Chen, S., and Bezdek, J. C. (1989). Pool2: A generic system for cognitive map development and decision analysis. *IEEE Trans. SMC* **19,** 31–39.

INFLUENCE OF HUNTINGTON'S DISEASE ON THE HUMAN AND MOUSE PROTEOME

Claus Zabel and Joachim Klose

Institute for Human Genetics
Charité—University Medicine Berlin
Berlin, Germany 13353

I. Introduction

Neurodegenerative diseases are inherited or sporadic conditions characterized by an increasing dysfunction of the nervous system. Often these disorders are
accompanied by an atrophy of the affected central and peripheral structures of
the nervous system. The most common neurodegenerative disorder is Alzheimer's disease. Of all people older than age 65, 7–10% of individuals (and 40% of
those older than age 80) are affected (Price and Sisodia, 1998). Parkinson's
disease, another common neurodegenerative disease, affects approximately one
million people in the United States (Olanow and Tatton, 1999). Apart from these
common neurodegenerative disorders there are rare disorders that are often
caused by a single defective gene. Some of these disorders are caused by the
extension of labile trinucleotide repeats that occur in exons as well as introns
of genes. Examples of the occurrence of the trinucleotide in an intron are
the fragile X syndrome and myotonic dystrophy (Gusella and MacDonald,

241

1996). If the trinucleotide occurs in an exon, it codes in some disorders such as Huntington's disease (HD) for the amino acid glutamine (Gusella and MacDonald, 1996; Zoghbi and Orr, 2000).

II. Neurodegenerative Disorders Caused by Elongated Poly-Glutamine Repeats

The number of known neurodegenerative diseases caused by an extension of a polyglutamine repeat is ever increasing. At least nine so-called polyglutamine diseases have been found (Bates, 2003). These diseases include spinobulbar muscular atrophy, spinocerebral ataxia, and HD (Zoghbi and Orr, 2000). HD affects approximately 1 in 10,000 individuals (Vonsattel and DiFiglia, 1998). It affects approximately 30,000 American citizens and is therefore one of the most common monogenetically inherited neurodegenerative diseases (McMurray and McMurray, 2001).

A. Huntington's Chorea

Huntington's disease is an autosomal dominant inherited disorder that usually presents in midlife and causes death 15–20 years after the first symptoms occur (Telenius et al., 1993). The disease-triggering mutation consists of an unstable, elongated CAG trinucleotide repeat at the 5' end of the HD gene IT15 first exon. The cytosine-adenine-guanine (CAG) repeat codes for a chain of glutamines (HDCRG, 1993). The number of polyglutamine repeats in the gene product of IT15, Huntingtin (Htt) (HDCRG, 1993), is one of the most important factors that determine the time of onset of the disorder. Individuals with 6–35 glutamines are not affected. Those with 36–39 have an increased risk of acquiring the disease, and repeats of 40 and above always cause the disease (Bates, 2003). If at least one of the alleles of the IT15 gene trespasses the threshold of 36 repeats, then the disease may occur (McMurray and McMurray, 2001; Wanker, 2000). The larger the number of the polyglutamine repeats, the earlier the age of onset (Telenius et al., 1993). The most severely affected neurons are the medium spiny neurons in the striatum of the brain (Sharp and Ross, 1996). The disease-causing protein of HD, Htt, is ubiquitously expressed in the body. Why it selectively causes the death of medium spiny neurons is not known. Nonetheless, several functions were already assigned to Htt. It was proposed to be involved in vesicle transport (Li et al., 2000), and had a role in the endosomal lysosomal pathway (Velier et al., 1998) and the regulation of the production of a growth factor that is derived from the neocortex, that is, brain-derived neurotrophic factor (BDNF) (Zuccato et al., 2001). BNDF is necessary for the survival of striatal neurons, which die in people who have HD. Recently it has been shown that Htt with an expanded polyglutamine repeat inhibited histone acetylation. This was done by directly inhibiting histone acetylases or by their recruitment into aggregates (Bates, 2001; Steffan *et al.*, 2001). In accordance with these results it could be shown that histone deacetylase inhibitors reduced the toxicity of expanded polyglutamine repeats (McCampbell *et al.*, 2001). The regulation of normal Htt fragment aggregation could be facilitated by Arfaptin 2 (Peters *et al.*, 2002). A potential function of Htt could be the inhibition of cell death by interaction with Hip-1. The extension of the polyglutamine repeat results in a reduction of binding efficiency to Hip-1. As a consequence, unbound Hip-1 can interact with the protein, Hippi, which may result in the recruitment of caspase 8. By means of the extrinsic receptor mediated cell death pathway, of which caspase 8 is a part, apoptosis could be triggered (Gervais *et al.*, 2002). Apoptosis is a process in which a prior defined sequence of biochemical and morphological alterations is triggered, allowing a cell to die without negatively affecting its neighbors (Mattson, 2000). The afore-mentions data show that there are many hints as to a possible function of Htt *in vivo*. When looking for a definitive answer, though, there is still a long way to go, because experiments so far were conducted mainly *in vitro*. Therefore the suggested functions merely present possibilities but not definitive answers.

B. PROTEOMICS WITH HUNTINGTON'S CHOREA

Even though there has been an extensive search for the function of the disease causing Htt, it is most probably not the protein alone that is responsible for the disease. Therefore it is important to identify as many changes during the pro-gression of disease as possible on the RNA, as well as on the protein level. In the last few years many studies have been performed that deal with the identification of as many mRNA alterations as possible during HD progression. The technique employed was the use of cDNA chips (Chan *et al.*, 2002; Luthi-Carter *et al.*, 2000, 2002a,b). Extensive studies on alterations of the mRNA level were carried out on oligonucleotide microarrays with one of the mouse models of HD, R6/2. Of the altered mRNA detected by means of those arrays, a selection was uniformly confirmed by northern blot (Luthi-Carter *et al.*, 2002a,b). In one paper (Luthi-Carter *et al.*, 2002a), selected alterations were also confirmed on the protein level in which, in all but one case (7/8), the expression change had the same direction on the mRNA and the protein level (Luthi-Carter *et al.*, 2002a). Apart from valuable information on the identity of the altered singular protein, some patterns in differential mRNA expression became clear as well (e.g., the changes of mRNAs regulated by the transcription factor Sp) (Luthi-Carter *et al.*, 2002a). To comple-ment these encouraging datasets on the mRNA level, a characterization of the proteome (the expressed genome) of this mouse model (R6/2) was carried out. Differential protein expression and post-translational modifications that went undetected by means of the mRNA analysis are accessible by a proteomics study. Their characterization is the next logical step after mRNA analysis.

1. *Proteomics in Neurodegenerative Diseases*

Before beginning a proteomics study it is important to consider some points with regard to planning and execution. The proteome of the tissue to be investigated consists of proteins that are expressed over time (Swinbanks, 1995). Protein expression depends on the developmental state of the tissue, and when studying a disorder, on the presence or absence of disease and its progression. To draw conclusions about the pathological changes that result in disease, it is important to have a reference tissue free of disease. To judge whether a proteomics study will be feasible is therefore dependent on the availability of the conditions "healthy" (normal) and "disease." Conclusions drawn solely on the grounds of the disease-affected tissue are not possible because there is no means to detect changes.

2. *Limiting Diversity in a Proteomics Study*

When choosing a species to be investigated, one should be aware of the advantages and limitations of that species, especially with regard to the information one will be able to obtain when carrying out a proteomics study. When investigating HD by means of postmortem tissues obtained from humans, the data obtained will be directly relevant for the human disorder. Because of their limited complexity, histological and morphological investigations yield good results with human sample material (DiFiglia *et al.*, 1997; Gutekunst *et al.*, 1999). If proteins from tissue are to be separated by large gel, two-dimensional gel electrophoresis (2DE), several thousand protein spots with intensities varying several orders of magnitude are generated on a single gel, resulting in a highly complex pattern (Klose, 1999c; Klose and Kobalz, 1995). Several factors may be responsible for spots found to be differentially expressed after comparing two different conditions (HD versus control). Disease unrelated protein polymorphisms within a species e.g., due to mutations, altered structure, or post-translational modifications are but one group. Physiological alterations, caused by metabolism, as well as limited reproducibility within the method used, constitute other categories. Finally, it is possible that the differences found are caused by the disorder under study. Post-translational processing and modifications are especially responsible for the increase in diversity when comparing RNA versus protein level. In humans this diversity is still increased by heterogeneity within the species. This problem of high variability in protein expression within the species *Homo sapiens* due to polymorphisms within the species naturally persists, even though highly reproducible large gel 2DE was used for the study (Klose, 1999c; Klose and Kobalz, 1995). This heterogeneity does not exist in animal models, in which inbreeding is the rule rather than the exception. Inbred animals have a homogenous genome that produces the same proteins with identical polymorphisms in each animal. Most often, differences between two proteomes to be compared, such as disease versus healthy control, are quantitative (spot intensity) and not qualitative (changing location of one or more spots [mobility variants]) in nature. This is an observation that was also made for the heterozygosity within a species in mice (Klose, 1999b), in which the differences within two mouse species were also characterized by quantitative differences between protein spots rather than their additional presence or their absence. These discrepancies might very well mask alterations in protein expression that are present because of disease. Again, this heterozygosity within a species can be omitted by using an inbred animal model for the disease under study, which drastically reduces the heterogeneity between two samples.

3. Selection of the Appropriate Model System

An important point for the study of HD is the selection of an appropriate inbred animal model to investigate all aspects of the disease, especially its progression over time. For the selection the question to be answered by the experiments has to be taken into account. When a neurodegenerative disease such as HD is investigated, it is important that the brain of the model animal (e.g., mouse) is relatively similar to the human brain, although the generation time should be significantly shorter. Therefore the mouse was selected as a good compromise in the study at hand. Figure 1 shows a relatively high degree of similarity of the protein spot pattern in equivalent sections of large 2D gels between the two species of mouse (Mus musculus) and human (Homo sapiens). A major advantage of a (mouse) model is that it can, in contrast to humans, be experimentally manipulated in a targeted manner, which simplifies the verification of complex hypothesis. The inbred model system selected shows a good reproducibility of most of the spot pattern between control and transgenic animals (see Fig. 1). This is important because it serves as internal standard for staining intensity and 2DE run reproducibility. Therefore, even if the number of differentially expressed spots is modest and the degree of variation is small, differences can still be readily detected. A different picture presents itself if one considers humans. The comparison of human HD and control samples yielded many differences that varied between sample pairs (see Fig. 1). The comparison of two controls or two HD brains also yielded many differences that equaled the number of the spots between HD and control (data not shown). The limitation of the mouse model system, however, is that the results obtained have to be verified in the human system.

4. Availability of Samples from Mouse and Humans

The access to suitable human sample material, contrasting blood or urine, is a problem not to be underestimated. Genetic disorders such as HD are rare, and the availability of sample material is limited; each individual sample is precious.

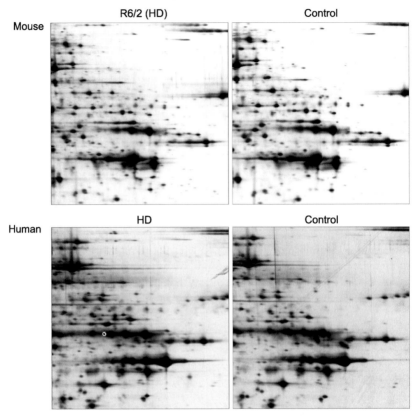

Fig. 1. Pattern reproducibility beyond species barriers, comparison of the reproducibility of the species mouse and human. 2D-gel sections from the basic side (pH range 6.0–9.5) of representative sample pairs of the species Homo sapiens (human) and Mus musculus (mouse) show clear pattern similarities. Note the high degree of similarity between the mouse R6/2 (HD) and control sample pair. The sample pair from the mouse was from 8-week-old mice. The human sample pair was taken from postmortem anterior cingulate cortex samples. At time of death the patients were 61 (HD) and 62 (control) years old.

Requests for human sample material from the brain to a tissue bank are honored only after supplying data from studies with an animal model showing promising results that justify the request. Another problem with human material is that it is mostly collected from the final stage of the disease. Samples from individuals who died before the final stage of the disease are extremely rare and highly sought after. These individuals are most likely victims of accidents and have to be diagnosed with HD before death to even be considered to belong to the group of postmortem donors. A person who meets these requirements is rare.

The number of suitable samples is decreased further by that fact that many brains are stored for extended periods at $4\,^\circ$C and/or conserved by means of formalin and then frozen. This is detrimental to the proteins in the sample. They can be modified or degraded during the time span at $4\,^\circ$C, and formalin can modify the proteins. Because of the limited sample availability at early stages, HD time course studies are nearly impossible. Interesting HD cases with juvenile or even child-age onset—displaying a very severe progression and early death and large alterations in protein expression—are also extremely rare. In addition to this limitation, there is a high demand for just these samples. Strict ethical guidelines in many countries demand special permission for the utilization of human material. To get this permission is time consuming, and when obtained, the research with human material does not warrant meaningful results. The availability of mouse material is due to almost indefinite breeding capacity, no sample limitation, and the optimal sample acquisition by removal shortly after death and immediate freezing, far superior to human material. Getting permission to conduct animal experiments even with transgenics is much easier and less time consuming. Another advantage is that mice are raised in the exact same location, control, and transgenic/test animals alike, drastically reducing differences in the proteome caused by the environment.

5. What Type of Information Can be Obtained by a Proteomics Study?

When carrying out a proteomics study in the context of investigating the mechanisms at work in any neurodegenerative disorder, one has to be aware of the results that might be obtained. After investigating the proteome at different time points during the progression of the disorder, one gets an expression pattern of different proteins during disease progression relative to the expression of those proteins in controls. Investigating different tissues increases the knowledge about protein expression by the variable tissue. Therefore one gets data on expression of many proteins over time in different tissues, and how protein expression varies among tissues. To increase the information obtained by the study even further, the samples can be fractionated before separation, according to different biochemical features such as hydrophobicity, subcellular localization, and many more (Dreger, 2003; Klose, 1999a). As a proteomics study is carried out today, it lays the foundation for further, more classical biochemical investigations that give information about possible interaction partners and protein function, as well as bioinformatics studies of known domains. When all the information has been gathered, it may yield a clue about the function of the proteins that were identified to be differentially expressed in HD. Although the proteomics study is a nonhypothesis-driven approach that widens one's horizon with ideas about what additional proteins might be involved in HD, it still needs support from more classical methods to generate meaningful results about HD (e.g., new starting points but no endpoints for investigation are generated).

III. Approach for an HD Proteomics Study

HD was already investigated by mouse models (Mangiarini *et al.*, 1996; Reddy *et al.*, 1998; Schilling *et al.*, 1999) and in humans (DiFiglia *et al.*, 1997). The changes on the RNA and protein level described so far are not conclusive to describe the dysfunction of neurons that contributes to the mechanism that leads to their decline and death (Turmaine *et al.*, 2000). Because of this fact, proteins that act outside the presently known metabolic pathways involved in the disease still have to be identified. The goal of an HD proteomics study is to identify proteins relevant to disease by first investigating the brain proteome of a well-established mouse model (R6/2) (Mangiarini *et al.*, 1996). This is accomplished by separating soluble, membrane, and DNA associated mouse brain proteins by large gel 2DE. Brain regions obtained postmortem from humans affected by HD will be scanned for differential expressions of candidate proteins from the murine system. An investigation of additional tissues in the mouse model was carried out to define the tissue expression profile of the proteins previously identified in the brain and to scan for additional proteins affected by HD not seen in the brain.

IV. Materials and Methods

In the field of proteomics the method applied for the study of a given proteome determines much about the outcome of the study. In our laboratory we have developed the large gel 2DE for years and have gained a large amount of experience with it. The 2DE method is one of the few available that is able to quantify changes on the protein level, including post-translational modifications. This technique has already been described in detail elsewhere (Klose, 1999c; Klose and Kobalz, 1995). Therefore the technique is introduced only where we emphasize points important for our comparative proteomics study.

Many differences seen in a biological system are very small or even minute. Therefore it is of utmost importance to create and compare only large 2D gels with very high reproducibility. This is achieved by treating the gels to be compared in the same way (i.e., sample preparation and electrophoresis runs are carried out in parallel, as was the staining procedure), and only gels run in such a way are compared. Reproducibility issues arise if gels are used from different runs (Molloy *et al.*, 2003). A standardized sample preparation protocol is essential for high-quality 2D gels (Klose, 1999a). For quantitative analysis, silver-stained gels were evaluated because of high sensitivity (Klose, 1999c). For protein identification, Coomassie Brilliant Blue G250 stained gels were used because of their superior compatibility with mass spectrometry (Scheler *et al.*, 1998).

V. Proteomics Study of HD

To investigate HD the proteome of brain, heart, liver, and testes of the Htt exon 1 transgenic mouse model R6/2 and of control mice of the same gender, age, and genetic background was compared by large gel 2DE. Depending on the type of tissue used, 4, 8, or 12 gel pairs were studied. Many thousand protein spots per time point investigated were compared. The exact number of spots per large 2D gel differed among the tissues investigated (liver ~9000, brain ~8000, heart ~5000, and testes ~10,000). To address the question of whether the results obtained are relevant to humans, the proteome of three brain regions with approximately 4000–5000 spots per gel were evaluated. Only spot differences that differed in all gel pairs of a time point investigated were taken into account. The evaluation of the spot pattern visible on the 2D gels resulted in the identification of five differentially expressed proteins belonging to three different protein families. In human tissue the differential expression of one protein identified in the mouse model could be confirmed.

A. Investigation of the Brain Proteome in Mice and Humans

After the evaluation of the total brain proteome of the mouse, it became clear that, interestingly, only a very small number of proteins were differentially expressed between R6/2 and control mice. The spot pattern of sample pairs showed hardly any difference, even close to terminal disease (Fig. 2). After evaluation of all spots, significant disease-relevant differences on the level of expression of only three proteins were detected. The difference in expression of one of those proteins became obvious only after studying further tissues. The localization of the protein spots in the 2D gel, the identification and subcellular distribution, and their expression during disease progression will be described in the following sections, and an attempt will be made to answer the question: How relevant are these results for the human disease?

1. *Differential Protein Expression Close to Terminal Disease in the Mouse Brain*

At the beginning of the study we intended to identify disease-specific differences in the brain proteome close to terminal disease (12 weeks) in transgenic R6/2 mice, a stage in which the largest differences in expression were to be expected between diseased and healthy tissue. To compensate for existing, small variations, only sample pairs were compared to each other that were run in parallel in the first and second dimension of the large gel 2DE.

a. R6/2 Mouse Brains Show Differential Expression of only Three Proteins Close to Terminal Disease. Three different fractions of the brain with proteins enriched from the cytoplasm, the membrane, and chromatin (Klose, 1999a) were

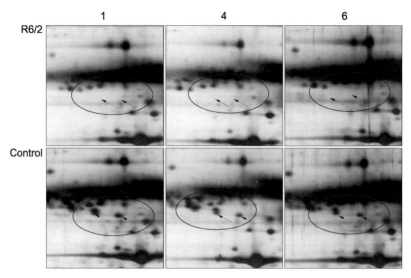

FIG. 2. Expression of AAT 1-5 seen in the cytoplasmic extract from mouse brains affected by HD close to terminal disease. Sample pairs 1, 4, and 6 from mice at 12 weeks of age are shown (See Table I). Three examples demonstrate the absence (arrows) of the AAT 1-5 spots in transgenic mice. The circles highlight the area in the gel sections of each sample pair where the AAT 1-5 spot group is absent in R6/2 mice. (Used with permission of the publisher from Zabel, C., Chamrad, D. C., Priller, J., Woodman, B., Meyer, H. E., Bates, G. P., and Klose, J. (2002). Alterations in the mouse and human proteome caused by Huntington's disease. *Mol. Cell Proteomics* **1**, 366–375, Fig. 1A.)

investigated from 12-week-old mice. The fractionation and independent separation of the protein fractions with 2DE made it possible to resolve and investigate a larger number of proteins than would have been possible using a total extract. The results obtained with each of the a fore mentioned fractions will now be shown in detail.

i. α1-Antitrypsin 1-5 is no longer detectable in the cytoplasmic fraction of R6/2 mouse brain extracts. In the pH range of 3.5–6.0 the 2D gels of R6/2 mice missed a three spot group in all eight HD/control sample pairs (See Fig. 2). All three spots in the spot group on the acidic side of the 2D gel were identified by mass spectrometry and belong to one of five existing murine isoforms of the serine protease inhibitor α1-antitrypsin 1-5 (AAT 1-5; database entry alpha1-antitrrypsin 1-5 precursor; Swiss Prot. #Q00898). The observed isoelectric point (pI) of 5.3 (determined from the 2D gel) for AAT 1-5 coincides well with 5.4 of the one calculated. The observed molecular weight of 61 kDa differs by 15 kDa from the one calculated (46 kDa).

ii. AAT 1-5 in the membrane and nuclear fraction. In addition to the cytoplasmic fraction of the mouse brain, two more fractions were investigated. Proteins solubilized by urea and detergent extraction (fraction 2) constitute the membrane fraction. DNA-binding proteins were released by DNAse (fraction 3) and encompass the nuclear fraction. The differences in the distribution pattern of proteins among these three fractions are shown in detail elsewhere (Klose, 1999a). No more differentially expressed proteins could be identified in the two additional fractions. AAT 1-5 could, in contrast to the cytoplasmic fraction (see Fig. 2), only be found in very small amounts in the membrane fraction, which could hint at a potential partial membrane association of the protein or a small overlap with the cytoplasmic fraction because of the fractionation procedure (Fig. 2 versus Fig. 3). In the nuclear fraction the protein was detectable in trace amounts in control gels and not detectable in R6/2 gels, which argues again for an almost exclusive cytoplasmic localization (Fig. 4).

   b. Reduced Expression of Contrapsin in R6/2 Mouse Brains. A spot group identified in the pH region of 3.5–6 with an average molecular weight of 70 kDa and a pI of nearly five could be assigned to the protein contrapsin (CTS, database entry contraspin; Swiss Prot. #Q62257) by mass spectrometry. The molecular weight of 70 kDa was 23 kDa higher than the one calculated (46.6 kDa). This spot group was mostly absent in R6/2 gels (six out of eight) but present in all control gels close to terminal disease. With one exception, where the expression was the same, it was always higher or much higher in the control brain (Fig. 5 and Table I). Contrapsin was not detected in the membrane and nuclear fractions of R6/2 and control mice (data not shown).

   c. Murine Brains Close to Terminal Disease Show a Reduced Expression of αB-Crystallin.

   i. Reduced expression of αB-crystallin in the cytoplasmic/nucleoplasmic fraction. In the pH region between 6.0–9.5 there was a quantitative difference in the expression of one spot detected in all eight sample pairs studied (Fig. 6; see Table I). Mass spectrometry determined the protein that this spot represents is αB-crystallin (ABC) (database entry alphaB-crystallin; Swiss Prot. #P23927). The molecular weight was determined to be 23 kDa by sodium dodecyl sulfate polyacrylamide gel electrophoresis (SDS-PAGE) in the second dimension. This differs from the calculated value (20.5 kDa) by only 2.5 kDa. The pI was determined to be 7.5 by means of isoelectric focusing (IEF) in the first dimension of the large 2D gel. This meant a difference of 0.6 pH units to the one calculated. This alteration in pI could be an indication of a post-translational modification to the protein.

   ii. Reduced expression of ABC close to terminal disease in R6/2 mice was also seen in the membrane and nuclear fraction. ABC was also detected in the membrane and the nuclear fraction. The expression of the protein did not decrease as compared to the cytoplasmic/nucleoplasmic fraction. As has been already seen in the cytoplasmic/nucleoplasmic fraction, the expression of ABC was lower in samples from R6/2 mice (Figs. 7 and 8).

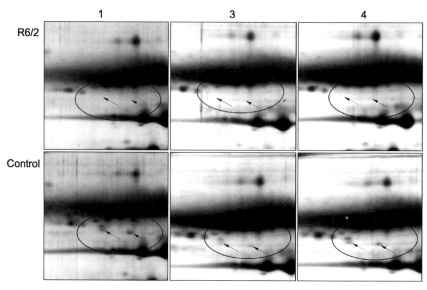

Fig. 3. Expression of AAT 1-5 in the membrane fraction close to terminal disease. Gel sections of three representative sample pairs (1, 3, and 4) show a weak expression of AAT 1-5 in control mice. Expression is absent in R6/2 mice.

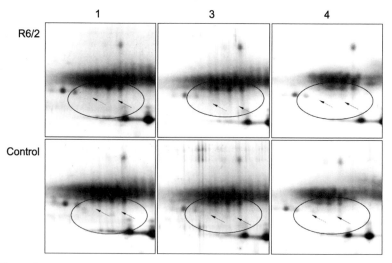

Fig. 4. Expression of AAT 1-5 in the nuclear fraction close to terminal disease. Gel sections of three representative sample pairs show no expression of AAT 1-5 in R6/2 and control mice at the age of 12 weeks. A very small amount of AAT 1-5 was expressed in the control mice, although this is hardly detectable in the figure.

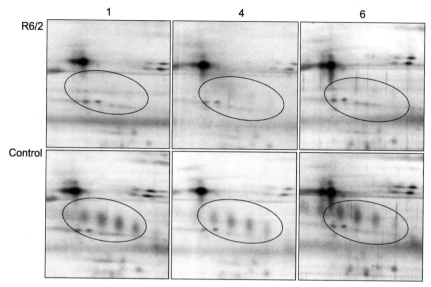

FIG. 5. 2D gel sections displaying CTS expression in the cytoplasmic extract of the brain close to terminal disease. Sample pairs 1, 4, and 6 from mice at 12 weeks of age are shown (see Table I). All three examples demonstrate a reduced level of CTS expression in transgenic mice.

2. Expression of AAT 1-5, CTS, and ABC During Disease Progression

The expression of AAT 1-5, CTS, and ABC in the cytoplasmic/nucleoplas-leoplasmic fraction of three selected time points in the disease progression—early (4 weeks), advanced (8 weeks), and close to terminal disease (12 weeks)—was probed to receive an overview with regard to their expression during disease progression.

a. Reduction of AAT 1-5 Expression with Disease Progression. In the early stage of the disease (e.g., 4 weeks), R6/2 mice showed heterogeneous AAT 1-5 expression (see Table I). One R6/2 mouse expressed the protein at a level that was seen in 12-week-old control mice, whereas other R6/2 mice showed no detectable expression. The expression of AAT 1-5 in control mice was heterogeneous as well. This indicates that AAT 1-5 was expressed in R6/2 mice at a level very close to control mice. After the disease progressed for 4 more weeks (8 weeks), AAT 1-5 could be detected in five out of eight R6/2 mice only at very low levels, whereas control mice at the same age displayed a high expression level of the protein (Fig. 9; Table I). The decrease in expression of all the spots in the three spot group was simultaneous, which suggested that a common pathway was responsible. As has already been discussed, there was no detectable expression of AAT 1-5 in R6/2 mice close to terminal disease (12 weeks). The expression in control mice at the same age was high (see Figs. 2 and 9 and Table I).

TABLE I
AAT, CTS, AND ABC EXPRESSION OVER TIME

Animals (no.)[a]	AAT 1-5		CTS		ABC	
	R6/2	Control	R6/2	Control	R6/2	Control
4 Weeks						
1	++	−	+	+	+	+
2	++	+	+	−	+	+
3	++	+++	−	+	+	+
4	++	+	−	+	+	+
5	+	+	+	+	+	+
6	+	+	+	+	+	+
7	+	−	−	+	+	+
8	+	+	−	+	+	+
9	+	+	+	−	+	+
10	+	++	−	−	+	+
11	−	+	+	−	+	+
12	−	−	+	+	+	+
8 Weeks						
1	++	+++	−	+	+	++
2	+	++	−	+	+	++
3	+	+++	+	+	+	++
4	+	++	+	+	+	++
5	+	+++	(+)	+	+	++
6	−	++	−	+	+	++
7	−	++	−	+	+	++
8	−	+++	(+)	+	+	++
12 Weeks						
1	−	+++	−	+(+)	+	+++
2	−	+++	−	+	+	+++
3	−	+++	+	+	+	+++
4	−	+++	(+)	++	+	+++
5	−	+++	−	++	+	+++
6	−	+++	−	++	+	+++
7	−	+++	−	+	+	+++
8	−	+++	−	+	+	+++

[a]Declaration of symbols: spot is present (+++) spot intensity of control mice at 12 weeks of age; spot is present, but the intensity is reduced (++); spot is present, but the intensity is severely reduced (+); spot is not detectable (−). (Used with permission of the publisher from Zabel, C., Chamrad, D. C., Priller, J., Woodman, B., Meyer, H. E., Bates, G. P., and Klose, J. (2002). Alterations in the mouse and human proteome caused by Huntington's disease. *Mol. Cell Proteomics* **1,** 366–375, modified from Table I.)

b. Reduction of CTS Expression with Disease Progression. The decrease in expression of CTS during the progression of disease mirrored the one seen in AAT 1-5. The CTS expression in R6/2 and control mice at 4 weeks was heterogeneous (see Table I). After the disease advanced, there was a reduced CTS expression at

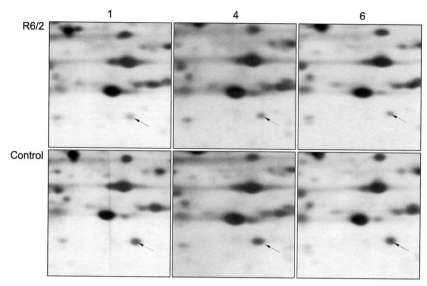

Fig. 6. 2D gel sections displaying ABC expression in the cytoplasmic extract of the brain close to terminal disease. Sample pairs 1, 4, and 6 from mice at 12 weeks of age are shown (see Table I). All three examples demostrate a reduced level of ABC expression in transgenic mice. (Used with permission of the publisher from Zabel, C., Chamrad, D. C., Priller, J., Woodman, B., Meyer, H. E., Bates, G. P., and Klose, J. (2002). Alterations in the mouse and human proteome caused by Huntington's disease. *Mol. Cell Proteomics* **1**, 366–375, Fig. 1B.)

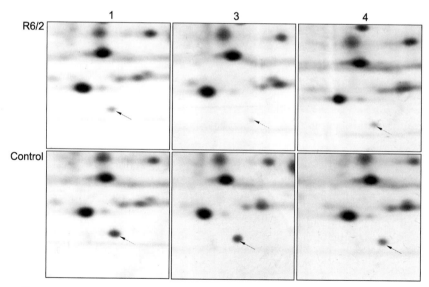

Fig. 7. ABC expression in the membrane fraction close to terminal disease. 2D gel sections from three representative sample pairs (1, 3, and 4) show a reduced expression of ABC at 12 weeks of age.

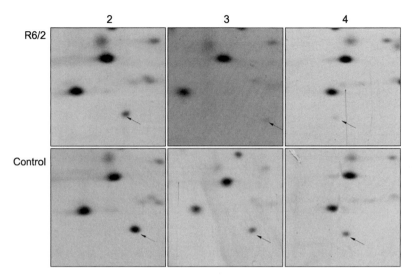

Fig. 8. ABC expression in the nuclear fraction close to terminal disease. 2D gel sections of three representative sample pairs (2, 3, and 4) show a reduced expression of ABC at 12 weeks of age.

8 weeks (Fig. 10 see Table I). Four out of eight R6/2 mice showed no CTS expression; whereas all control mice showed CTS expression. Close to terminal disease at 12 weeks of age, six out of eight R6/2 mice showed no CTS expression, whereas the expression was robust in control mice of the same age (see Fig. 10 and Table I). Therefore CTS decreased in expression during disease progression in a way similar to AAT 1-5 (compare Figs. 2 and 10 and Table I).

   c. Reduced Expression of ABC with Disease Progression. With age, the amount of ABC expressed was steadily increasing in control mice (Fig. 11; Table I). The increase was homogenous in all mice investigated (see Table I). Contrasting this increase, the amount of ABC in R6/2 mice remained constant at best at an expression level close to that at 4 weeks of age (see Fig. 11 and Table I). Contrasting the results with AAT 1-5 and CTS, there was no heterogeneity in ABC expression observed during disease progression at each time point (see Table I). The expression pattern observed hints at a decreased production and/or or increased consumption of ABC.

3. Gender-Specific Expression of AAT 1-5 and CTS

   The gender specificity of the expression of AAT 1-5, CTS, and ABC was investigated in the brain and in brain regions using C57Bl/6 mice. At this point it is important to note that the 2D-gel spot pattern of the CBAxC57Bl/6 mice (genetic background of the transgenic R6/2 mice and their controls) and C57Bl/6 mice coincided very well and that the positions and intensities of the

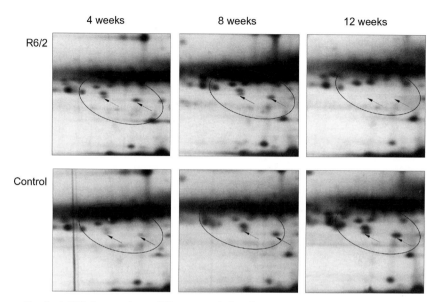

Fig. 9. AAT 1-5 expression at different ages during disease progression in the brain. The three spot group that belongs to AAT 1-5 is highlighted by a circle and the spots indicated by arrows. One representative sample pair from Table I is shown for each time point. (Used with permission of the publisher from Zabel, C., Chamrad, D. C., Priller, J., Woodman, B., Meyer, H. E., Bates, G. P., and Klose, J. (2002). Alterations in the mouse and human proteome caused by Huntington's disease. *Mol. Cell Proteomics* **1,** 366–375, Fig. 2.)

spots (control animals) of the three proteins of interest (AAT 1-5, CTS, and ABC) were nearly identical in both mouse strains.

    a. Lower Level of Expression of AAT 1-5 in Female than Male Mice. All results presented so far were obtained with male mice. Therefore female brains were studied. On the level of the whole brain there was no AAT 1-5 expression detectable in female C57B1/6 mice (Table II). This was later confirmed for female CBAxC57B1/6 mice (data not shown). An investigation of different brain regions obtained from three female C57B1/6 mice revealed that AAT 1-5 was expressed in medium to low quantities in certain brain regions. The region with the highest expression of AAT 1-5 was the trigeminal nerve, but other regions such as the pituitary, the motor cortex, the hippocampus, the bulb olfactory, and the cerebellum showed expression of the serine protease inhibitor (SERPIN) as well. Large brain areas such as the cortex, the midbrain, and the cerebellum expressed AAT 1-5 at very low levels or not at all (see Table II). The large contribution of those brain regions to the mass of the whole tissue extract could have diluted the AAT 1-5 present so much that it was no longer detectable by silver staining (detection limit: 2 ng).

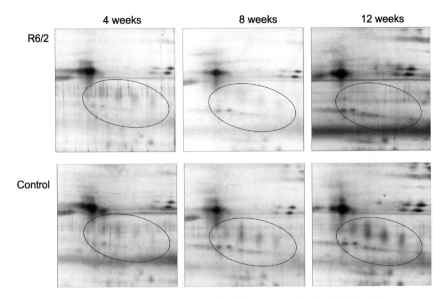

Fig. 10. CTS expression at different ages during disease progression in the brain. The spot group that belongs to CTS is highlighted by a circle in each gel section. One representative sample pair from Table I is shown for each time point.

b. CTS Expression in Female Mice Was Detected in Two Brain Regions. As in the case of AAT 1-5, there was an unsuccessful demonstration of CTS expression on the whole tissue level of the brain (data not shown). CTS was expressed in 2 of 12 brain regions. Similar to AAT 1-5, the trigeminal nerve showed the highest expression of CTS. Again, large brain regions such as cortex, midbrain, and cerebellum showed no expression of CTS (see Table II).

c. Expression Level of ABC is the Same in Female and Male Mice. ABC was expressed at the same level in the whole brains of female and male mice (data not shown). Brain regions showed a homogenous expression, except in the trigeminal nerve (very high) and the pituitary (low) (see Table II).

4. *Altered Protein Expression at Terminal Disease in Humans with HD*

The expression of the three proteins (AAT, CTS, and ABC), in which the expression was reduced in R6/2 as compared to control mice, was now investigated in three human brain regions. The postmortem tissue was collected from individuals with HD and age- and sex-matched controls.

a. Altered Expression of AAT in HD Postmortem Tissue. In HD a group of six spots was found on the gel half with the low pH range (3.5–6), whereas in control gels there were only three spots detectable in the same area (Fig. 12). This indicates

4 weeks   8 weeks   12 weeks

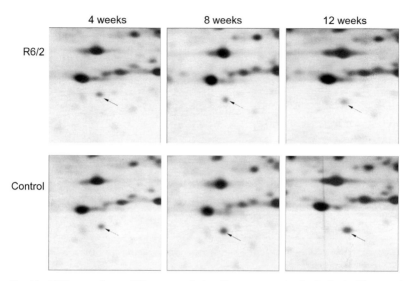

R6/2

Control

Fɪɢ. 11. ABC expression at different ages during disease progression in the brain. The spot that belongs to ABC is indicated by an arrow. One representative sample pair from Table I is shown for each time point. (Used with permission of the publisher from Zabel, C., Chamrad, D. C., Priller, J., Woodman, B., Meyer, H. E., Bates, G. P., and Klose, J. (2002). Alterations in the mouse and human proteome caused by Huntington's disease. *Mol. Cell Proteomics* **1,** 366–375, Fig. 2B.)

that a spot duplication, probably caused by a conformational change or post-translational modifications that do not alter the charge of the protein, might have taken place. This altered expression was detected in the striatum and parietal lobe of a female individual and a male individual who were affected by HD (see Fig. 12; data not shown). Two of four anterior cingulate cortex postmortem tissue samples of females with HD showed the same spot duplication (Figs. 12 and 13). The age, gender, and grading for disease severity (Vonsattel and DiFiglia, 1998; Vonsattel *et al.*, 1985) for each human sample are provided in Table III. The four most intensively stained spots were identified with mass spectrometry. They belong to AAT (database entry alpha1-antitrypsin precursor; Swiss Prot. #P01009), a protein of the same family of SERPINS as AAT 1-5 that was determined to be differentially expressed in the mouse brain. The average pI of the AAT spot group was determined to be approximately 4.7 (determined by IEF, first dimension of 2DE), and the molecular weight was found to be approximately 40 kDa, as determined by mobility in the SDS-PAGE dimension of 2DE. The spot pattern differed by 0.6 pH units from the calculated pI of 5.3 and had a 20-kDa lower molecular weight than that found with the mouse AAT 1-5, although it is a lot closer to the calculated molecular weight of AAT (46 kDa). Both differences might indicate AAT processing during HD. In the case of the anterior

TABLE II

DISTRIBUTION OF AAT, CTS, AND ABC IN DIFFERENT BRAIN REGIONS OF FEMALE MICE

Brain region[a]	AAT 1-5	CTS	ABC
Trigeminal nerve	++	++	++++[b]
Pituitary gland	++	+	+
Motor cortex	+	−	+++
Hippocampus	+	−	+++
Olfactory bulb	+	−	++
Cerebellum	−	−	+++
Striatum	−	−	+++
Frontal cortex	−	−	+++
Midbrain	−	−	+++
Rhombencephalon	−	−	+++
Thalamus	−	−	+++
Septum	−	−	+++

[a]The motor cortex includes amygdala and area entorhinalis. The area indicated as thalamus includes the hypothalamus as well.

[b]++++ indicates higher expression of ABC in this brain region than was found on the tissue level in brain and heart. (Used with permission of the publisher from Zabel, C., Chamrad, D. C., Priller, J., Woodman, B., Meyer, H. E., Bates, G. P., and Klose, J. (2002). Alterations in the mouse and human proteome caused by Huntington's disease. *Mol. Cell Proteomics* **1**, 366–375, Table II, bottom.)

cingulate cortex samples the double spot pattern was also observed in one control brain region (see Fig. 13). The brain where the brain region was obtained from was affected by "fresh blood in the subarachnoid space of the cerebellum" and neuronal changes in the cerebral cortex that are "consistent with (a) terminal hypoxic ischemic episode: scattered neurons are shrunken, eosinophilic with scalloped cytoplasmic membrane, prominent processes and small dark nuclei." There was no gliosis observed in the cortex. The brain was diagnosed with an "encephalopathy of hypoxic-ischemic type, acute, moderate" (neuropathology report supplied for brain B3813 by the Harvard Brain Tissue Resource Center, Belmont, Mass.). Although there was no readily observable gliosis, a huge difference in expression of the glial fibrillary acidic protein was detected between the HD and the control brain region. The control showed excessive glial fibrillary acidic protein (GFAP) expression, whereas the HD sample showed almost none (see Fig. 13, sample pair 2). Because GFAP is a widely accepted gliosis marker, gliosis was most likely present in this brain, although at a subvisual level. Two of the three remaining control brain regions were normal. The third (B4625) showed a "poorly differentiated tumor" consistent with a metastatic melanoma that affected several brain regions including the cortex and brainstem. This brain showed no increased GFAP and no spot duplication (see Fig. 13, sample pair 4).

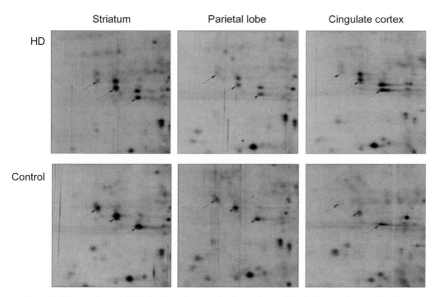

FIG. 12. Expression of AAT in three human brain regions of individuals affected by HD. Gel sections from three brain regions are shown: striatum, parietal lobe, and cingulate cortex from postmortem tissue of individuals with the disease, and age- and sex-matched controls are shown. The striatum and parietal lobe sample are from patients 93 (HD) and 104 (control), the cingulate cortex samples are from patients B3703 (HD) and B3700 (control) (also see Table III for details). Arrows indicate the spot pattern of interest. (Used with permission of the publisher from Zabel, C., Chamrad, D. C., Priller, J., Woodman, B., Meyer, H. E., Bates, G. P., and Klose, J. (2002). Alterations in the mouse and human proteome caused by Huntington's disease. *Mol. Cell Proteomics* **1,** 366–375, Fig. 4.)

b. ABC Expression in Human Brain Regions Was Not Detectable. The isoform of ABC that decreased in expression in the HD mouse model R6/2 during disease progression could not be detected in the human brain regions investigated by silver staining (results not shown). This was most likely due to an expression that was too low to be detected in the human brain, because this spot was already found in human heart by 2DE (Jungblut *et al.*, 1999). The pI and the molecular weight of the murine and human ABC spot are nearly identical (Jungblut *et al.*, 1999).

B. EXPRESSION OF THE DISEASE RELEVANT PROTEINS IN DIFFERENT TISSUES

In R6/2 mice, protein aggregates were found that contain the N-terminal fragment of the HD-causing protein Htt as intranuclear inclusions in various tissues apart from the central nervous system (Sathasivam *et al.*, 1999). Therefore it was interesting if the expression of the differentially expressed proteins found in

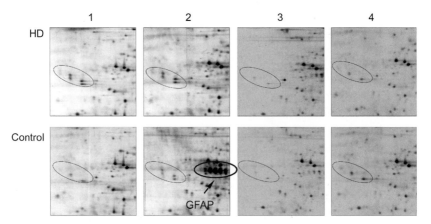

FIG. 13. Expression of AAT in the anterior cingulate cortex in HD postmortem brains. The sample pairs (HD/control) 1 (B3703/B3700), 2 (B4226/B3813), 3 (B4356/B3959), and 4 (B4381/B4625) are shown (for details, see Table III). The brain areas were obtained from females with HD and age and sex matched controls with age around 60 years. The circle indicates the spot group of interest. In sample pair 2 the strongly increased GFAP expression is indicated.

the brain (AAT, CTS, and ABC) was also disease specifically altered in other tissues. When investigating the brain, a tissue was chosen that had developed mainly from ectoderm, one of the three embryonic germ layers. When selecting the other tissues, at least one representative of the mesoderm (heart) and endoderm (liver) was chosen. Because R6/2 mice have reproductive difficulties (Mangiarini *et al.*, 1996) and testes showed the highest degree of atrophy out of six tissues investigated (brain, muscle, testes, liver, kidney, and spleen) (Davies *et al.*, 1997; Sathasivam *et al.*, 1999), they were also selected, an additional tissue created from mesoderm.

1. Initial Expression Analysis of AAT 1-5, CTS, and ABC in Different Tissues and Brain Regions

AAT 1-5 and CTS were expressed in the heart, liver, and testes of male CBA × C57B1/6 mice apart from the brain (Table IV). ABC was found to be expressed only in the brain and heart of C57B1/6 mice (Figs. 6 and 14; data not shown).

2. Differential Protein Expression in the Heart in R6/2 and Control Mice

Following the promising initial studies in the brain the cytoplasmic/nucleoplasmic fraction of protein extracts from the heart of R6/2 mice were investigated for altered protein expression of the three proteins that were differentially expressed—AAT 1-5, CTS and ABC. Furthermore, a scan for additional proteins, which showed disease-specific altered expression, was carried out.

TABLE III

HUMAN BRAIN REGION SAMPLES IN DETAIL

Brain no.	Source of tissue	Brain region	Grade of severity[a]	Age at removal (yr)	Gender	Frozen after (hr)
56[b]	LMU[c]	Str, Ptl;	2–3	56	F	56
93	LMU	Str; Ptl;	2–3	61	M	9
99	LMU	Str, Tha;	0	55	F	14
104	LMU	Str; Ptl;	0	59	M	?
B3703	HBTRC	ACC	4	61	F	25
B4226	HBTRC	ACC	4	62	F	28
B4356	HBTRC	ACC	4	61	F	24
B4381	HBTRC	ACC	4	55	F	23
B3700	HBTRC	ACC	0	62	F	16
B3813	HBTRC	ACC	0	58	F	20
B3959	HBTRC	ACC	0	59	F	18
B4625	HBTRC	ACC	0	53	F	24

[a]Grade of severity of the disease according to Vonsattel (Vonsattel and DiFiglia, 1998; Vonsattel et al., 1985).

[b]Sample pairs were created from brains no. 56 and 99, as well as 93 and 104.

[c]LMU, Institute for Neuropathology, "Ludwig Maximilian" University, Munich, Germany; HBTRC, Harvard Brain Tissue Resource Center, McLean Hospital, Belmont, Mass.; Str, striatum; Ptl, parietal lobe; ACC, anterior cingulate cortex; F, female; M, male; ?, unknown.

a. Reduced Expression of AAT in the Heart of R6/2 Mice. AAT 1-5 displayed a strongly reduced expression in the heart of R6/2 mice close to terminal disease (see Fig. 14). The number of spots that cosegregated increased from three to five (Fig. 14A and E). Contrasting the three spot group, which was already identified in the brain and was unambiguously linked to AAT 1-5 by mass spectrometry in the heart as well, the other two spots could not be identified by mass spectrometry, because they contained a mixture of several proteins. One of these proteins was protein disulfide isomerase (PDI; database entry Swiss Prot. #P09103). Although PDI was also identified for two spots at the same location when the two altered spots were absent, it is still hard to tell if all five spots belong to the same protein. Apart from AAT 1-5, another AAT isoform, AAT 1-4 (database entry alpha1-antitrypsin 1-4 precursor, Swiss Prot. #Q00897), with two protein spots was identified (Fig. 14B). This isoform was slightly lower expressed in R6/2 mice close to terminal disease. As was already the case for AAT 1-5, the molecular weight of AAT 1-4, (60 kDa), determined by electrophoretic mobility, was approximately 14 kDa higher than the one calculated.

b. Reduced CTS Expression in the Heart of R6/2 Mice. CTS showed strongly reduced expression in the heart, as was already detected in the brain (Figs. 14C and D). In addition to the CTS spot group that was found in the brain (pI approximately 5 and 70 kDa; Fig. 14C), an additional group of six spots was

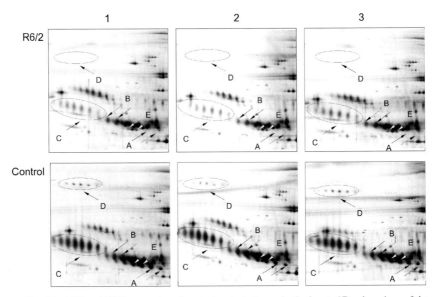

Fig. 14. AAT and CTS expression close to terminal disease in the heart. 2D gel sections of the low pH range of three representative sample pairs (1, 2, and 3) from cytoplasmic extracts of mice at 12 weeks of age are shown. Arrows and circles indicate the areas of interest. AAT 1-5 (A), AAT 1-4 (B), CTS 70-kDa isoform (C), CTS 170-kDa isoform (D) and unidentified spots (E) are marked.

absent in R6/2 mice close to terminal disease (Fig. 14D). The pI was nearly the same as in the previous group, but the molecular weight was approximately 170 kDa. Because the molecular weight was determined by electrophoretic mobility in the second dimension (SDS-PAGE), the higher molecular weights were harder to determine exactly due to the logarithmic scaling. Deviations of the molecular weight from 170 kDa were therefore very well possible. Thus this additional spot pattern could very well be a CTS dimer that would have had an observed molecular weight of 140 kDa, twice the weight of the 70-kDa isoform.

c. Unaltered ABC Expression in the Heart of R6/2 Mice. ABC was expressed at a high level in hearts of R6/2 and control mice at 12 weeks of age. The localization of the single ABC spot was identical in the brain and in the heart. The spot intensities were practically identical in R6/2 and control mice close to terminal disease, indicating no differential ABC expression in the heart (data not shown).

d. Expression of AAT 1-5 and CTS during Disease Progression. At 8 weeks, there was a slight decrease in AAT 1-5 and CTS expression in at least one out of four sample pairs. A pronounced decrease in expression was only seen at 12 weeks of age, close to terminal disease (See Table IV).

3. Reduced Expression of AAT and CTS in the Testes of R6/2 Mice

Studying the brain and heart proteome yielded two proteins, AAT 1-5 and CTS, which were down-regulated in both tissues in R6/2 mice. The levels of AAT 1-4 and ABC were reduced in heart or brain, respectively, during disease progression. The testes were now probed for similar alterations in expression. The severe weight loss of this tissue during disease progression (Sathasivam *et al.*, 1999) made the occurrence of further differentially expressed proteins highly likely.

a. Reduced Expression of AAT in the Testes of R6/2 mice. As has already been shown in the heart, there was a simultaneous reduction of at least five protein spots in the testes in the low pH range (Fig. 15). Three of them could be unanimously identified to belong to AAT 1-5. Two of them cosegregate with the three spot group but are part of a protein mixture of more than one protein. AAT 1-4 showed a reduced expression in R6/2 mice in three out of four samples (see Fig. 15). A higher AAT 1-4 expression in one R6/2 mouse (see Fig. 15, sample pair 4) could be due to the fact that the testes of this R6/2 mouse showed the highest degree of atrophy. Both testes had a remaining weight of 20 mg and the control testes had 262 mg. The average testes weight was 253 mg with a standard deviation of 23.7 mg in control mice. This means that the R6/2 testes had only 7.6% (w/w) of the control weight, therefore approximately 92% (w/w) were lost by atrophy. The protein composition of the residual tissue could have changed significantly. The testes of the R6/2 mouse with the second lowest weight that still showed a difference in AAT 1-4 expression had a weight of 34 mg, nearly 1.7-fold the weight of the lightest testes with no expression difference. An increased level of AAT 1-5 and CTS was not detected in sample pair 4. (see Table IV).

b. Reduced CTS Expression in the Testes of R6/2 Mice. CTS (70 kDa spot group) expression was also strongly reduced in the testes of R6/2 mice close to terminal disease (see Fig. 15). The 170-kDa isoform could not be detected in three out of four sample pairs and was therefore not evaluated. In the control testes (sample pair one) that showed CTS (170 kDa) expression, the spot intensities were already close to the detection limit of silver staining. Therefore the reduced expression of one as compared to two isoforms of CTS could be reliably detected in the testes. This could be a result of the generally higher expression level of CTS in the heart as compared to the testes (compare Fig. 15 to Fig. 14).

c. Reduction of AAT and CTS Expression during Disease Progression. Similar to the heart, the expression of AAT and CTS decreased slightly in R6/2 mice at the age of 8 weeks. A pronounced change in expression was observed only at 12 weeks of age close to terminal disease (see Table IV). Therefore a combined decrease of AAT 1-5 and CTS was now seen in three tissues: brain, heart, and testes, close to terminal disease (see Figs. 2, 14, and 15 and Table IV).

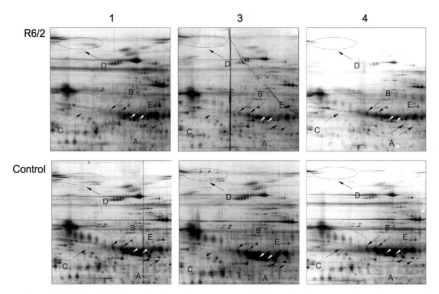

Fɪɢ. 15. AAT and CTS expression close to terminal disease in the testes. 2D gel sections of the low pH range of three representative sample pairs (1, 3, and 4) from cytoplasmic extracts of mice at 12 weeks of age are shown. Arrows and circles indicate the areas of interest. AAT 1-5 (A), AAT 1-4 (B), CTS 70-kDa isoform (C), CTS 170-kDa isoform (D) and unidentified spots (E) are marked.

4. Reduced Expression of AAT and CTS in the Liver

When investigating the proteome of the brain (ectoderm) and the mesoderm tissues, heart, and testes, a total of four proteins that were differentially expressed in at least one of those tissues, AAT 1-4, AAT 1-5, CTS, and ABC could be identified. In spite of the high degree of atrophy and weight loss during disease progression in the testes, there were no additional consistently differentially expressed proteins identified. This supports the conclusion that the proteins so far identified in the context of the disease are not due to gross tissue alterations (e.g., by atrophy), as was observed in testes (Sathasivam *et al.*, 1999). The investigation of the liver from the endoderm completed the study of the three germ layers.

a. Reduced Expression of AAT in the Liver of R6/2 Mice. In the liver there was a clearly visible, reduced expression of AAT 1-4 and a strongly reduced expression of AAT 1-5 (Fig. 16). In the heart and testes five spots cosegregated in expression, but only three could be identified as AAT 1-5. In the liver the three spot group of AAT 1-5 was again no longer detectable close to terminal disease, as was already seen in the heart and testes (compare Figs. 14 to 16). Contrasting the heart, the additional two spots were not altered in expression in the liver (compare Fig. 16E

TABLE IV

Expression of AAT 1-5 (top) and CTS (bottom) in Different Tissues over Time

Animal	R6/2				Control			
	Brain	Heart	Liver	Testes	Brain	Heart	Liver	Testes
8 weeks								
1[a]	[b]++	+++	+++	+++	+++	+++	+++	+++
2	+	+++	+++	+++	++	+++	+++	+++
3	+	++	++	++	+++	+++	+++	+++
4	−	+++	++	+++	++	+++	+++	+++
12 weeks								
1	−	−	−	−	+++	+++	+++	+++
2	−	−	−	−	+++	+++	+++	+++
3	−	−	−	−	+++	+++	+++	+++
4	−	−	−	−	+++	+++	+++	+++
8 weeks								
1	−	+++	++	++	++	+++	++	++
2	−	+++	++	++	++	+++	++	+
3	+	+	+	+	++	++	++	++
4	++	++	++	++	++	+++	++	++
12 weeks								
1	−	+	−	−	++	+++	++	++
2	++	+	−	+	+++	+++	++	++
3	−	+	−	+	++	+++	++	++
4	−	+	−	+	++	+++	++	++

[a]AAT 1-5 is identical with the three spot pattern found in all four tissues (see Fig. 2, arrows).
[b]For declaration of symbols see Table I. (Used with permission of the publisher from Zabel, C., Chamrad, D. C., Priller, J., Woodman, B., Meyer, H. E., Bates, G. P., and Klose, J. (2002). Alterations in the mouse and human proteome caused by Huntington's disease. *Mol. Cell Proteomics* **1,** 366–375, modified from Table III, top.)

to Figs. 14 and 15). As has already been mentioned before, the location of those two spots holds more than one protein. This expression difference gave an indication that the five cosegregating spots in the heart and testes might actually not belong to the same protein. This adds to the importance of studying more than one tissue to uncover differences in expression pattern among organs.

b. Reduced Expression of CTS in the Liver of R6/2 Mice. In the liver the expression of the 70-kDa isoform of CTS was robust in control mice but almost undetectable in R6/2 mice. The overall expression level of the 70-kDa CTS isoform in controls was comparable to testes but much lower than in the heart (compare Fig. 16 to Figs. 14 and 15). The 170-kDa isoform that was clearly visible in the heart and barely detectable in testes in only one sample pair, was not observed in

R6/2

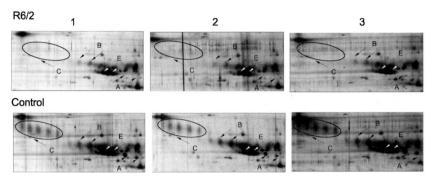

FIG. 16. AAT and CTS expression close to terminal disease in the liver. 2D gel sections of the low pH range of three representative sample pairs (1, 2, and 3) from cytoplasmic extracts of mice at 12 weeks of age are shown. Arrows and circles indicate the areas of interest. AAT 1-5 (A), AAT 1-4 (B), CTS 70-kDa isoform (C), and unidentified spots (E, white arrows) are marked. The CTS 170-kDa isoform was not, detected in the liver. (Used with permission of the publisher from Zabel, C., Chamrad, D. C., Priller, J., Woodman, B., Meyer, H. E., Bates, G. P., and Klose, J. (2002). Alterations in the mouse and human proteome caused by Huntington's disease. *Mol. Cell Proteomics* **1**, 366–375, Fig. 3A.)

R6/2

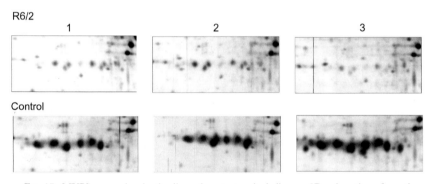

FIG. 17. MUPS expression in the liver close to terminal disease. 2D gel sections from three representative sample pairs (1, 2, and 3) are displayed. Cytoplasmic extracts from mouse liver at 12 weeks of age were used. (Used with permission of the publisher from Zabel, C., Chamrad, D. C., Priller, J., Woodman, B., Meyer, H. E., Bates, G. P., and Klose, J. (2002). Alterations in the mouse and human proteome caused by Huntington's disease. *Mol. Cell Proteomics* **1**, 366–375, Fig. 3B.)

any control, much less in any R6/2 sample pair of the liver (see Figs. 14 and 15; data not shown).

c. Strongly Reduced Expression of Major Urinary Proteins in the Liver of R6/2 Mice. An extraordinary, although liver-specific, difference in protein expression was found with a pattern of at least nine strongly reduced spots (Fig. 17). The spots in this pattern belong to the major urinary proteins (MUPs; database entry

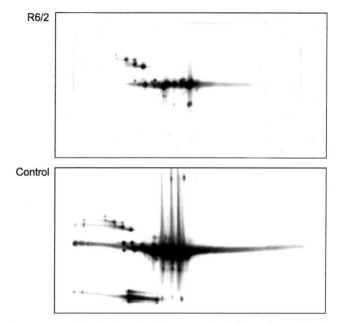

Fig. 18. MUPS expression in the urine close to terminal disease. Two gel sections show a representative example of a urine sample from R6/2 and control mice at 12 weeks of age. A strong reduction of MUPS (almost all spots shown) can be seen. The R6/2 urine sample was stained much longer than the control sample, that is, until background staining was clearly visible. This was done because no reference spots for equal staining intensity were available on the 2D gels.

MUP1_mouse, Swiss Prot. #P11588). The exact MUPs isoform for each spot could not be determined by means of mass spectrometry, because the differences between the isoforms are only minor and the necessary sequence coverage to distinguish them from each other was not reached. The pI identified by mobility in the first dimension (IEF) ranged between 4.9 and 5.3, and the molecular weight was determined to be approximately 22 kDa by mobility in the SDS-PAGE (second dimension). Those values correlate well with data from the literature. The pI was already shown to be between 4.6 and 5.3, depending on the MUPs isoform (Clissold and Bishop, 1982). The calculated molecular weight was approximately 21 kDa (data sheets to the Swiss Prot. entry MUP_1 [P11588]). Complementing the results from the liver, a strongly reduced expression of MUPs was also found in the urine of R6/2 mice close to terminal disease at 12 weeks (Fig. 18).

d. Expression of AAT, CTS, and MUPs During Disease Progression. During disease progression the expression of AAT and CTS differed between R6/2 and control mice only close to terminal disease at 12 weeks of age but hardly at 8 weeks

TABLE V
EXPRESSION OF MUPS OVER TIME

Animals (no.)	R6/2	Control
8 weeks		
1	+++[a]	+++
2	+++	+++
3	+++	+++
4	+++	+++
12 weeks		
1	+	+++
2	+	+++
3	+	+++
4	+	+++

[a]Abbreviations, see Table I. (Used with permission of the publisher from Zabel, C., Chamrad, D. C., Priller, J., Woodman, B., Meyer, H. E., Bates, G. P., and Klose, J. (2002). Alterations in the mouse and human proteome caused by Huntington's disease. *Mol. Cell Proteomics* **1**, 366–375, Table III, bottom.)

(see Table IV). MUPs expression was unaltered at 8 weeks and strongly reduced at 12 weeks of age (Table V).

C. SUMMARY OF THE RESULTS OBTAINED FROM THE STUDY OF DIFFERENT TISSUES

In this study, tissue from three different germ layers—ectoderm (brain), mesoderm (heart and testes), and endoderm (liver)—was investigated. An important point made by the proteomics study of those tissues is that the expression of the SERPINS AAT 1-5 and CTS was gender specific and was highly reduced in the brain much earlier (8 weeks) than in other tissues (12 weeks) (see Table IV). The chaperone ABC showed lower expression in the brain of R6/2 mice but not in the heart (Fig. 6 and data not shown). It was not detectable in testes and liver (data not shown). The proteins that showed a decreased expression belong to three different protein families: three SERPINS (AAT 1-4, AAT 1-5, and CTS), one chaperone (ABC), and one lipocalin (MUPS) (Flower *et al.*, 2000).

VI. Discussion

When comparing the proteomes of HD exon 1 transgenic mice (R6/2) with control mice, there were very few but disease specific differences in the protein spot pattern. The largest part in a large gel 2D pattern was identical. The lack of expression differences was not expected in such a severe phenotype as is seen in R6/2 mice close to terminal disease (Mangiarini *et al.*, 1996). The differences that did exist were quite reproducible and usually severe at 12 weeks of age. Close to terminal disease, the expression of AAT 1-5 was no longer detectable by silver staining (2 ng). The expression of the 70-kDa isoform of CTS was strongly reduced in all tissues studied close to terminal disease. Both proteins decreased in the brain almost 4 weeks earlier than in the other tissues. AAT 1-4 showed reduced expression in heart, testes, and liver, although a severe reduction occurred only in the liver. The expression of ABC was strongly reduced in the brain but not heart. It was not detectable in testes and liver. The study of the liver revealed the very strong decrease of MUPs in R6/2 mice close to terminal disease. This finding stresses the importance of investigating tissues other than those primarily affected by a disease to cover the full area of influence of the disorder under study. Investigations on human samples collected postmortem from different brain regions showed a disease specific alteration of expression in the protein AAT. This alteration was detected in all three brain regions. The observation bridges the mouse model with the human disease by showing altered expression of closely related proteins in both species.

A. Integrating the Results into HD Pathology

The initial interpretation of data obtained by the proteomics study was primarily restricted to cluster analysis and literature search. The identification of proteins differentially expressed close to terminal disease, and the resolution of their expression in time as well as tissue, were important means of this proteomics study to provide a much-needed initial framework to the expression data. By grouping proteins of similar kind (family) and/or expression in time, cluster analysis provides valuable clues as to what kind of pathways may be involved. Three clusters could be built from the five proteins differentially expressed. The first obvious cluster was that all proteins were down-regulated in their expression. The second one found includes three proteins that belong to the SERPIN family: AAT 1-4, AAT 1-5, and CTR. Finally, two proteins of the same family (AAT 1-5 and CTS) were strongly down-regulated in the brain earlier than in the other tissues studied. By literature research, known functions can be exploited to obtain clues about the function of the differentially expressed proteins in the disease under study. The protein functions characterized in most of the protein studies were determined within a certain context (e.g., a disease or a cellular function). The protein therefore may very well play a role in this context, although it might have many other functions not observable in the problem under study. Therefore it is important to keep an open mind about possible other functions of a protein that are not described in the literature but that might fit a lot better in the context of the own proteomics study;

for example, a protein might be a chaperone and be involved in protein folding. Let us assume this function is known from the literature. It might as well be important in cell death, which is not known but important in the context of the study at hand. Therefore, although literature data contain valuable information, it is important that it is still incomplete. Because of this, it is very important to form a testable hypothesis with the proteomics results obtained, in combination with cluster analysis and literature data, and carry out an independent experiment to verify one's conclusions drawn from the proteomics study. After those more general considerations, the next sections will provide some examples on how proteomics results may be integrated to develop testable hypotheses.

1. Role of AAT in the Body

AAT is a protein that is mainly produced in the liver and participates in the acute phase response (Baumann and Gauldie, 1994). It is secreted to prohibit lasting tissue damage (Baumann and Gauldie, 1994). In the brain, AAT is expressed mainly by astrocytes (Gollin et al., 1992).

2. Characterization and Evaluation of SERPIN Expression during HD in Mice and Humans

Based on literature data on the progression of the disease in the mouse model R6/2 (Carter et al., 1999; Li et al., 1999a; Lione et al., 1999), the decrease of AAT 1-5 and CTS (Takahara and Sinohara, 1982) at the age of 8 weeks in the brain seemed to be a later event that coincided with an increase in severity of the disease.

When considering all four tissues studied, there was a decrease of three SERPINS (AAT 1-4, AAT 1-5, and CTS) in the mouse model during disease progression, indicating that a pathway might be involved that uses SERPINS of varying substrate specificities. The concerted decrease of these three SERPINS told nothing about the reason of the disease; that is, if it caused or contributed to the disease or if it was the effect of some bystander process occurring during disease progression. An interesting hint as to why both SERPINS were down-regulated might come from the fact that after orchiectomy, male mice show a decreased expression of AAT and CTS (Yamamoto and Sinohara, 1984). Testosterone administration restored the levels of both proteins to normal in castrated mice (Yamamoto and Sinohara, 1984). It is further known that C57B1/6 mice possess five AAT isoforms (Goodwin et al., 1997) and the serum levels of two of them, including AAT 1-5 (and AAT 1-7) but not AAT 1-4, are influenced by androgens such as testosterone (Barbour et al., 2002). It has already been shown that the testes of R6/2 mice display excessive atrophy close to terminal disease (Sathasivam et al., 1999). Because the testes are the main site of testosterone synthesis, the levels of AAT 1-5 and CTS are expected to drop during disease progression, due to the lack of testosterone production. This example shows the value of literature data and the availability of data on more than one protein at a time to develop and solidify a hypothesis.

Humans possess only one AAT isoform. Its reactive center specificity differs from AAT 1-5, thereby most likely changing its protease specificity (Goodwin *et al.*, 1997). The primary target of human AAT is neutrophil elastase (Travis and Salvesen, 1983). In humans with HD AAT expression of this one isoform was altered. Contrasting sex-specific differential expression of AAT 1-5 in the mouse, the altered expression was seen in both genders. The spot pattern of AAT in humans was different than in mice as well (pI and molecular weight). The increased molecular weight of AAT in the mouse, determined by SDS-PAGE, was probably due to its conformation. It could be argued that the protein was not fully denatured in SDS and retained at least some of its globular shape. This shape led to a reduced SDS binding, decreasing the charge of the protein and therefore causing lower mobility (Finotti and Pagetta, 1997). AAT is a member of the SERPIN family of proteins that employ a unique suicide substrate-like inhibitory mechanism (Silverman *et al.*, 2001). SERPINS display a native strain that is important for their function (Seo *et al.*, 2002). This strain is lost as part of their suicide inhibitory mechanism (Huntington *et al.*, 2000; Seo *et al.*, 2002). The lost strain causes a high degree of conformational disorder by relaxation of the protein (Huntington *et al.*, 2000; Seo *et al.*, 2002). The protein in a relaxed state could be more accessible to SDS and therefore more susceptible to denaturation. Therefore a decrease in the observed molecular weight to a level close to the one calculated might be possible. In addition to that the molecular weight after removal of the leader sequence of the precursor protein and the removal of the digopeptide cut off during the suicide inhibition by the protease, the molecular weight calculated by the ProtParam Tool (http://us.expasy.org/cgi-bin/protparam) was 40.2 kDa, nearly the molecular weight determined by SDS-PAGE for human AAT.

The theoretical pI calculated by the same program was 5.16, which is still significantly higher than the pI of 4.7, as determined in the 2DE gel. There had to be an addition of negative charges or a removal of positive charges. Phosphorylation could have contributed to an increase in negative charge without increasing the molecular weight much. Because the phosphorylation status of the proteins in the spot group was not studied, this remains speculative. Therefore some clue about the reduced molecular weight as compared to the mouse model could be gained from the study of the literature, but the reasons for the significantly higher observed pI remain elusive. A detailed scan for protein modifications might shed light on the subject.

3. Reduced Expression of the Chaperone ABC in a Transgenic Mouse Model for HD

In the study at hand the reduced ABC expression at the age of 8 weeks (see Fig. 11 and Table I) coincides with the increased emergence of neuropil aggregates in R6/2 mice (Li *et al.*, 1999a). It is interesting that the reduced expression of ABC was observed in the brain but not in the heart of R6/2 mice (See Fig. 6

and data not shown). Note that in the heart the spots surrounding the unaltered ABC spot show no difference in silver staining as well, serving as an internal standard for 2DE quality. Those observations argue for the same expression level of ABC in R6/2 and controls (data not shown). This could mean that different tissues are differentially affected by the disease, or that the heart contains and/or produces enough ABC to compensate for any loss during disease progression. ABC is expressed in a variety of tissues (Bhat and Nagineni, 1989; Bhat et al., 1991; Dubin et al., 1989). It was already known that heart and skeletal muscle show high expression of ABC mRNA (Dubin et al., 1989; Iwaki et al., 1989). On the protein level, expression was demonstrated to be high in the human (Jungblut et al., 1999) and murine heart (Zabel et al., 2002) and moderate in the mouse brain (Zabel, 2003). It was shown that the concentration of ABC increased in Alexander's disease (Iwaki et al., 1989) and in cardiovascular diseases in which fast post-translational modifications may occur as well (Arrell et al., 2001). The decreased expression seen in the mouse model (R6/2) might have at least two reasons: Because disease in general means stress for the affected tissue, it might be possible that in the case of HD the level of ABC increased initially as a protective response against cellular stress but that the protein was used up quickly in the attempt to reduce aggregation. Another possibility may be that the disease progressed so quickly (approximately 8 weeks versus 15–20 years) that there was no chance for ABC to accumulate. ABC might play a protective role because it is already known that molecular chaperones, including heat shock proteins, prevent misfolding and aggregation of newly synthesized mutant proteins and stress-denatured proteins, and thereby reduce the burden on the ubiquitin-proteasome pathway (Glover and Lindquist, 1998; Johnson and Craig, 1997). It is also known that Htt interacts with heat shock proteins in a length-dependent manner (Jana et al., 2000). Because ABC belongs to the family of small heat shock proteins, it might also interact with mutated proteins such as Htt. A role in protection against aggregates is supported by the known disaggregation capability of ABC (Koyama and Goldman, 1999). Another protective role of ABC might be its binding to procaspase 3 and partially processed procaspase 3, thereby blocking apoptosis (Kamradt et al., 2001; Mao et al., 2001b).

The calculated molecular weight of 20.1 kDa coincided well with the 22 kDa determined by SDS-PAGE. The same molecular weight was already determined for human ABC by SDS-PAGE (Muchowski et al., 1997). Mouse and human ABC show 97.7% identity on the amino acid level, as determined by Sim-Prot (http://us.expasy.org/tools/sim-prot.html). Therefore the mouse ABC should also have shown a molecular weight of 22 kDa in SDS-PAGE, which was the case. There was an increase of 0.7 pH units between the calculated (6.8) and the IEF determined pI value (7.5). ABC contains three potential phosphorylation sites (Kato et al., 1998). It contains one probable acetylation and one glycosylation site. (Compare database entries in Swiss Prot. alphaB-crystallin for human:

P02511 and mouse: P23927.) The post-translational modifications listed were either neutral (acetylation) or shift the protein to a more acidic pI due to addition of negative charges (phosphorylation). With the data available, we were therefore unable to explain this pI shift. Studies on post-translational modifications were again hampered by insufficient sequence coverage. In a proteomics study of the human heart the pI determined for ABC was approximately 7.4 (Jungblut *et al.*, 1999). This correlates well with the pI of 7.5 determined in this study for the mouse. In another heart proteomics investigation in the rat the pI was determined to be approximately 7.8 (Li *et al.*, 1999b), again closely matching the result obtained. Therefore, although the reason for the altered pI is unknown, the pI shift seems to be reproducible between species in 2DE.

4. Reduced MUPs Expression—A General Indicator of Disease?

The expression of a group of proteins, the MUPs, with no known homolog in humans, was strongly reduced in the liver and urine of 12 week-old mice close to terminal disease (see Figs. 17 and 18). It is already known that MUPs show a liver-specific expression (Cavaggioni and Mucignat-Caretta, 2000). The expression is significantly higher in male mice than in female mice (Wicks, 1941). The MUPs possess a molecular weight of approximately 20 kDa and form β-barrel structures, enclosing a hydrophobic cavity (Bacchini *et al.*, 1992). 2,3-Dihydro-exo-brevicomin and 2-sec-butyl-4,5-dihydrothiazole are examples of compounds that bind to this cavity (Brennan, 2001). The binding to MUPs allows those volatile ligands to be released from the urine over an extended period (Brennan, 2001). The release of those ligands communicates the state of aggression of one male to another (Hurst *et al.*, 2001) and stimulates estrus in females (Marchlewska-Koj *et al.*, 2000).

R6/2 mice reproduce only a short time after reaching sexual maturity (Mangiarini *et al.*, 1996) at 6–7 weeks of age (Pomeroy *et al.*, 1990). This loss of bodily function coincides well with reduced MUPs expression and testes weight loss. MUPS expression starts to decrease in R6/2 mice at 8 weeks of age (see Table V), only 1 week after reaching sexual maturity (Pomeroy *et al.*, 1990). The testes were already shown to severely lose weight at approximately the same time (Sathasivam *et al.*, 1999). Recognition as an individual mouse seems also to be dependent on MUPs, so that a reduction of those proteins in the urine could result in a perturbed social interaction of the mice (Beynon and Hurst, 2003; Hurst *et al.*, 2001). It was also observed that MUPs expression decreased in an experimental model for stroke (Sironi *et al.*, 2001). This could mean that the expression of MUPs is sensitive to a large number of diseases and that their down-regulation contributes to the regulation of proliferation in mice. MUPs are easily accessible for analysis through the urine. Therefore they could be utilized as a marker for testing pharmacological substances on their efficacy for HD treatment, at least in the R6/2 mouse model.

B. An Altered Strategy for Proteomics Studies

One of the core results was the high degree of similarity between the R6/2 and control proteome in all tissues studied, except the testes, close to terminal disease. It will be important to determine the reason for this unexpected similarity. It is conceivable that this similarity was based on a lack of sensitivity (e.g., most of the altered proteins were not detected). Another possibility is that changes were occurring in many proteins, but that they were too small in magnitude to be detectable by the means used in this study (e.g, manual detection by eye). It is already known from the literature that many proteins interact with huntingtin (Harjes and Wanker, 2003). These proteins could interact differentially with mutant and wild type Htt (Gervais *et al.*, 2002; Zuccato *et al.*, 2003). Aberrant interactions would also be very hard to study by the approach used, in which only the protein expression differences on the whole organ level were detectable.

1. *Lack of Sensitivity of the Proteomics Approach Used*

When looking at the proteins found to be differentially expressed in this study, it was obvious that no low-abundance proteins such as transcription factors and their silencers were found, although these classes were already implicated in the pathology of HD in the literature (Dunah *et al.*, 2002; Freiman and Tjian, 2002; Zuccato *et al.*, 2001, 2003). AAT is a protein highly expressed in the liver and blood (Kalsheker *et al.*, 2002; Travis and Salvesen, 1983). The expression of CTS is highly expressed in the serum of male mice (Kueppers and Mills, 1983; Yamamoto and Sinohara, 1984). ABC shows high expression in the lens (de Jong *et al.*, 1993). It has also been demonstrated to be highly expressed in heart and skeletal muscle on the mRNA level (Dubin *et al.*, 1989; Iwaki *et al.*, 1989). MUPs show a high expression in the mouse liver and urine (Beynon and Hurst, 2003). In summary, all proteins identified to be differentially expressed argue that only middle, to high abundant proteins were detected. Because low abundance proteins can not be amplified like DNA or RNA, it will be important to enrich them by other means. Because proteins are not distributed equally in a tissue or a cell's organelles, compartments containing high amounts of specific proteins could be enriched and fraction specific proteins, now present in high abundance, could be detected. Fluorescence dyes or even radio labeling could also be used to increase sensitivity. Although a protein is ubiquitously expressed, changes in protein expression could also be localized (e.g., to a specific brain region). It might therefore be useful to determine the differences between certain subproteomes such as brain regions, which are mainly affected by the disease. Although this would not change the sensitivity to detect proteins per se, changes of already detectable proteins might become more pronounced and therefore visible by large gel 2DE.

The use of subproteomes implies that a larger amount of tissue is needed. If, for example, the striatum or even a certain region of it is of interest, one still needs one whole brain to get just two of those regions. Therefore a lot of brains are needed to accumulate enough material of just this one region. Because human material is scarcely available, the need for a readily available model system emerges. In the case of this study it was the R6/2 mouse model. It has already been shown that the R6/2 mouse model does to some degree recapitulate the striatum specific neurodegeneration seen in humans with HD (Turmaine *et al.*, 2000; Vonsattel and DiFiglia, 1998; Vonsattel *et al.*, 1985), although at an age right before death and therefore older than the 12 weeks studied. Before this time point, actual neurodegeneration, including cell death, was not observed (Turmaine *et al.*, 2000). In spite of those difficulties it is still easier to breed enough mice to obtain the needed tissue than try to use human material.

2. Covering the Full Spectrum of all Protein Classes

It is now well established that hydrophobic proteins escape the separation capability of classical large gel 2DE with complex protein mixtures (Santoni *et al.*, 2000). Another problem of the proteomics of whole tissues is that aberrant protein interactions that do not necessarily result in a change in overall protein concentration are not detected (Dreger, 2003). It is therefore important to use additional techniques such as separation by liquid chromatography in combination with mass spectrometry or 2DE, employing two different detergents (Dreger, 2003). Another method for the comparison of complex protein mixtures is ICAT (isotope-coded affinity tags) (Gygi *et al.*, 1999). Proteins that are to be compared are labeled with tags having a fixed mass difference but are otherwise identical. This is done by substituting hydrogen atoms with deuterium atoms. Unfortunately, even if using all the methods described and many more available not described here, it is still not possible to cover all proteins in the HD proteome. Still, a proteomics study might give useful starting points for the identification of pathways involved in the disease. The determination of all the members of those pathways will then be subject to classical biochemical studies.

VII. Conclusion

The main success of this proteomics study was to build a bridge from the mouse model to the human disease by identifying differentially expressed proteins of the same family in humans and mice (e.g., AAT 1-4, AAT 1-5 [mouse], and AAT in humans).

In addition, a differential expression of protein classes previously not implicated in HD but in other neurodegenerative diseases such as Alzheimer's disease

[AAT (Gollin *et al.*, 1992), ABC (Mao *et al.*, 2001a; Renkawek *et al.*, 1994)] and Parkinson's disease (ABC) (Braak *et al.*, 2001; Renkawek *et al.*, 1999) has been found. Although it seems that the differences in SERPIN, ABC, and MUPs expression are not causative in nature for the disease, they still add some pieces to the puzzle of HD, increasing the pool of altered proteins available. The in-depth study of the role of different tissue in HD by a proteomics approach was a first step to tackle the complete HD proteome on a more global level than merely the brain furthering our understanding of all implications of the disorder for the affected individual. Much has been learned from this study in terms of sensitivity of the chosen approach, the way a study has to be planned, and which refinements are necessary in the future.

Acknowledgments

We would like to thank Gillian P. Bates for providing the mouse tissue samples from the R6/2 mouse model and for valuable discussions of the results, and Ben Woodman for his expertise in handling the tissues. We are grateful to Helmut E. Meyer and Maik Wacker for protein identifications. We are indebted to the Harvard Brain Tissue Resource Center, supported in part by PHS grant number MH/NS 31862, for providing the anterior cingulate cortex tissue and ongoing support. We very much appreciate the help of Dr. Schwegler for dissecting the brain regions used for the protein expression study. We thank Anj Mahal for the genotyping of mice and acknowledge the excellent technical support by Marion Hermann and Yvonne Kläre with the large 2D gels.

References

Arrell, D. K., Neverova, I., and Van Eyk, J. E. (2001). Cardiovascular proteomics: Evolution and potential. *Circ. Res.* **88,** 763–773.

Bacchini, A., Gaetani, E., and Cavaggioni, A. (1992). Pheromone binding proteins of the mouse, Mus musculus. *Experientia* **48,** 419–421.

Barbour, K. W., Goodwin, R. L., Guillonneau, F., Wang, Y., Baumann, H., and Berger, F. G. (2002). Functional diversification during evolution of the murine alpha(1)-proteinase inhibitor family: Role of the hypervariable reactive center loop. *Mol. Biol. Evol.* **19,** 718–727.

Bates, G. (2003). Huntingtin aggregation and toxicity in Huntington's disease. *Lancet* **361,** 1642–1644.

Bates, G. P. (2001). Huntington's disease. Exploiting expression. *Nature* **413,** 691, 693–694.

Baumann, H., and Gauldie, J. (1994). The acute phase response. *Immunol. Today* **15,** 74–80.

Beynon, R. J., and Hurst, J. L. (2003). Multiple roles of major urinary proteins in the house mouse, Mus domesticus. *Biochem. Soc. Trans.* **31,** 142–146.

Bhat, S. P., Horwitz, J., Srinivasan, A., and Ding, L. (1991). Alpha B-crystallin exists as an independent protein in the heart and in the lens. *Eur. J. Biochem.* **202,** 775–781.

Bhat, S. P., and Nagineni, C. N. (1989). alpha B subunit of lens-specific protein alpha-crystallin is present in other ocular and non-ocular tissues. *Biochem. Biophys. Res. Commun.* **158,** 319–325.

Braak, H., Del Tredici, K., Sandmann-Kiel, D., Rub, U., and Schultz, C. (2001). Nerve cells expressing heat-shock proteins in Parkinson's disease. *Acta. Neuropathol. (Berl.)* **102,** 449–454.

Brennan, P. A. (2001). The vomeronasal system. *Cell Mol. Life Sci.* **58,** 546–555.

Carter, R. J., Lione, L. A., Humby, T., Mangiarini, L., Mahal, A., *et al.* (1999). Characterization of progressive motor deficits in mice transgenic for the human Huntington's disease mutation. *J. Neurosci.* **19,** 3248–3257.

Cavaggioni, A., and Mucignat-Caretta, C. (2000). Major urinary proteins, alpha(2U)-globulins and aphrodisin. *Biochim. Biophys. Acta* **1482,** 218–228.

Chan, E. Y., Luthi-Carter, R., Strand, A., Solano, S. M., Hanson, S. A., *et al.* (2002). Increased huntingtin protein length reduces the number of polyglutamine-induced gene expression changes in mouse models of Huntington's disease. *Hum. Mol. Genet.* **11,** 1939–1951.

Clissold, P. M., and Bishop, J. O. (1982). Variation in mouse major urinary protein (MUP) genes and the MUP gene products within and between inbred lines. *Gene* **18,** 211–220.

Davies, S. W., Turmaine, M., Cozens, B. A., DiFiglia, M., Sharp, A. H., *et al.* (1997). Formation of neuronal intranuclear inclusions underlies the neurological dysfunction in mice transgenic for the HD mutation. *Cell* **90,** 537–548.

de Jong, W. W., Leunissen, J. A., and Voorter, C. E. (1993). Evolution of the alpha-crystallin/small heat-shock protein family. *Mol. Biol. Evol.* **10,** 103–126.

DiFiglia, M., Sapp, E., Chase, K. O., Davies, S. W., Bates, G. P., *et al.* (1997). Aggregation of huntingtin in neuronal intranuclear inclusions and dystrophic neurites in brain. *Science* **277,** 1990–1993.

Dreger, M. (2003). Subcellular proteomics. *Mass Spectrom. Rev.* **22,** 27–56.

Dubin, R. A., Wawrousek, E. F., and Piatigorsky, J. (1989). Expression of the murine alpha B-crystallin gene is not restricted to the lens. *Mol. Cell Biol.* **9,** 1083–1091.

Dunah, A. W., Jeong, H., Griffin, A., Kim, Y. M., Standaert, D. G., *et al.* (2002). Sp1 and TAFII130 transcriptional activity disrupted in early Huntington's disease. *Science* **296,** 2238–2243.

Finotti, P., and Pagetta, A. (1997). Albumin contamination of a purified human alpha 1-antitrypsin preparation does not affect either structural conformation or the electrophoretic mobility of the inhibitor. *Clin. Chim. Acta* **264,** 133–148.

Flower, D. R., North, A. C., and Sansom, C. E. (2000). The lipocalin protein family: Structural and sequence overview. *Biochim. Biophys. Acta* **1482,** 9–24.

Freiman, R. N., and Tjian, R. (2002). Neurodegeneration. A glutamine-rich trail leads to transcription factors. *Science* **296,** 2149–2150.

Gervais, F. G., Singaraja, R., Xanthoudakis, S., Gutekunst, C. A., Leavitt, B. R., *et al.* (2002). Recruitment and activation of caspase-8 by the Huntingtin-interacting protein Hip-1 and a novel partner Hippi. *Nat. Cell Biol.* **4,** 95–105.

Glover, J. R., and Lindquist, S. (1998). Hsp104, Hsp70, and Hsp40: A novel chaperone system that rescues previously aggregated proteins. *Cell* **94,** 73–82.

Gollin, P. A., Kalaria, R. N., Eikelenboom, P., Rozemuller, A., and Perry, G. (1992). Alpha 1-antitrypsin and alpha 1-antichymotrypsin are in the lesions of Alzheimer's disease. *Neuroreport* **3,** 201–203.

Goodwin, R. L., Barbour, K. W., and Berger, F. G. (1997). Expression of the alpha 1-proteinase inhibitor gene family during evolution of the genus Mus. *Mol. Biol. Evol.* **14,** 420–427.

Gusella, J. F., and MacDonald, M. E. (1996). Trinucleotide instability: A repeating theme in human inherited disorders. *Annu. Rev. Med.* **47,** 201–209.

Gutekunst, C. A., Li, S. H., Yi, H., Mulroy, J. S., Kuemmerle, S., *et al.* (1999). Nuclear and neuropil aggregates in Huntington's disease: Relationship to neuropathology. *J. Neurosci.* **19,** 2522–2534.

Gygi, S. P., Rist, B., Gerber, S. A., Turecek, F., Gelb, M. H., and Aebersold, R. (1999). Quantitative analysis of complex protein mixtures using isotope-coded affinity tags. *Nat. Biotechnol.* **17,** 994–999.

Harjes, P., and Wanker, E. E. (2003). The hunt for huntingtin function: Interaction partners tell many different stories. *Trends Biochem. Sci.* **28,** 425–433.

HDCRG (1993). A novel gene containing a trinucleotide repeat that is expanded and unstable on Huntington's disease chromosomes. The Huntington's Disease Collaborative Research Group. *Cell* **72,** 971–983.

Huntington, J. A., Read, R. J., and Carrell, R. W. (2000). Structure of a serpin-protease complex shows inhibition by deformation. *Nature* **407,** 923–926.

Hurst, J. L., Payne, C. E., Nevison, C. M., Marie, A. D., Humphries, R. E., *et al.* (2001). Individual recognition in mice mediated by major urinary proteins. *Nature* **414,** 631–634.

Iwaki, T., Kume-Iwaki, A., Liem, R. K., and Goldman, J. E. (1989). Alpha B-crystallin is expressed in non-lenticular tissues and accumulates in Alexander's disease brain. *Cell* **57,** 71–78.

Jana, N. R., Tanaka, M., Wang, G., and Nukina, N. (2000). Polyglutamine length-dependent interaction of Hsp40 and Hsp70 family chaperones with truncated N-terminal huntingtin: Their role in suppression of aggregation and cellular toxicity. *Hum. Mol. Genet.* **9,** 2009–2018.

Johnson, J. L., and Craig, E. A. (1997). Protein folding *in vivo*: Unraveling complex pathways. *Cell* **90,** 201–204.

Jungblut, P. R., Zimny-Arndt, U., Zeindl-Eberhart, E., Stulik, J., Koupilova, K., *et al.* (1999). Proteomics in human disease: cancer, heart and infectious diseases. *Electrophoresis* **20,** 2100–2110.

Kalsheker, N., Morley, S., and Morgan, K. (2002). Gene regulation of the serine proteinase inhibitors alpha1-antitrypsin and alpha1-antichymotrypsin. *Biochem. Soc. Trans.* **30,** 93–98.

Kamradt, M. C., Chen, F., and Cryns, V. L. (2001). The small heat shock protein alpha B-crystallin negatively regulates cytochrome c- and caspase-8-dependent activation of caspase-3 by inhibiting its autoproteolytic maturation. *J. Biol. Chem.* **276,** 16059–16063.

Kato, K., Ito, H., Kamei, K., Inaguma, Y., Iwamoto, I., and Saga, S. (1998). Phosphorylation of alphaB-crystallin in mitotic cells and identification of enzymatic activities responsible for phosphorylation. *J. Biol. Chem.* **273,** 28346–28354.

Klose, J. (1999a). Fractionated extraction of total tissue proteins from mouse and human for 2-D electrophoresis. *Methods Mol. Biol.* **112,** 67–85.

Klose, J. (1999b). Genotypes and phenotypes. *Electrophoresis* **20,** 643–652.

Klose, J. (1999c). Large-gel 2-D electrophoresis. *Methods. Mol. Biol.* **112,** 147–172.

Klose, J., and Kobalz, U. (1995). Two-dimensional electrophoresis of proteins: an updated protocol and implications for a functional analysis of the genome. *Electrophoresis* **16,** 1034–1059.

Koyama, Y., and Goldman, J. E. (1999). Formation of GFAP cytoplasmic inclusions in astrocytes and their disaggregation by alphaB-crystallin. *Am. J. Pathol.* **154,** 1563–1572.

Kueppers, F., and Mills, J. (1983). Trypsin inhibition by mouse serum: Sexual dimorphism controlled by testosterone. *Science* **219,** 182–184.

Li, H., Li, S. H., Cheng, A. L., Mangiarini, L., Bates, G. P., and Li, X. J. (1999a). Ultrastructural localization and progressive formation of neuropil aggregates in Huntington's disease transgenic mice. *Hum. Mol. Genet.* **8,** 1227–1236.

Li, H., Li, S. H., Johnston, H., Shelbourne, P. F., and Li, X. J. (2000). Amino-terminal fragments of mutant huntington show selective accumulation in striatal neurons and synaptic toxicity. *Nat. Genet.* **25,** 385–389.

Li, X. P., Pleissner, K. P., Scheler, C., Regitz-Zagrosek, V., Salnikow, J., and Jungblut, P. R. (1999b). A two-dimensional electrophoresis database of rat heart proteins. *Electrophoresis* **20,** 891–897.

Lione, L. A., Carter, R. J., Hunt, M. J., Bates, G. P., Morton, A. J., and Dunnett, S. B. (1999). Selective discrimination learning impairments in mice expressing the human Huntington's disease mutation. *J. Neurosci.* **19,** 10428–10437.

Luthi-Carter, R., Hanson, S. A., Strand, A. D., Bergstrom, D. A., Chun, W., *et al.* (2002a). Dysregulation of gene expression in the R6/2 model of polyglutamine disease: Parallel changes in muscle and brain. *Hum. Mol. Genet.* **11,** 1911–1926.

Luthi-Carter, R., Strand, A., Peters, N. L., Solano, S. M., Hollingsworth, Z. R., *et al.* (2000). Decreased expression of striatal signaling genes in a mouse model of Huntington's disease. *Hum. Mol. Genet.* **9,** 1259–1271.

Luthi-Carter, R., Strand, A. D., Hanson, S. A., Kooperberg, C., Schilling, G., *et al.* (2002b). Polyglutamine and transcription: gene expression changes shared by DRPLA and Huntington's disease mouse models reveal context-independent effects. *Hum. Mol. Genet.* **11,** 1927–1937.

Mangiarini, L., Sathasivam, K., Seller, M., Cozens, B., Harper, A., *et al.* (1996). Exon 1 of the HD gene with an expanded CAG repeat is sufficient to cause a progressive neurological phenotype in transgenic mice. *Cell* **87,** 493–506.

Mao, J. J., Katayama, S., Watanabe, C., Harada, Y., Noda, K., *et al.* (2001a). The relationship between alphaB-crystallin and neurofibrillary tangles in Alzheimer's disease. *Neuropathol. Appl. Neurobiol.* **27,** 180–188.

Mao, Y. W., Xiang, H., Wang, J., Korsmeyer, S., Reddan, J., and Li, D. W. (2001b). Human bcl-2 gene attenuates the ability of rabbit lens epithelial cells against H2O2-induced apoptosis through down-regulation of the alpha B-crystallin gene. *J. Biol. Chem.* **276,** 43435–43445.

Marchlewska-Koj, A., Cavaggioni, A., Mucignat-Caretta, C., and Olejniczak, P. (2000). Stimulation of estrus in female mice by male urinary proteins. *J. Chem. Ecol.* **26,** 2355–2366.

Mattson, M. P. (2000). Apoptosis in neurodegenerative disorders. *Nat. Rev. Mol. Cell Biol.* **1,** 120–129.

McCampbell, A., Taye, A. A., Whitty, L., Penney, E., Steffan, J. S., and Fischbeck, K. H. (2001). Histone deacetylase inhibitors reduce polyglutamine toxicity. *Proc. Natl. Acad. Sci. USA* **98,** 15179–15184.

McMurray, S. E., and McMurray, C. T. (2001). Huntington's disease. A sports star and a cook. *Lancet* **358**(Suppl), S38.

Molloy, M. P., Brzezinski, E. E., Hang, J., McDowell, M. T., and VanBogelen, R. A. (2003). Overcoming technical variation and biological variation in quantitative proteomics. *Proteomics* **3,** 1912–1919.

Muchowski, P. J., Bassuk, J. A., Lubsen, N. H., and Clark, J. I. (1997). Human alphaB-crystallin. Small heat shock protein and molecular chaperone. *J. Biol. Chem.* **272,** 2578–2582.

Olanow, C. W, and Tatton, W. G. (1999). Etiology and pathogenesis of Parkinson's disease. *Annu. Rev. Neurosci.* **22,** 123–144.

Peters, P. J., Ning, K., Palacios, F., Boshans, R. L., Kazantsev, A., *et al.* (2002). Arfaptin 2 regulates the aggregation of mutant huntingtin protein. *Nat. Cell Biol.* **4,** 240–245.

Pomeroy, S. L., LaMantia, A. S., and Purves, D. (1990). Postnatal construction of neural circuitry in the mouse olfactory bulb. *J. Neurosci.* **10,** 1952–1966.

Price, D. L., and Sisodia, S. S. (1998). Mutant genes in familial Alzheimer's disease and transgenic models. *Annu. Rev. Neurosci.* **21,** 479–505.

Reddy, P. H., Williams, M., Charles, V., Garrett, L., Pike-Buchanan, L., *et al.* (1998). Behavioural abnormalities and selective neuronal loss in HD transgenic mice expressing mutated full-length HD cDNA. *Nat. Genet.* **20,** 198–202.

Renkawek, K., Stege, G. J., and Bosman, G. J. (1999). Dementia, gliosis and expression of the small heat shock proteins hsp27 and alpha B-crystallin in Parkinson's disease. *Neuroreport* **10,** 2273–2276.

Renkawek, K., Voorter, C. E., Bosman, G. J., van Workum, F. P., and de Jong, W. W. (1994). Expression of alpha B-crystallin in Alzheimer's disease. *Acta. Neuropathol. (Berl.)* **87,** 155–160.

Santoni, V., Molloy, M., and Rabilloud, T. (2000). Membrane proteins and proteomics: Un amour impossible? *Electrophoresis* **21,** 1054–1070.

Sathasivam, K., Hobbs, C., Turmaine, M., Mangiarini, L., Mahal, A., *et al.* (1999). Formation of polyglutamine inclusions in non-CNS tissue. *Hum. Mol. Genet.* **8,** 813–822.

Scheler, C., Lamer, S., Pan, Z., Li, X. P., Salnikow, J., and Jungblut, P. (1998). Peptide mass fingerprint sequence coverage from differently stained proteins on two-dimensional electrophoresis patterns by matrix assisted laser desorption/ionization-mass spectrometry (MALDI-MS). *Electrophoresis* **19,** 918–927.

Schilling, G., Becher, M. W., Sharp, A. H., Jinnah, H. A., Duan, K., *et al.* (1999). Intranuclear inclusions and neuritic aggregates in transgenic mice expressing a mutant N-terminal fragment of huntingtin. *Hum. Mol. Genet.* **8,** 397–407.

Seo, E. J., Lee, C., and Yu, M. H. (2002). Concerted regulation of inhibitory activity of alpha 1-antitrypsin by the native strain distributed throughout the molecule. *J. Biol. Chem.* **277,** 14216–14220.

Sharp, A. H., and Ross, C. A. (1996). Neurobiology of Huntington's disease. *Neurobiol. Dis.* **3,** 3–15.

Silverman, G. A., Bird, P. I., Carrell, R. W., Church, F. C., Coughlin, P. B., *et al.* (2001). The serpins are an expanding superfamily of structurally similar but functionally diverse proteins. Evolution, mechanism of inhibition, novel functions, and a revised nomenclature. *J. Biol. Chem.* **276,** 33293–33296.

Sironi, L., Tremoli, E., Miller, I., Guerrini, U., Calvio, A. M., *et al.* (2001). Acute-phase proteins before cerebral ischemia in stroke-prone rats: Identification by proteomics. *Stroke* **32,** 753–760.

Steffan, J. S., Bodai, L., Pallos, J., Poelman, M., McCampbell, A., *et al.* (2001). Histone deacetylase inhibitors arrest polyglutamine-dependent neurodegeneration in Drosophila. *Nature* **413,** 739–743.

Swinbanks, D. (1995). Government backs proteome proposal. *Nature* **378,** 653.

Takahara, H., and Sinohara, H. (1982). Mouse plasma trypsin inhibitors. Isolation and characterization of alpha-1-antitrypsin and contraspin, a novel trypsin inhibitor. *J. Biol. Chem.* **257,** 2438–2446.

Telenius, H., Kremer, H. P., Theilmann, J., Andrew, S. E., Almqvist, E., *et al.* (1993). Molecular analysis of juvenile Huntington disease: The major influence on (CAG)n repeat length is the sex of the affected parent. *Hum. Mol. Genet.* **2,** 1535–1540.

Travis, J., and Salvesen, G. S. (1983). Human plasma proteinase inhibitors. *Annu. Rev. Biochem.* **52,** 655–709.

Turmaine, M., Raza, A., Mahal, A., Mangiarini, L., Bates, G. P., and Davies, S. W. (2000). Nonapoptotic neurodegeneration in a transgenic mouse model of Huntington's disease. *Proc. Natl. Acad. Sci. USA* **97,** 8093–8097.

Velier, J., Kim, M., Schwarz, C., Kim, T. W., Sapp, E., *et al.* (1998). Wild-type and mutant huntingtins function in vesicle trafficking in the secretory and endocytic pathways. *Exp. Neurol.* **152,** 34–40.

Vonsattel, J. P., and DiFiglia, M. (1998). Huntington disease. *J. Neuropathol. Exp. Neurol.* **57,** 369–384.

Vonsattel, J. P., Myers, R. H., Stevens, T. J., Ferrante, R. J., Bird, E. D., and Richardson, E. P., Jr. (1985). Neuropathological classification of Huntington's disease. *J. Neuropathol. Exp. Neurol.* **44,** 559–577.

Wanker, E. E. (2000). Protein aggregation and pathogenesis of Huntington's disease: Mechanisms and correlations. *Biol. Chem.* **381,** 937–942.

Wicks, L. F. (1941). Sex and proteinuria of mice. *Proc. Soc. Exp. Biol. Med.* **48,** 395–400.

Yamamoto, K., and Sinohara, H. (1984). Regulation by sex hormones of serum levels of contraspin and alpha 1-antiprotease in the mouse. *Biochim. Biophys. Acta* **798,** 231–234.

Zabel, C. (2003). Veränderungen im Proteom von Maus und Mensch durch Huntington's Chorea. Ph. D. Thesis.

Zabel, C., Chamrad, D. C., Priller, J., Woodman, B., Meyer, H. E., *et al.* (2002). Alterations in the mouse and human proteome caused by Huntington's disease. *Mol. Cell Proteomics* **1,** 366–375.

Zoghbi, H. Y., and Orr, H. T. (2000). Glutamine repeats and neurodegeneration. *Annu. Rev. Neurosci.* **23,** 217–247.

Zuccato, C., Ciammola, A., Rigamonti, D., Leavitt, B. R., Goffredo, D., *et al.* (2001). Loss of huntingtin-mediated BDNF gene transcription in Huntington's disease. *Science* **293,** 493–498.

Zuccato, C., Tartari, M., Crotti, A., Goffredo, D., Valenza, M., *et al.* (2003). Huntingtin interacts with REST/NRSF to modulate the transcription of NRSE-controlled neuronal genes. *Nat. Genet.* **35,** 76–83.

SECTION V
OVERVIEW OF THE NEUROPROTEOME

PROTEOMICS—APPLICATION TO THE BRAIN

Katrin Marcus, Oliver Schmidt, Heike Schaefer, Michael Hamacher,
André van Hall, and Helmut E. Meyer

Medical Proteom-Center
Ruhr University of Bochum
Bochum, Germany 44780

I. Introduction

The term *proteomics* was first described in the mid-1990s by Marc Wilkins (Wilkins *et al.*, 1996) and has prompted the scientific community to reemphasize the importance of protein analysis of a cell, tissue, or organism as a whole as a complement of the genome. The proteome describes the entirety of proteins expressed by a cell at a single time point. Proteomics investigations also aim to determine protein localization, modifications, interactions, and protein function (Fig. 1). Postgenomic biology offers a conceptually novel opportunity to understand disease mechanisms in that it attempts to progress from current reductionist approaches to an integrated understanding of biological systems. Recent advances/developments in molecular biology, instrument technology, and bioinformatics enable us to simultaneously analyze the entire complement of genes expressed in a particular cell or tissue. These advances have created unique opportunities in the field of medicine, where the results from gene expression studies are expected to help identify cellular alterations that are associated with disease etiology, progression, outcome, and response to therapy. This occurs at levels of complexity, ranging from molecules and molecular machines, via protein networks, to the molecular topology of the cell—of particular importance, for cells of the nervous system—to the network of cellular cross talks. The recent observation that many

287

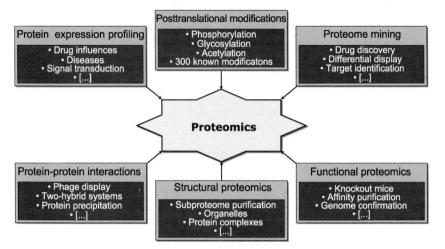

Fɪɢ. 1. Overview over the variety of research fields in proteomics. Proteomics today represents a substantial, interdisciplinary area in research, combining the fundamental natural sciences such as biology, chemistry, and biochemistry. The main goal of proteomics is to obtain a comprehensive overview about the processes in a cell, tissue, or organism to be able to explain the regulatory mechanisms in detail, which are the causes of disease.

proteins work in form of protein complexes clearly shows that proteins exert their function in concert with other proteins. Recent research in proteomics (e.g., genome-wide studies of protein-protein interaction, analysis of the cellular protein topology, and theories on proteome evolution) suggests, however, that even pathways and complexes represent only elements of a cell-wide protein network. How this network is organized in the cell, how complex it is, how it is regulated, and what "network" means in terms of the various mechanisms that may relate one protein to another one are fundamental questions that have to be elucidated. As such, the integration of expert clinical phenotyping, and molecular, cellular, developmental, and evolutionary biology, using genomic, transcriptomic, and proteomic approaches is essential for getting complementary insights into a host of biological processes and improved understanding of the regulation of these processes.

II. Potential of Proteomics

Proteomics can be viewed as an experimental approach to explain the information contained in the genomic sequences in terms of the structure, function, and control of biological processes and pathways. The proteome indicates the quantitative expression profile of a cell, an organism, or a tissue under exactly defined conditions. In contrast to the temporally constant genome, the proteome is dependent on intracellular and extracellular parameters, dynamics, and variables. The analysis of a proteome represents an important supplementation to the genome analysis. The human genome encodes in the order of approximately 100,000 proteins, although the number of genes in the genome is substantially lower, with current estimates of nearly 38,000 genes. It is now well appreciated that one gene may produce a variety of protein products in consequence of alternative splicing of the pre-mRNA and post-translational modifications. An additional introduction of post-translational modifications such as gylcosylation, phosphorylation, acetylation, ubiquitination, sulfation, farnesylation, or controlled proteolysis contributes to a complex protein pattern. In total, there are approximately 300 different post-translational modifications that have been reported (Aebersold and Goodlett, 2001), affecting protein conformation, stability, localization, binding interactions, and function. The majority of proteins is modified after translation, often at more than one site. In most of the cases the site(s) of modification are not predictable from the amino acid sequence. It might be possible to identify a putative consensus sequence for a special protein kinase from the genetic sequence, for example, but whether or not this site is utilized under given conditions can not be predicted from the DNA level.

Additionally, several researchers demonstrated in the past that there is only a poor correlation between mRNA and the corresponding gene product levels (Anderson and Seilhammer, 1997; Gygi *et al.*, 1999a). Gygi and co-workers (1999a) determined the relationship between mRNA and protein expression level for selected expressed genes in *Saccharomyces cerevisiae* to be insufficient to predict the protein expression levels from quantitative mRNA data. More than 150 protein spots were identified by capillary liquid chromatography-tandem mass spectrometry (LC-MS/MS) and quantified by metabolic labeling and scintillation counting. The corresponding mRNA levels were determined by serial analysis of gene expression (SAGE). It was found that the protein expression levels coded for by mRNA with comparable abundance varied by as much as thirtyfold, and that the mRNA levels coding for proteins with comparative expression levels varied by as much as twentyfold. Consequently, proteome analysis must incorporate analysis of protein expression patterns, protein quantitation, and post-translational modifications.

III. Methods in Proteome Analysis

The description of a biological system requires the characterization of a complex mixture of thousands of proteins. To get a wide and preferably complete overview of the proteins present in the respective cell system a suitable analysis strategy adapted to the respective sample must be established. The proteome studies today are driven by a four-stage process: protein preparation, protein separation, protein quantification, and mass spectrometric (MS) analysis. Separation is done either directly on the protein basis using two-dimensional polyacrylamide gel electrophoresis (2D-PAGE), one-dimensional polyacrylamide gel electrophoresis (1D-PAGE), or comprehensive one-dimensional or multidimensional liquid phase based separation techniques (1D/MD-LC). Multidimensional separation typically relies on using two or more independent physical properties of the sample to fractionate the mixture into individual components. When the separation properties are completely independent, the combined separation methods are considered "orthogonal." The number of individual components that can be resolved by a given separation method is defined as the peak capacity. Typically components that are not separated in the first dimension are resolved in the second. A mathematical model exists that shows—if a multidimensional separation is orthogonal—the total peak capacity being a product of each individual separation step (Giddings, 1987). The combination of two or more independent separation dimensions provides the possibility for better resolution of complex protein/peptide mixtures and additionally increases the loading capacity of the system. As a consequence, the sensitivity of the method is increased, allowing the detection of low-abundant proteins/peptides in complex mixtures. For quantification analysis several approaches are described, such as metabolic isotope labeling or chemical labeling. A comprehensive overview for the actual quantification methods is given by Lill (2003) and Moritz and Meyer (2003). Although a high-resolution separation of proteins or peptides is necessary and new pre fractionation and/or separation methods for complex protein/peptide mixtures are published almost monthly (Isaaq *et al.*, 2002; Jiang *et al.*, 2004; von Horsten, 2003; overview: Dreger, 2003; Righetti, 2003), the gains in dynamic range and sensitivity needed for the detection of low-abundance proteins is ultimately limited by the MS instrumentation. Hence new developments in MS instrumentation today focus primarily on methods that introduce as many peptide ions into the mass spectrometer as possible, as well as ways to manipulate the ion population so that lower-abundance species can be measured exclusively in a complex mixture. It becomes more and more apparent that in the near future the most powerful technology for the comprehensive analysis of complex protein mixtures will be a combination of multidimensional fractionation and advanced MS instrumentation. A comprehensive overview about proteomics and its technologies and applications is given in Graves and Haystead (2002).

A. Protein/Peptide Separation

1. *2D-PAGE*

At present, 2D-PAGE (a combination of isoelectric focusing and SDS-PAGE) using carrier-ampholytes (Klose, 1975) or immobilized pH-gradients (Görg *et al.*, 1985) in the first dimension is the method of choice for separating complex mixtures with up to 10,000 different protein species (Fig. 2). It is the only known method that immediately leads from thousands of proteins to various functional data, data concerning protein up-/down-regulation, presence/absence, formation of isoforms, cleavage products, polymorphisms, and post-translational modifications. Although 2D-PAGE still provides an unparalleled resolving power, the following are some restrictions that limit the use of 2D-PAGE:

- The loading capacity is limited to a protein amount of 1 mg at most.
- Automation is difficult, and there is no simple way for online coupling to mass spectrometric detection.
- Hydrophobic and membrane proteins exhibit incomplete solubility in the 2D-PAGE system and therefore are often not present in the 2D gel.
- Highly acidic and basic proteins, as well as very small and large proteins, are difficult to resolve.
- The dynamic range is limited to 10^2–10^3 in protein abundance.

These drawbacks necessitate the application of alternative techniques and have stimulated, in particular, the development of several LC-based technologies.

2. Liquid chromatography

Liquid chromatography more and more evolves to a highly qualified technology for the separation of complex protein and peptide mixtures. It circumvents most of the afore-mentioned limitations concerning 2D-PAGE. The possibility of multimodular combinations of different chromatographic steps such as ion exchange chromatography (IEX), chromatofocusing (CF), size-exclusion chromatography (SEC), reverse phase (RP) chromatography, affinity chromatography (AC), etc. provides numerous options for the comprehensive protein/peptide separation (Fig. 3). Most of the single dimension separations lack sufficient resolution capability to resolve complex biological protein samples or cellular extracts. Separations employing multiple dimensions offer better promise for such applications. In the past, several promising approaches have been published, including combinations of SEC-RPLC, strong cation exchange (SCX)-RPLC, SEC-CE (capillary electrophoresis), AC-RPLC, CF-RPLC, etc. A comprehensive overview is given by Wang and Hanash (2003) and Link (2002). Most LC-based proteomics studies today deal with the analysis of peptides rather than proteins because of their higher solubility in a wide variety of solvents and their improved separation properties. Indeed the sample complexity of digested proteins is enormously increased and a tremendous number of different peptides must be separated (Righetti et al., 2003a) resulting in a lack of resolving power of the method. Several approaches tried to overcome this problem by performing MD-LC separation of intact proteins (Lubman et al., 2002; Opiteck et al., 1998; Wagner et al., 2002), showing very promising results.

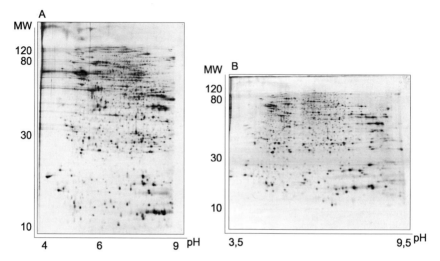

FIG. 2. Two-dimensional polyacrylamide gel electrophoresis (2D-PAGE) of mouse brain extracts performed in our laboratory. (A) Carrier ampholyte based large-scale gel of whole mouse brain extract (100 μg), according to Klose (1975). The first dimension was run using a 20-cm homemade gel, pH 3–10, and the second dimension on a 15% SDS gel. Several thousand proteins were detected after visualization by silver staining. (B) IPG gel of whole mouse brain extract (100 μg), according to Görg (1985). The first dimension was run using a 24-cm IPG strip (Amersham Biosciences, Freiburg, Germany), pH 3–10, and the second dimension on a 13% SDS gel. Approximately 1,000 proteins were detected after visualization by silver staining. (See Color Insert.)

Our own results clearly demonstrate the gel-based separation and the LC-based separation methods to be highly complementary. When analyzing the same mouse brain sample with either multi-dimensional liquid chromatography (MD-LC) or 2D-PAGE, different sets of proteins were identified (unpublished results).

B. Protein Quantification

In addition to the initial identification and characterization of proteins, a key parameter in proteomics analysis is the ability to quantify proteins of interest. In proteomics analyses, quantitation remains a highly important component of target validation and of the determination of post-translational effects affecting the production and function of the corresponding protein. Most proteomics applications are concerned with relative abundances, in which the protein/ peptide patterns of two or more independent samples are compared. In the last years several techniques for quantitative proteomics were developed, each exhibiting its individual strengths and failings. The reviews of Lill (2003) and Moritz

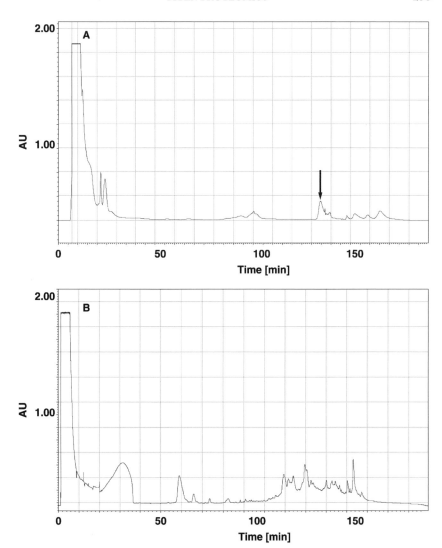

FIG. 3. Two-dimensional LC-based separation of mouse brain proteins. For the protein separation, the PF2D system (Beckman Coulter, Krefeld, Germany) was used in our laboratory. (A) UV chromatogram of the chromatofocusing (first separation dimension) of 3.5-mg whole mouse brain proteins. The fractions were collected automatically, and the fraction marked with an arrow was subjected to the second separation dimension. (B) UV chromatogram of the reversed phase LC (second separation dimension) of the fraction, marked with an arrow. The separation capacity of the 2D-LC set-up can be clearly demonstrated.

(2003) provide a broad summary of state-of-the-art quantification methods. Some of the most used techniques are described briefly in the next paragraphs.

1. *2D-PAGE and 2D-DIGE*

The proteins are visualized using nonspecific staining techniques, following separation by 2D-PAGE (Heukeshoven and Dernick, 1985; Lopez *et al.*, 2000; Neuhoff *et al.*, 1988). After staining, the gel images are quantitated by densitometry, whereby differences in staining intensity correlate with differences in protein abundance. Significant improvements have been made in the 2D-PAGE technology with the development of two-dimensional fluorescence difference gel electrophoresis (2D-DIGE). The DIGE system (Amersham Biosciences, Freiburg, Germany) uses prelabeling of protein samples with size- and charge-matched spectrally resolvable CyDye DIGE fluors (Fig. 4). The internal standard is labeled with one of the CyDye DIGE fluors (Cy2), whereas the experimental and control samples are labelled with Cy3 and Cy5 CyDye DIGE fluors, respectively. The internal standard and both samples are, subsequently, combined before being separated in the same 2D gel. Different excitation and emission wavelengths are used for successive scanning of each particular sample. Differentially expressed proteins can be excised from the gel, and after proteolytic digestion, can be identified by mass spectrometry (see Section on mass spectometry, later in this chapter).

2. *Metabolic* (in vivo) *Labeling* ($^{14}N/^{15}N$, $^{12}C/^{13}C$, H/D)

For metabolic *in vivo* labeling, isotopic tags (generally stable-isotope species of a chosen amino acid) are incorporated in proteins during the processes of cellular metabolism and during the protein biosynthesis, introducing the exogenous added amino acids in the nascent protein. The proteins of cultivated cells are labeled with either heavy or light isotopes of nitrogen, carbon, or hydrogen. After protein or peptide separation, light and heavy forms can be differentially detected and integrated by MS methods (see Section on mass spectometry, later in this chapter). The quotient of the resulting integrals represents the difference in the quantity of the analyzed protein (Fig. 5). Several studies have been reported describing the use of selected stable, isotope-incorporated amino acids as tools for quantifying protein/peptide levels between two given cell lines (Ong *et al.*, 2002; Zhu *et al.*, 2002). The metabolic labeling procedure is one of the most accurate methods for the quantitation of proteins from a cell line, because every protein produced by the cell will contain the isotopically labeled amino acid. Indeed the metabolic labeling is limited to cell culture samples and is not amenable to other samples of interest, such as clinical tissue. For these applications, chemical *in vitro* labeling has to be used.

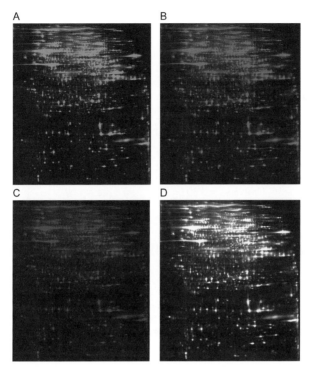

Fɪɢ. 4. Differential proteomics analysis of the right and left side of a mouse brain using the 2D-DIGE system (Amersham Biosciences, Freiburg, Germany). The figure shows the theoretical images of three gels after scanning for Cy2, Cy3, and Cy5 fluorescence. For each gel, both sides of the brain (sample A and B, labeled with Cy3 and Cy5) are run alongside the internal standard (labeled with Cy2) over the same first and second dimension. The internal standard is a pool of all samples included in the study (sample A and B). (A) Carrier-ampholyte based large-scale gel of protein extract of the left side of mouse brain (100 μg), labeled with Cy3. (B) Carrier ampholyte based large-scale gel of a protein extract of the right side of mouse brain (100 μg) labeled with Cy5. (C) Carrier-ampholyte based large-scale gel of an internal standard (100 μg mixture of sample A and B), labeled with Cy2. (D) Overlay of all three theoretical gel images. (See Color Insert.)

3. Chemical Labeling (^{18}O, ICAT)

In those cases in which the metabolic tagging fails, the procedure of chemical labeling offers an excellent alternative. In general, two different methods are distinguished, as follows:

- Labeling during proteolysis (^{18}O incorporation), and
- Labeling by the introduction of isotopic tags.

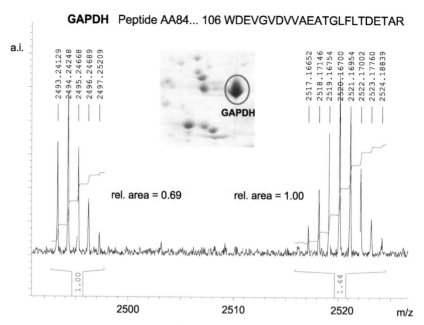

FIG. 5. Differential MS-spectrum after metabolic (*in vivo*) labeling (^{14}N/^{15}N) of *E. coli* cell cultures. Two different states of an *E. coli* cell culture were labeled metabolically with either ^{14}N or [15]N. After combination of both samples and cell lysis, 2D-PAGE was performed according to Görg. The red, marked spot was excised from the gel, digested with trypsin, and analyzed by MALDI-MS. The resulting MS-spectrum shows the signals of both peptides [14]N(WDEVGVDVVAEATGLFLTDE-TAR) and [15]N(WDEVGVDVVAEATGLFLTDETAR) of GAPDH. The quantity ratio of both samples was determined by the integration of the ion signals of the peptide pair. (See Color Insert.)

In the case of quantifying on the basis of peptides, the proteins have to be proteolytically digested before analysis. During proteolysis, an oxygen atom is incorporated from the solvent into the C-terminus of the resulting peptide by the protease (Yao *et al.*, 2003). This phenomenon can be used for relative quantification, and in several studies heavy (^{18}O) and light (^{16}O) isotopic oxygen incorporation during the protein cleavage were applied in parallel for differential analysis (Mirgorodskaya *et al.*, 2002; Yao *et al.*, 2001). For this purpose one set of proteins is cleaved in "heavy" water ($H_2^{18}O$) and the other set is cleaved in parallel in "light" water ($H_2^{16}O$). Subsequent MS analysis results in the detection of a peptide mass difference of 2 Daltons (Da).

For differential isotopic labeling, different tags are used in a variety of applications today. A favorite target for chemical labeling is the thiol group of cysteine. Labeling of cysteine residues is achieved by iodoacetamide derivatives.

The proteins are labeled using isotope-coded affinity tag (ICAT) reagents in an alkylation step and can be either separated by SDS-PAGE or are proteolytically digested and analyzed by mass spectrometry (see next Section; Gygi et al., 1999b). The original ICAT reagents contain a biotin tag for the affinity enrichment of labeled peptides or proteins. For differential analysis, protein sample A is labeled with the "heavy" ICAT reagent and sample B with the "light" one. Different types of reagents are employed, such as deuterated (D_8)/nondeuterated (D_0) (Griffin et al., 2001) or $^{12}C/^{13}C$ (Applied Biosystems, Framingham, Mass.) tags.

In the last years some more labeling procedures were developed for differential quantitative analysis, such as lysine-specific labeling (Berger et al., 2001; Peters et al., 2001), labeling of the N-terminus (Munchbach et al., 2000), phosphoserine and phosphothreonine-specific labeling (Oda et al., 2001; Zhou et al., 2001), etc. (For more details see Lill, 2003; Moritz and Meyer, 2003).

4. *Mass Spectrometry*

In the past the identification of proteins was either done using specific antibodies or N-terminal Edman-sequencing. Today mass spectrometry (MS) represents one of the most important tools in proteomics. The main advantages of MS, compared to other methods in protein identification, include in a short analysis time, the high sensitivity (up to the attomole range), and the potential for automation. After separation and detection, the proteins of interest are analyzed by MS methods. This technique identifies a protein not by analyzing it directly but by analyzing the peptides derived from proteolytic digestion with a protease, usually trypsin (Fig. 6). For a sensitive detection and identification of the proteins or peptides, respectively, different types of high-sensitive mass spectrometers (e.g., time-of-flight [TOF], triple quadrupole, or iontrap mass spectrometers) with various ionization types (e.g., matrix-assisted laser desorption ionization [MALDI] and electrospray-ionization [ESI]) are used today (Fenn, 1989; Karas et al., 2000). Generally the resulting peptides are separated by liquid chromatography or are directly analyzed by mass spectrometry (Aebersold and Goodlett, 2001). Within the mass spectrometer, the peptides are ionized, separated, and identified by a detector.

Since the introduction of MS in proteomics, peptide mass fingerprinting (PMF) analysis became the method of choice in high-throughput protein identification (Shevchenko et al., 1996). In this approach the protein of interest is analyzed after proteolytic or chemical digestion. If the number of peptides for PMF analysis is not sufficient or the complete genome sequence of the analyzed species is unknown, fragmentation analysis (PFF) (MALDI postsource decay [Spengler and Kirsch, 1992]; ESI-MS/MS) can be performed for a more detailed and specific analysis. With these techniques individual peptides are separated and fragmented within the mass spectrometer. The received data of

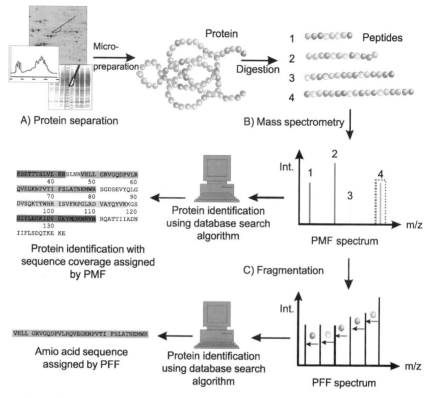

FIG. 6. Overview of common proteomics strategies for protein identification. (A) Protein separation can be done using different separation techniques such as 2D-PAGE, 1D-PAGE, and LC-based methods. In the case of gel-based separation the proteins are subsequently recovered from the gel, washed, and proteolytically or chemically digested. After LC-based separation, generally an in-solution digest is performed. (B) For protein identification, the peptides are first analyzed by peptide mass fingerprinting (PMF). Searching sequence databases with a search algorithm, the proteins are identified because of high mass accuracy and sufficient sequence coverage. (C) If the number of proteolytic peptides is not sufficient for PMF analysis, fragmentation analysis (PFF) (MALDI post-source decay [Spengler and Kirsch, 1992]; ESI-MS/MS) can be performed for a more detailed and specific analysis. Therefore the parent mass of an interested peptide (#4) is selected and the fragmentation is detected using the MS/MS mode of a mass spectrometer. The sequence of the peptide is also determined via a database search using specific search algorithms. (See Color Insert.)

the PMF and/or MS/MS analyses are evaluated automatically via search algorithms, comparing measured data with theoretically estimated data from protein- and DNA-databases. More detailed information about mass spectrometry in proteomics is reviewed in Gevaert and Vanderkerckhove (2000), Aebersold and Goodlett (2001), Aebersold and Mann (2003), Ashcroft (2003).

IV. Proteome Analysis in Neurosciences

The systematic separation, identification, and characterization of proteins of the nervous system offer a basis for research trying to elucidate the mechanisms of neurodegenerative diseases. These studies of neurodegenerative diseases, on the basis of molecular phenotypes, will lead to a new understanding of neurodegeneration. Taken together the study of the genome, transcriptome, and proteome provides complementary insights into a host of biological processes and affords a greater understanding of the regulation of these processes.

Parkinson's disease (PD) and Alzheimer's disease (AD) are the most prevalent neurodegenerative disorders affecting the aging human brain. Risk assessment of these diseases is difficult and prophylaxis not established, because the primary conditions causing these diseases remain unknown, and reliable tools for their early diagnosis are missing. Current therapeutic interventions fail to halt or neutralize the basic disease mechanisms, which lead to chronically and severely disabling states. Despite the fact that numerous outstanding groups are presently investigating both disorders, as well as normal aging processes, the elucidation of their central molecular mechanisms is still in its infancy. The lack of knowledge regarding the basic disease-initiating cellular and molecular mechanisms is an obstacle to the development of rational strategies for prevention and treatment.

Elucidation of degenerative disease mechanisms on the one hand, and aging processes on the other, will allow the identification of common features that will lead to a cross-fertilization of insights and development of new strategies for therapy.

Interactions between genetic and environmental factors are expected to determine the risk, penetrance, onset, and progression of neurodegenerative diseases, as well as the onset and progression of normal aging. Because of their inherent complexity, classical strategies alone for elucidating the genetic contribution to disease (linkage analysis, positional cloning, hypothesis driven reductionist approaches) are likely to be inadequate. The progress made thus far in understanding the primary causes of neurodegenerative diseases has been limited almost exclusively to rare, monogenetic subtypes among the diseases.

Several proteomics approaches were described for the analysis of brain samples. Present studies in this field of research are now providing the first idea about the huge diversity of proteins expressed in the nervous system and how the variation in protein composition is in response to injury and/or disease. In 1990, Matsuoka and co-workers demonstrated an automated high-resolution two-dimensional chromatographic system (strong anion exchange [SAX]-RPLC) for the fractionation of peptides from brain extracts (Matsuoka *et al.*, 1990), demonstrating the huge complexity of brain proteins. In the following years many 2D-PAGE–based studies, concerning different model animals followed by mass spectrometry were published (e.g., initiating proteome maps of the whole mouse and rat brain) (Fountoulakis *et al.*, 1999, 2000; Gauss *et al.*, 1999; Klose *et al.*, 2002). Gauss and co-workers fractionated the total protein of the mouse brain into three fractions: supernatant, pellet extract, and rest pellet suspension, resulting in a 2D pattern with approximately 8500 protein spots. By comparing the two-dimensional patterns from C57BL/6 mice with those of another mouse species (Mus spretus), more than 1000 genetically variant spots were detected. Fountoulakis and co-workers (1999) described a two-dimensional database of rat brain proteins including approximately 200 different proteins. Additional age studies of newborn and adult rat brains showed differences in the protein expression profile. Single subfractions such as the cerebellum from rat (Taoka *et al.*, 2000), pig (Friso and Wikstrom, 1999), and mouse (Beranova-Giorgianni *et al.*, 2002) were also analyzed by 2D-PAGE and mass spectrometry, each comprising several thousands of proteins. In the study by Taoka several proteins were detected with expression rates specific for either mature or immature cerebellum. Some proteins were identified by mass spectrometry and found to fulfill defined roles in the development of the nervous system. Also, a preliminary 2D map of the human brain was established in the late 1990s by the group of Fountoulakis (Langen *et al.*, 1999), with 400 visible protein spots comprising approximately 200 different proteins. The establishment of comprehensive brain proteome maps proves to be a useful reference database for the study of changes in protein expression levels associated with development and aging, as well as neurodegenerative disorders. The generation of free radicals and the degree to which they cause oxidative injury play an important role in the process of aging and various age-related degenerative diseases. It is widely accepted that the protein oxidation generation is tightly linked to pathological processes during the course of age-related neurological disorders. Protein carbonylation content is widely used as a marker for the level of protein oxidation. Specifically carbonylated proteins of mouse brain in the process of aging were analyzed by Soreghan and co-workers in 2003. One hundred carbonylated proteins were identified to potentially play a role in the process of aging and in the progress of age-related neurological diseases. Some other proteins such as tau and ubiquitin are well known to be involved in neurodegenerative diseases. Abnormal tau expression and hyperphosphorylation have been implicated in the pathogenesis of several human neurodegenerative disorders including AD, Down syndrome, Pick's disease, and others (Adamec *et al.*, 2001; Hutton *et al.*, 2001; Pickering-Brown *et al.*, 2000; van Leeuwen *et al.*, 1998). Glycogen synthase kinase-3β (GSK-3β) was proved to be the serine/threonine kinase capable of phosphorylating tau. Proteomics studies with GSK-3β

transgenic mice compared to normal mice resulted in the identification of 51 proteins whose expression rates significantly changed proteins. A significant reduction in the relative abundance in cytoskeletal proteins and proteins involved in energy metabolism, and an increase in protein amount involved in signal transduction and oxidative stress was observed in GSK-3β transgenic mice. The comparison of protein patterns in tau and GSK-3β transgenic mice showed the same changes in expression levels, indicating the involvement of tau and GSK-3β in neurodegeneration (Tilleman et al., 2002).

Our own proteomics analyses of mouse brains concerning protein linkage to their genes (Klose et al., 2002) resulted in the detection of approximately 1300 polymorphic proteins, indicating that single proteins may act as polygenic traits. Genetic analysis of proteomes may detect the types of polymorphism that are most relevant in disease-association studies. Hence in the last few years more and more proteomics studies dealt with brain samples from patients with neurodegenerative diseases. Several comparative proteome studies of post-mortem human brain material were performed in the last years, comparing the diseased protein expression patterns with the patterns of normal control brains.

AD is the neurodegenerative disease most investigated by proteomics approaches. Besides the well-defined pathophysiological hallmarks, AD is associated with synapse loss, oxidative stress, decreased protein turnover, and increased protein misfolding. The expression alterations observed in many proteins involved in a number of pathways help to find new perusable mechanisms responsible for the development of AD. A broad overview about proteomics in AD is given in Butterfield et al. (2003). Schonberger and co-workers (2001) found significant differences in the brain of Alzheimer's patients compared to age-matched nondemented control tissue after 2D-PAGE and N-terminal sequencing. In severely injured brain regions, between 40 and 80 proteins were found to be differentially expressed in various brain regions (temporal cortex, entorhinal cortex, and hippocampus) of diseased tissue compared to control brains. Even in relatively spared regions such as cerebellum, cingulated gyrus, and sensorimotor cortex differentially expressed proteins were detected. This study clearly demonstrates the complexity of interrelated disease mechanisms at work in a complex, multifactorial disease and proves proteomics is a very good tool to develop important new insights into pathogenic mechanism in the dementias. Additionally, the accumulation of glycolytic enzymes such as α- and γ-enolase and glyceraldehydes-3-phosphate dehydrogenase proves the glucose metabolism to be involved in AD. In Butterfield's group, different proteomics studies resulted in a deeper insight into the mechanisms of AD (Castegna et al., 2002, 2003). In these studies, proteomics techniques were used for the detection and identification of oxidized and nitrated proteins in AD. Several specific targets of protein oxidation in AD brain, creatine kinase BB, glutamine synthase, and ubiquitin

carboxy-terminal hydrolase L-1 were identified as potentially involved in neurodegeneration in AD brain. Other reports were published analyzing cerebrospinal
fluid (CSF) of AD patients compared to normal CSF. Because the CSF is in direct
contact with the brain extracellular space, biochemical changes in the brain are
reflected in CSF. As AD pathology is restricted to the brain, CSF is the obvious
source of biomarkers for AD. The group of Kaj Blennow identified several
proteins, including proapolipoprotein, apolipoprotein E, β-2 microglobulin, reti-
nol-binding protein, transthyretin, alpha-1 antitrypsin, cell cycle progression
8 protein, and ubiquitin with significantly altered expression levels in CSF of
AD patients using mini 2D-PAGE in combination with mass spectrometry
(Davidsson et al., 2002; Puchades et al., 2003). Our own work revealed two
different proteins with changing expression levels in the brains of Huntington's
diseased mice and human postmortem tissue (Zabel et al., 2002). In our effort to
identify proteins involved in processes upstream or downstream of the disease-
causing huntingtin, we studied the proteome of a well-established mouse model,
as well as human postmortem brain. In the mouse brain the expression levels
of α1-antitrypsin and αB-crystallin were found to decrease over the course of
the disease. In three brain regions obtained from human Huntington's disease
patients the α1-antitrypsin expression levels were also altered, demonstrating
the involvement of these proteins in this disease. Crystallins are small heat shock
proteins with chaperone function that prevent heat- and oxidative stress-induced
aggregation of proteins. The importance of crystallins in the process of aging is
demonstrated in one of our studies: The proteomic analysis of the eye lens
protein αA-crystallin as a model system for aging processes showed significant time-dependent changes in the 2D protein pattern (Schäfer et al., 2003;
and unpublished results) (Fig. 7). Post-translational modifications including
Ser/Thr-phosphorylation have been shown to change the intrinsic charge and
hydrophobicity of the protein, resulting in an inhibition of chaperone function.
Expression of αA-crystallin has also been described in brain (Deretic et al., 1994).
The extent of αA-crystallin modification is correlated with aging, which indicates
a potential role of this protein in age-related diseases. The understanding of the
complex networks in the nervous system, its function, the mechanisms of signaling pathways and cellular interactions, and, of course, the comprehension of
the effects of changes in the balance of these events is a daunting task today.
The technical developments in the field of proteomics facilitate the generation
of advances in our understanding of protein expression, function, and organization in signaling processes and regulatory networks, providing deeper insight
in how cellular proteomes are regulated in the nervous system in health and
disease.

Nevertheless, new and better technologies in the field of proteomics have to
be developed, and already existing ones must be further advanced.

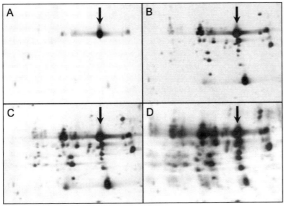

A   embryo day 18
B   4 week old mice
C   14 week old mice
D   100 week old mice

Fig. 7. Gel section of separated lenticular proteins. Lenticular proteins of four different age brackets are separated by large 2D-PAGE. The sections show the region of separated αA-crystallin. (A) αA-crystallin 2D-PAGE pattern of mice embryo lenses, day 18. Three spots were visualized. The most intensive spot is the origin αA-crystallin spot. This spot is marked with an arrow in all four detailed gel pictures. (B) αA-crystallin 2D-PAGE pattern of mice embryo lenses, 4 weeks. The number of protein spots in the gel increased, and several distinct spots can be observed. (C) αA-crystallin 2D-PAGE pattern of mice embryo lenses, 14 weeks. The number of protein spots with lower molecular weight increased, indicating an increased time-dependent protein degradation. (D) αA-crystallin 2D-PAGE pattern of mice embryo lenses, 100 weeks. An explicit intensity increase of protein spots was observed, especially in the more acidic area of the gel. This was an indication for extensive phosphorylation of αA-crystallin during aging. Extensive protein degradation at the C-terminus as well as phosphorylation was confirmed in the subsequent MS analyses (Schäfer *et al.*, 2003).

V. Administrative Realization of Neuroproteomics

As already mentioned, in the course of the so-called post genomic era it becomes more and more visible that the genetic information alone will not lead to a profound understanding of most diseases, and thus probably will not lead to therapeutic approaches.

Estimating 10,000 to 100,000 protein species per tissue, it is obvious that the analysis of even one organ is one of the biggest approaches in scientific history, especially in regard to such complex tissues as brain. Thus the scientific community has to collaborate in large consortia and has to develop useful standards and standard operation procedures (SOPs). In contrast to the Human Genome Organization (HUGO), where each participating country deciphered a chromosome on its own, it is difficult to distribute tasks when analyzing proteomes. As a consequence, the work is focused on whole human organs during aging and/or pathogenesis.

The work in large consortia *per se* is different to smaller networks in regard to the administrative, distributive, or bioinformatics challenges, for example. Due to the increasing complexity of modern science (e.g., international networking) and the urgent need to present scientific research to the funding organization as well as to the public, it is highly advisable to implement an administration into medium-scale and large projects. As the experiences made in major projects (e.g., the NGFN Human Brain Proteome Project [HBPP]) clearly showed, the support of a common administration staff leads to a relief of the scientific members and to an optimization of the scientific output (increasing added value and optimized utilization concepts).

The organization and the feedback of teamwork, as well as the flow of information within the network, are an essential part of the administration work. Additionally, interactions between the consortium and other national and international research projects, research institutions and private enterprises are managed (by arranging project meetings). Furthermore, the composition of progress reports and final reports on schedule, the organization and calling of coordination meetings, the coordination and active participation in public relations (e.g., conferences, seminars, TV, radio, journals) for the project team, the planning and realization of training courses concerning technologies and topics provided by the consortium members, and the publication of the subproject results obtained at the respective time point have to be seen as several of the assigned administration tasks. Moreover, the existing homepages for the national and international initiatives have to be cultivated so that they will serve not only as an information platform, but also as an interchange and communication portal.

In the following section the efforts of the German Human Brain Proteome Project (NGFN HBPP), as well as the HBPP initiative of the Human Proteome Organization (HUPO), are briefly described to elucidate the teamwork of numerous lab groups as an example of how to establish synergistic networks to approach such huge projects.

A. NGFN HBPP

In 2001 the German Federal Ministry of Education and Research (BMBF) funded the so-called "Nationales Genomforschungsnetz" (NGFN-1) for 3 years with approximately 180 million €. One of the largest applications is the Human Brain Proteome Project (NGFN HBPP), with 10,5 million € consisting of three companies: Protagen AG, Dortmund, Scienion AG, and MicroDiscovery GmbH, (Berlin), and nine academic groups consisting of the Medical Proteom-Center (Ruhr-University of Bochum), the Institute of Human Genetics, (Charité Berlin), the Innovationskolleg Theoretical Biology (Humboldt-University Berlin), the BIA Research Laboratory (University of Kassel), Department of Chemical

Biology (GBF Braunschweig), the Mucosa Research Group (Clinic of the University of Kiel), as well as the Automation Group, the Mass Spectrometry Group, and the Protein Group of the Max-Planck-Institute for Molecular Genetics, Berlin.

Focused on improvement of technologies, the consortium started a long-ranging brain analysis approach with the aim to characterize the human and mouse brain proteomes. The data gained (e.g., identified proteins, mRNA profiles, protein/protein interactions, validated targets) is used to compare mouse models and relevant human tissues for neurodegenerative diseases. Further aims are the validation of the identified protein targets, the mRNA-profiling of the identical samples that are used for proteome analysis, the identification of protein/protein interactions, and the development of UniClone sets (non-redundant cDNA expression library) from the adult human brain. To reach these aims the essential technological methods had to be improved and new technologies had to be identified.

The interest of the consortium in developing and testing new tools for proteome analysis is directed to solutions for particular technical problems concerning sample preparation, the 2D-PAGE-system, protein quantification, and the development of UniClone sets from human brain to be used for creating clinically relevant biochips. Furthermore, all these techniques will be combined to develop a fully integrated Proteomic-Workstation, in which samples are prepared and processed automatically. Another practiced technology is the use of 2D/3D Bio-chips on which the samples are immobilized for further analyses. In bioinformatics the important goal is to build up the project database in which all data files provided by the project partners will be stored link variation in protein expression to particular genes in order to elucidate the regulatory network acting between the genome and the proteome.

It is proposed to create new insights for drug development concerning neurodegenerative diseases such as Huntington's chorea, PD, AD, and multiple sclerosis. Besides basic research the consortium is focused on the further development of marketable technology products of the aforementioned fields. Thus the NGFN HBPP is an outstanding example for consortial teamwork to approach neuroproteomic section challenges. In the following the consequential continuation of these network activities to international cooperation is shown.

B. HUPO HBPP

In 2001 the international Human Proteome Organization was established by colleagues working in the protein field according to the HUGO genome work. More than 35 well-known scientists are shaping the ongoing scope of HUPO in the official councils (for further information, visit www.hupo.org). The overall goals of HUPO include the following:

- Consolidation of national and regional proteome organizations into a worldwide organization (HUPO).
- Engagement in scientific and educational activities to encourage the spread of proteomics technologies and to disseminate knowledge pertaining to the human proteome and that of model organisms.
- Assistance in the coordination of public proteome initiatives.

As already mentioned, scientists divided up single chromosomes between the national scientific consortia for sequencing of the human genome. In reference to proteomics, this approach is not feasible. Instead, several initiatives have been established under the roof of HUPO, such as the Human Plasma Proteome Project (HPPP), organized by American colleagues, or the Human Liver Proteome Project (HLPP), under the leadership of Chinese scientists.

Concerning the brain proteome, Profs. Helmut E. Meyer (Medical Proteom-Center, Ruhr-University of Bochum) and Joachim Klose (Institute of Human Genetics, Charité Berlin) agreed to start the International Human Brain Proteome Project (HUPO HBPP) in spring 2003. The inspiration and strategic considerations were taken in part from the NGFN HBPP, but it is to distinguish that the HUPO HBPP initiative is an open and independent project driven by more than 200 interested participants spread throughout the world. As a consequence of the enormous task of analyzing the human brain proteome, this step of international coordination is essential.

The overall aim of the HBPP was postulated as the defining and analysis of the normal brain proteome, including aging, polymorphisms, and modifications, as well as the identification of brain-derived proteins in body fluids. Disease-related proteins will be revealed in comparison with neurodegenerative diseases, validated and functionally characterized by techniques and methods available within the participating groups. These defined proteins might serve as early-onset markers and/or pharmacological targets. The focus will be on the analysis of AD, PD, and aging, including corresponding mouse models. In addition to AD/PD-associated brain regions, brain-derived proteins in liquor and plasma will be analyzed to identify early-onset markers of these diseases.

It is without question that a profound phenotyping of mouse models/patients, a complete characterization of tissue samples before proteome analysis, and a high degree of standardization are extremely important to obtain reliable results. Thus the following two pilot studies were initiated:

- A quantitative proteome and expression profiling analysis of normal mice brain of three different developmental stages (mice kindly provided by Prof. Gert Lubec, Vienna) has been started. With the help of this standardized study the quality of 2D-gel and non-2D-gel based quantitative proteome analysis of the participating groups will be studied, the brain proteome database will be filled with reliable data, and proteome and transcriptome will be compared.

• In addition, a quantitative proteome analysis of human brain from biopsy and autopsy tissue was designed to assess protein stability in postmortem tissue and to feed the brain proteome database with reliable data. (Samples provided by Dr. Albert Becker, Bonn, Germany and Prof. Hans Kretzschmar, Munich, Germany.)

The studies started in spring 2004 with 10 participating groups each and will end within a year, yielding the first results in early summer 2004.

In parallel, human brain material will be collected and delivered to interested groups. Brain tissue will be made available from such sources as the Brain-Net Europe (Prof. Hans Kretzschmar), the Hungarian Brain Bank (Prof. Miklos Palkovits, Budapest, Hungary/Bethesda, USA) and others. Collection of CSF and plasma samples from AD and PD patients will be organized and made available by Prof. Jens Wiltfang, Erlangen-Nuremberg, Germany.

The HUPO HBPP was introduced by Profs. Meyer and Klose at the Second HUPO World Congress in Montreal (Oct. 8–11, 2003) and will be presented in a symposium and a workshop at the Third HUPO World Congress in Beijing in October, 2004. In addition, collaboration with the International Society of Neuroscience is planned, covering combined symposia, sharing standards, and educational efforts. Further information is available at www.hbpp.org.

Thus, in general, it is to state that the work of the large consortia in modern research is not feasible without any administrative team.

References

Adamec, E., Chang, H. T., Stopa, E. G., Hedreen, J. C., and Vonsattel, J. P. (2001). Tau protein expression in frontotemporal dementias. *Neurosci. Lett.* **315,** 21–24.

Aebersold, R., and Goodlett, D. R. (2001). Mass spectrometry in proteomics. *Chem. Rev.* **101,** 269–295.

Aebersold, R., and Mann, M. (2003). Mass spectrometry-based proteomics. *Nature* **422,** 198–207.

Anderson, L., and Seilhammer, J. (1997). A comparison of selected mRNA and protein abundances in human liver. *Electrophoresis* **18,** 533–537.

Ashcroft, A. (2003). Protein and peptide identification: The role of mass spectrometry in proteomics. *Nat. Prod. Rep.* **20,** 202–215.

Berger, S. J., Lee, S. W., Anderson, G. A., Pasa-Tolic, L., Tolic, N., Shen, Y., Zhao, R., and Smith, R. D. (2001). High-throughput global peptide proteomic analysis by combining stable isotope amino acid labeling and data-dependent multiplexed-MS/MS. *Anal. Chem.* **74,** 4994–5000.

Beranova-Giorgianni, S., Pabst, M. J., Russell, T. M., Giorgianni, F., Goldowitz, D., and Desiderio, D. M. (2002). Preliminary analysis of the mouse cerebellum proteome. *Brain Res. Mol. Brain Res.* **98,** 135–140.

Butterfield, D. A., Boyd-Kimball, D., and Castegna, A. (2003). Proteomics in Alzheimer's disease: Insights into potential mechanisms of neurodegeneration. *J. Neurochem.* **86,** 1313–1327.

Castegna, A., Aksenov, M., Aksenova, M., Thongboonkerd, V., Klein, J. B., Pierce, W. M., Booze, R., Markesbery, W. R., and Butterfield, D. A. (2002). Proteomic identification of oxidatively modified proteins in Alzheimer's disease brain. Creatine kinase BB, glutamine synthase, and ubiquitin carboxy-terminal hydrolase L-1. *Free Radio. Bio. Med.* **33,** 562–571.

Castegna, A., Thongboonkerd, V., Klein, J. B., Lynn, B., Markesbery, W. R., and Butterfield, D. A. (2003). Proteomic identification of nitrated proteins in Alzheimer's disease brain. *J. Neurochem.* **85,** 1394–1401.

Davidsson, P., Westman-Brinkmalm, A., Nilsson, C. L., Lindbjer, M., Paulson, L., Andreasen, N., Sjogren, M., and Blennow, K. (2002). Proteome analysis of cerebrospinal fluid proteins in Alzheimer patients. *Neuroreport* **13,** 611–615.

Deretic, D., Aebersold, R. H., Morrison, H. D., and Papermaster, D. S. (1994). Alpha A-and alpha B-crystallin in the retina. Association with the post-Golgi compartment of frog retinal photoreceptors. *J. Biol. Chem.* **269,** 16853–16861.

Dreger, M. (2003). Subcellular proteomics. *Mass. Spectr. Rev.* **22,** 27–56.

Fenn, J. B. (1989). Electrosprayionization for mass spectrometry of large biomolecules. *Science* **246,** 64–71.

Fountoulakis, M., Schuller, E., Hardmeier, R., Berndt, P., and Lubec, G. (1999). Rat brain proteins: Two-dimensional protein database and variations in the expression level. *Electrophoresis* **20,** 3572–3579.

Fountoulakis, M., Hardmaier, R., Schuller, E., and Lubec, G. (2000). Differences in protein level between neonatal and adult brain. *Electrophoresis* **21,** 673–678.

Friso, G., and Wikstrom, L. (1999). Analysis of proteins from membrane-enriched cerebellar preparations by two-dimensional gel electrophoresis and mass spectrometry. *Electrophoresis* **20,** 917–927.

Gauss, C., Kalkum, M., Lowe, M., Lehrach, H., and Klose, J. (1999). Analysis of the mouse proteome. I. Brain proteins: Separation by two-dimensional electrophoresis and identification by mass spectrometry and genetic variation. *Electrophoresis* **20,** 575–600.

Gevaert, K., and Vandekerckhove, J. (2000). Protein identification methods in proteomics. *Electrophoresis* **21,** 1145–1154.

Giddings, J. C. (1987). Concepts and comparisons in multidimensional separation. *J. High Resolut. Chromatogr. Commun.* **19,** 319–323.

Görg, A., Postel, W., Günther, S., and Weser, J. (1985). Improved horizontal two-dimensional electrophoresis with hybrid isoelectric focusing in immobilized pH gradients in the first dimension and laying-on transfer to the second dimension. *Electrophoresis* **6,** 599–604.

Graves, P. R., and Haystead, T. A. J. (2002). Molecular biologists' guide to proteomics. *Microbiol. Mol. Biol. Rev.* **66,** 39–63.

Griffin, T. J., Gygi, S. P., Rist, B., and Aebersold, R. (2001). Quantitative proteomic analysis using a MALDI quadrupole time-of-flight mass spectrometer. *Anal. Chem.* **73,** 978–986.

Gygi, S. P., Rochon, Y., Franza, B. R., and Aebersold, R. (1999a). Correlation between protein and mRNA abundance in yeast. *Mol. Cell Biol.* **19,** 1720–1730.

Gygi, S. P., Rist, B., Gerber, S. A., Turecek, F., Gelb, M. H., and Aebersold, R. (1999b). Quantitative analysis of complex protein mixtures using isotope-coded affinity tags. *Nat. Biotech.* **17,** 994–999.

Heukeshoven, J., and Dernick, R. (1985). Simplified method for silver staining of proteins in polyacrylamide gels and the mechanisms of silver staining. *Electrophoresis* **6,** 103–112.

Hutton, M., Lewis, J., Dickson, D., Yen, S. H., and McGowan, E. (2001). Analysis of tauopathies with transgenic mice. *Trends Mol. Med.* **7,** 467–470.

Isaaq, H. J., Conrads, T. P., Janini, G. M., and Veenstra, T. D. (2002). Methods for fractionation, separation and profiling of proteins and peptides. *Electrophoresis* **23,** 3048–3061.

Jiang, L., He, L., and Fountoulakis, M. (2004). Comparison of protein precipitation methods for sample preparation prior to proteomic analysis. *J. Chromatogr. A.* **1023**, 317–320.

Karas, M., Gluckmann, M., and Schafer, J. (2000). Ionization in matrix-assisted laser desorption/ionization: singly charged molecular ions are the lucky survivors. *J. Mass Spectrom.* **35**, 1–12.

Klose, J. (1975). Protein mapping by combined isoelectric focusing and electrophoresis of mouse tissues. A novel approach to testing for induced point mutation in mammals. *Humangenetik* **26**, 231–243.

Klose, J., Nock, C., Herrmann, M., Stühler, K., Marcus, K., Blüggel, M., Krause, E., Schalkwyk, L. C., Rastan, S., Brown, S. D., Bussow, K., Himmelbauer, H., and Lehrach, H. (2002). Genetic analysis of the mouse brain proteome. *Nat. Genet.* **30**, 385–393.

Langen, H., Berndt, P., Roder, D., Cairns, N., Lubec, G., and Fountoulakis, M. (1999). Two-dimensional map of human brain proteins. *Electrophoresis* **20**, 907–916.

Lill, J. (2003). Proteomic tools for quantitation by mass spectrometry. *Mass Spectr. Rev.* **22**, 182–194.

Link, A. J. (2002). Multidimensional peptide separations in proteomics. *Trends Biotechnol* **20**, S8–S13.

Lopez, M. F., Berggren, K., Chernokalskaya, M., Lazarev, V., Robinson, M., and Patton, W. F. (2000). A comparison of silver stain and SYPRO Ruby Protein Gel Stain with respect to protein detection in two-dimensional gels and identification by peptide mass profiling. *Electrophoresis* **17**, 3673–3683.

Lubman, D. M., Kachman, M. T., Wang, H., Gong, S., Yan, F., Hamler, R. L., O'Neil, K. A., Zhu, K., Buchanan, N. S., and Barder, T. J. (2002). Two-dimensional liquid separations-mass mapping of proteins from human cancer cell lysates. *J. Chromatogr. B. Analyt. Technol. Biomed. Life Sci.* **782**(1–2), 183–196.

Matsuoka, K., Taoka, M., Isobe, T., and Okuyam, T. (1990). Automated high-resolution two-dimensional liquid chromatographic system for the rapid and sensitive separation of complex peptide mixtures. *J. Chromatogr. A.* **515**, 313–320.

Mirgorodskaya, O. A., Kozmin, Y. P., Titov, M. I., Korner, R., Sonken, C. P., and Roepstorff, P. (2002). Quantitation of peptides and proteins by matrix-assisted laser desorption/ionization mass spectrometry using 18O-labeled internal standards. *Rapid Commun. Mass Spectrom.* **14**, 1226–1232.

Moritz, B., and Meyer, H. E. (2003). Approaches for the quantification of protein concentration ratios. *Proteomics* **11**, 2208–2220.

Munchbach, M., Quadroni, M., Miotto, G., and James, P. (2000). Quantitation and facilitated the de novo sequencing of protein by isotopic N-terminal labeling of peptides with a fragmentation-directing moiety. *Anal. Chem.* **72**, 4047–4057.

Neuhoff, V., Arold, N., Taube, D., and Erhard, W. (1988). Improved staining of proteins in polyacrylamide gels including isoelectric focusing gels with clear background at nanogram sensitivity using Coomassie Brilliant Blue G-250 and R-250. *Electrophoresis* **9**, 255–262.

Oda, Y., Nagasu, T., and Chait, B. T. (2001). Enrichment analysis of phosphorylated proteins as a tool for probing the phosphoproteome. *Nat. Biotechnol.* **19**, 379–382.

Ong, S. E., Blagoev, B., Kratchmarova, I., Kristensen, D. B., Steen, H., Pandey, A., and Mann, M. (2002). Stable isotope labeling by amino acids in cell culture, SILAC, as a simple and accurate approach to expression proteomics. *Mol. Cell. Proteomics* **1**, 376–386.

Opiteck, G. J., Ramirez, S. M., Jorgenson, J. W., and Moseley, M. A. (1998). Comprehensive two-dimensional high-performance liquid chromatography for the isolation of overexpressed proteins and proteome mapping. *Anal. Biochem.* **258**(2), 349–361.

Peters, E. C., Horn, D. M., Tully, D. C., and Brock, A. (2001). A novel multifunctional labeling reagent for enhanced protein characterization with mass spectrometry. *Rapid Commun. Mass Spectrom.* **15**, 2387–2392.

Pickering-Brown, S., Baker, M., Yen, S. H., Liu, W. K., Hasegawa, M., Cairns, N., Lantos, P. L., Rossor, M., Iwatsubo, T., Davies, Y., Allsop, D., Furlong, R., Owen, F., Hardy, J., Mann, D., and Hutton, M. (2000). Pick's disease is associated with mutations in the tau gene. *Ann. Neurol.* **48,** 859–867.

Puchades, M., Hansson, S. F., Nilsson, C. L., Andreasen, N., Blennow, K., and Davidsson, P. (2003). Proteomic studies of potential cerebrospinal fluid protein markers for Alzheimer's disease. *Brain Res. Mol. Brain Res.* **118,** 140–146.

Righetti, P. G., Castagna, A., Antonucci, F., Piubelli, C., Cecconi, D., Campostrini, N., Zanusso, G., and Monaco, S. (2003a). The proteome: Anno Domini 2002. *Clin. Chem. Lab. Med.* **41**(4), 425–438.

Righetti, P. G., Castagna, A., Herbert, B., Reymond, F., and Rossier, J. S. (2003b). Prefractionation methods in proteome analysis. *Proteomics* **3,** 1397–1407.

Schäfer, H., Marcus, K., Sickmann, A., Herrmann, M., Klose, J., and Meyer, H. E. (2003). Identification of phosphorylation and acetylation sites in alphaA-crystallin of the eye lens (mus musculus) after two-dimensional gel electrophoresis. *Anal. Bioanal. Chem.* **376,** 966–972.

Schonberger, S. J., Edgar, P. F., Kydd, R., Faull, R. L., and Cooper, G. J. (2001). Proteomic analysis of the brain in Alzheimer's disease: Molecular phenotype of a complex disease process. *Proteomics* **1,** 1519–1528.

Shevchenko, A., Jensen, O. N., Podtelejnikov, A. V., Sagliocco, F., Wilm, M., Vorm, O., Mortensen, P., Boucheriie, H., and Mann, M. (1996). Linking genome and proteome by mass spectrometry: Large-scale identification of yeast proteins from two dimensional gels. *Proc. Natl. Acad. Sci. USA* **93,** 14440–14445.

Soreghan, B. A., Yang, F., Thomas, S. N., Hsu, J., and Yang, A. J. (2003). High-throughput proteomic-based identification of oxiatively induced protein carbonylation in mouse brain. *Pharm. Res.* **20,** 1713–1720.

Spengler, B., and Kirsch, D. (1992). Peptides sequencing by matrix assisted laser desorption mass spectrometry. *Rapid. Comm. Mass Spectrom.* **6,** 105–108.

Taoka, M., Wakamiya, A., Nakayama, H., and Isobe, T. (2000). Protein profiling of rat cerebella during development. *Electrophoresis* **21,** 1872–1879.

Tilleman, K., Stevens, I., Spittaels, K., Haute, C. V., Clerens, S., Van Den Bergh, G., Geerts, H., Van Leuven, F., Vandesande, F., and Moens, L. (2002). Differential expression of brain proteins in glycogen synthase kinase-3 transgenic mice: A proteomics point of view. *Proteomics* **2,** 94–104.

Van Leeuwen, F. W., De Kleijn, D. P. V., Van den Hurk, W. H., Neubauer, A., Sonnemans, M. A. F., Sluijs, J. A., Köycü, S., Ramdjielal, R. D. J., Salehi, A., Martens, G. J. M., Grosveld, F. G., Burbach, J. P. H., and Hol, E. M. (1998). Frameshift mutants of beta amyloid precursor protein and ubiquitin-B in Alzheimer's and Down patients. *Science* **279,** 242–247.

Von Horsten, H. H. (2003). An agarose gel subfractionation technique for the recovery of low-abundance proteins. *Anal. Biochem.* **316,** 139–141.

Wagner, K., Miliotis, T., Marko-Varga, G., Bischoff, R., and Unger, K. K. (2002). An automated on-line multi-dimensional HPLC system for protein and peptide mapping with integrated sample preparation. *Anal. Chem.* **74,** 809–820.

Wang, H., and Hanash, S. (2003). Multi-dimensional liquid phase based separations in proteomics. *J. Chromatogr. B.* **787,** 11–18.

Wilkins, M., Sanchez, J. C., Gooley, A. A., Appel, R. D., Humphrey-Smith, I., Hochstrasser, D. F., and Williams, K. L. (1996). Progress with proteome projects: Why all proteins expressed by a genome should be identified and how to do it. *Biotechnol. Genet. Eng. Rev.* **13,** 19–50.

Yao, X., Freas, A., Ramirez, J., Demirev, P. A., and Fenselau, C. (2001). Proteolytic 18O labeling for comparative proteomics: Model studies with two serotypes of adenovirus. *Anal. Chem.* **73,** 2836–2842.

Yao, X., Afonso, C., and Fenselau, C. (2003). Dissection of proteolytic [18]O labeling: Endoprotease-catalyzed ^{16}O-to-^{18}O exchange of truncated peptide substrates. *J. Proteome Res.* **2,** 147–152.

Zabel, C., Chamrad, D. C., Priller, J., Woodman, B., Meyer, H. E., Bates, G. P., and Klose, J. (2002). Alterations in the mouse and human proteome caused by Huntington's disease. *Mol. Cell Proteomics* **1,** 366–375.

Zhu, H., Pan, S., Gu, S., Bradbury, E. M., and Chen, X. (2002). Amino acid residue specific stable isotope labeling for quantitative proteomics. *Rapid Comm. Mass Spectrom.* **16,** 2115–2123.

Zhou, H., Ranish, J. A., Watts, J. D., and Aebersold, R. (2001). Quantitative proteome analysis by solid-phase isotope tagging and mass spectrometry. *Nat. Biotech.* **19,** 512–515.

INDEX

CONTENTS OF RECENT VOLUMES

Volume 52

Volume 53

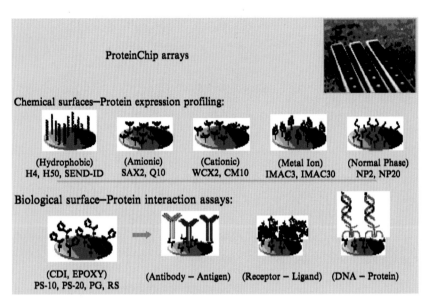

WALKER AND XU, FIG. 1. Many different surface chemistries are available with SELDI-TOF-MS technology.

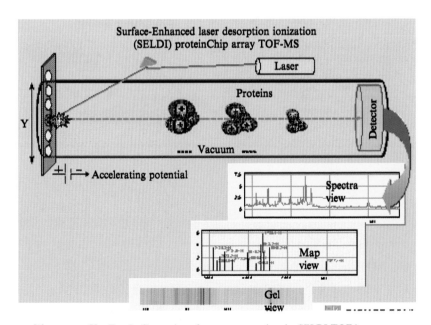

WALKER AND XU, FIG. 2. Generation of mass spectra using the SELDI-TOF instrument.

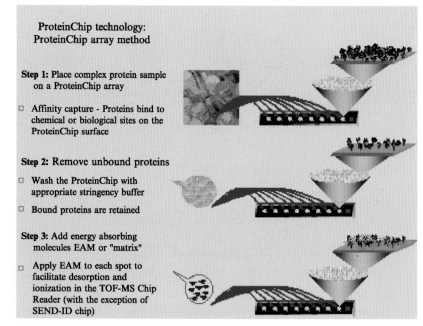

**ProteinChip technology:
ProteinChip array method**

Step 1: Place complex protein sample
on a ProteinChip array

☐ Affinity capture - Proteins bind to
chemical or biological sites on the
ProteinChip surface

Step 2: Remove unbound proteins

☐ Wash the ProteinChip with
appropriate stringency buffer

☐ Bound proteins are retained

Step 3: Add energy absorbing
molecules EAM or "matrix"

☐ Apply EAM to each spot to
facilitate desorption and
ionization in the TOF-MS Chip
Reader (with the exception of
SEND-ID chip)

WALKER AND XU, FIG. 3. Steps in the process of protein binding to the chip surface and being prepared for detection in the mass spectrometer.

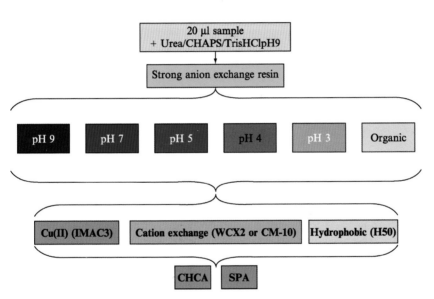

WALKER AND XU, FIG. 4. Fractionation and expression profiling for serum.

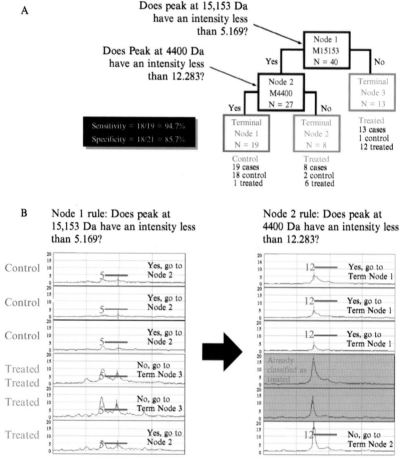

WALKER AND XU, FIG. 6. Classification tree sample. (A) Each node (blue square) is a decision point. Each sample is sifted down the tree based on how it answers the question in each node. For example, the first node asks the question, "Does peak at molecular weight 15,153 Da have a peak intensity less than 5.169?" If the answer is yes, the sample goes to the left node 2; otherwise, it goes to the right terminal node 3. Terminal nodes are stopping points, and the majority of samples determine the classification of each terminal node. In terminal node 3, there is 1 control and 12 treated samples; the control is misclassified and the treated samples are classified correctly. Sensitivity is calculated as the ratio of the number of correctly classified treated samples to the total number of treated samples. Similarly, specificity is calculated as the ratio of the number of control samples to the total number of controls. (B) How the rules in the classification tree manifest themselves in the raw data. In this subset of six spectra from the study used to generate the tree in (A), we can see how the classification tree uses peak intensities to classify each sample. (Reprinted with permission from Fung and Enderwick, 2002.)

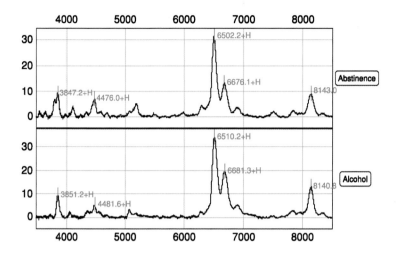

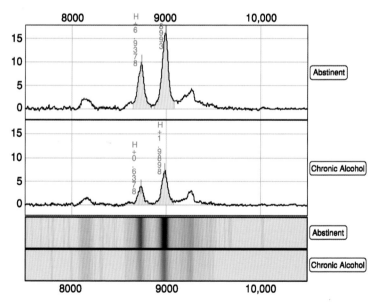

WALKER AND XU, FIG. 7. SELDI-TOF-MS analysis of serum protein profiles in drinking and nondrinking monkeys. Serum samples from cynomolgus macaques that had been self-administering large amounts of alcohol for nine months were compared to non drinking controls using the Ciphergen ProteinChip system. The majority of the proteins were unchanged, as illustrated by the profile in the upper panel (for a collection of proteins analyzed on a WCX weak cation exchange chip surface). On the other hand, proteins were identified on a number of surfaces that did appear to be dierentially regulated. In this case, hydrophobic proteins (analyzed on an H4 hydrophobic binding surface) were dierentially regulated. Proteins at approximately 9000 daltons appeared to be reduced by ethanol self-administration (lower panel). The bottom of the lower panel shows a "pseudo-gel" representation of the relative expression levels of the various proteins.

Differential expression of candidate autistic biomarkers: analysis of pH 5 eluted frac. (4) using WCX2 surface

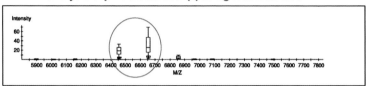

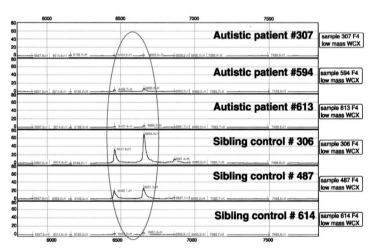

WALKER AND XU, FIG. 8. SEDLI-TOF-MS profiles. Fractionated serum samples from three autistic patients and three non autistic siblings were assayed on a weak cationic exchange surface and eluted at pH 5. Data presented here show that fraction 4 in two of the three control samples contains two proteins, at 6450 and 6650 daltons, that are absent in autistic samples.

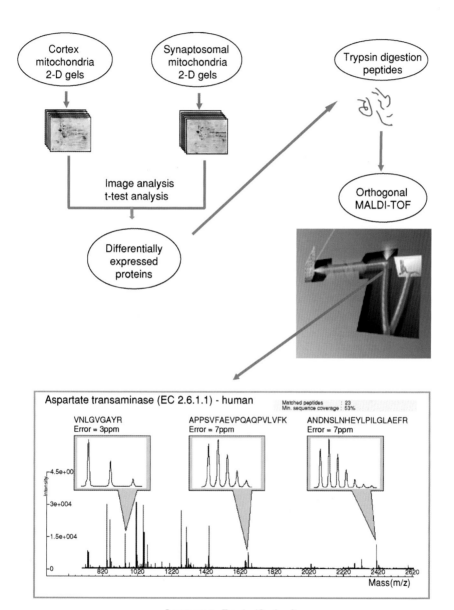

LOPEZ *ET AL.*, FIG. 1. *(Continued)*

Lopez *et al.*, Fig. 1. 2-D gel/MALDI-TOF-based strategy for the identification of differential protein expression in mitochondria isolated from mouse brain cortex and synaptosomes. Mitochondria and synaptosomes were prepared using a method from Lai and Clark (1976) with the following modifications. All animal procedures were carried out in accordance with approved IACUC (Institutional Animal Care and Use Committees) animal protocols at the Buck Institute in Novato, Calif. Cerebral hemispheres of wild-type mice at 18–21 days of age were harvested, cut into small pieces and homogenized with a Dounce homogenizer in cold H buffer (0.21 M mannitol, 70 mM sucrose, 1 mM EGTA, 0.1 (wt/vol) BSA, and 5 mM HEPES at pH 7.2) before being centrifuged at 1000 Xg for 10 minutes at 4 °C. The supernatant was centrifuged at 8500 Xg, and the pellet was carefully drained. The resuspended pellet was layered onto a step gradient of 15%, 12%, 9%, and 6% ficoll solution (wt/vol). After centrifugation at 75,000 Xg for 45 minutes at 4 °C, the synaptosomes and mitochondrial bands were removed. Mitochondria were washed twice in H buffer (−)BSA and stored at −20 °C until further use. The two synaptosomal bands were washed and the mitochondria present inside the synaptosomes were isolated via a method modified from those of Lai and Clark (1976) and Asakura *et al.* (1989). Briefly, the synaptosomes were osmotically shocked in water, then resuspended in a 3% ficoll solution and layered onto a 3–6% ficoll cushion. After centrifugation at 11,500 Xg for 30 minutes at 4 °C, the synaptic mitochondria in the pellet were washed before storage at −20 °C. Protein concentrations were estimated using the Bradford assay (Bio-Rad, Hercules, Calif.) according to the manufacturer's protocol. Proteins from the cortical and synaptosomal mitochondria were prepared and run on large-format 2-D gels (Lopez *et al.*, 2000). Five replicate gels were run from each sample. Gel images were acquired with a CCD camera imaging system (ProXPRESS, PerkinElmer, Boston) and analyzed (Progenesis Discovery, Nonlinear Dynamics Ltd, United Kingdom). Normalized spot volumes were exported into a customized Excel (Microsoft, Redmond, Wash.) template and used in heteroscedastic t-test calculations. The ratios of synaptosomal and cortex matched spots were calculated, and the candidate differentially expressed spots were validated for accurate matching and quantification by relocation on the original gel images in Progenesis. Validated protein spots were excised, digested with trypsin, and analyzed with prOTOF (PerkinElmer, Boston) orthogonal MALDI-TOF mass spectrometry. Peptide mass fingerprinting and protein identification was done using TOFWorks software (PerkinElmer).

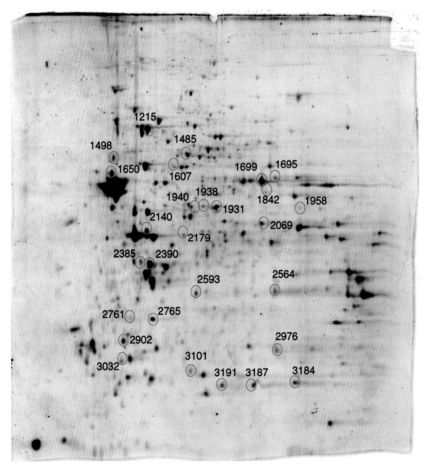

LOPEZ *ET AL.*, FIG. 2. 2-D gel image of cortical mitochondrial proteins with the differentially expressed spots indicated. Differentially expressed proteins in synaptosomal and cortex mitochondria (see Fig. 1) are indicated. The designated proteins were excised and subjected to trypsin digestion and subsequent peptide mass fingerprinting by orthogonal MALDI-TOF mass spectrometry (see description in Fig. 1 and Table I).

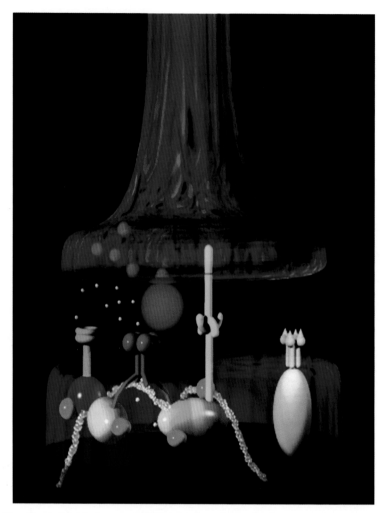

Husi, Fig. 1. Model of a synapse highlighting the various molecular components participating in synaptic function. Neurotransmitters (purple) are released from the presynaptic terminal and target postsynaptic receptors (turquoise and red), which are either channels for other small molecules such as calcium (gray), or are transmitting signals through other means such as G-proteins (blue). Other signaling machineries (green) then convey signals through specific pathways to downstream targets. Linkage between these molecules is by and large provided by cytoskeletal molecules (brown and white), and the presynaptic and postsynaptic side is tethered together by cadherins and other cell-adhesion–related molecules (yellow).

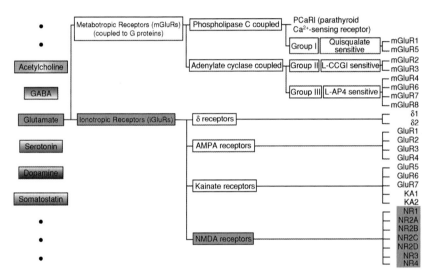

Husi, Fig. 2. The glutamate receptor family. Glutamate receptors are classified based on pharmacological properties and whether they contain seven transmembrane spanning regions and are coupled to G-proteins (metabotropic glutamate receptors), or whether they form Na^+/K^+- and/or Ca^{2+}-permeable channels (ionotropic glutamate receptors). The molecules belonging to the NMDA receptor family are highlighted in blue.

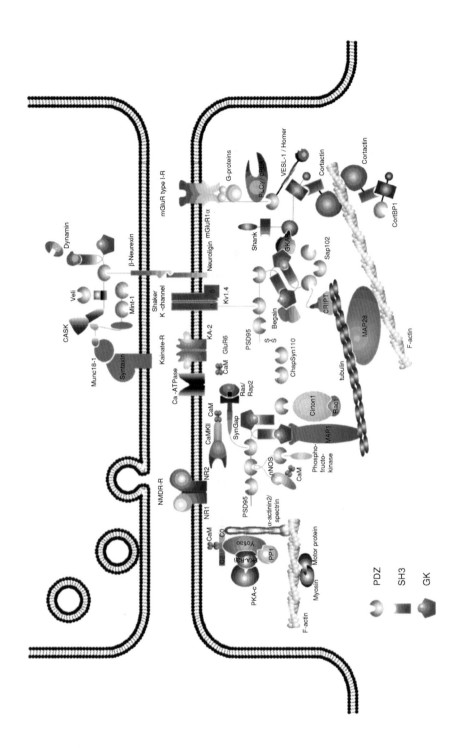

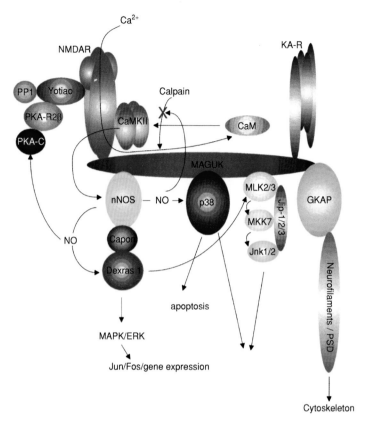

Husi, Fig. 4. Schematic representation of a potential signal-transduction pathway following NMDAR activation and Ca^{2+} influx by NRC tethered components. Ca^{2+} leads to activation of Calmodulin (CaM), which in turn activates CaMKII. Nitric oxide (NO) is produced by *neuronal nitric oxide synthase* (nNOS) after activation by CaMKII, and this potent messenger leads to activation of *protein kinase A* (PKA), *dexamethasone-induced RAS protein 1* (Dexras1), p38 *protein kinase*, and *mixed lineage kinase 2/3* (MLK2/3), as well as inhibition of Calpain and ultimately to downstream events, including gene expression.

Husi, Fig. 3. Schematic diagram of synaptic multiprotein complexes. Postsynaptic complexes of proteins associated with the NMDA receptor and PSD-95, found at excitatory mammalian synapses, are shown. Individual proteins are illustrated with arbitrary shapes, and known interactions are indicated. Proteins shown in color are those found in a proteomic screen, whereas those shown in gray are inferred from bioinformatic studies. The specific protein–protein interactions are predicted, based on published reports from yeast two-hybrid studies. Membrane proteins (e.g., receptors, channels, and adhesion molecules) are attached to a network of intracellular scaffold, signaling, and cytoskeletal proteins, as indicated.

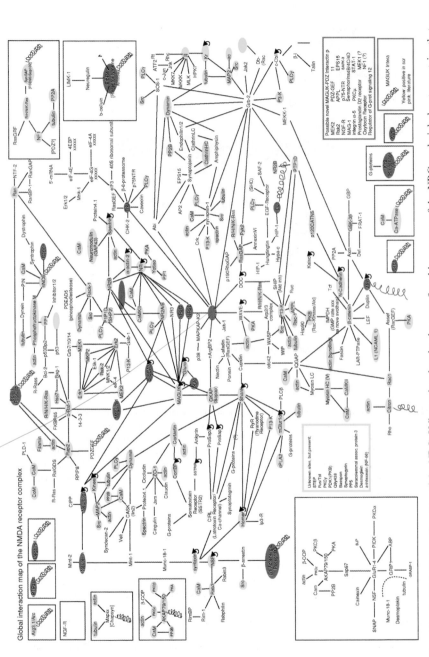

HUSI, FIG. 6. Global interaction map of the NRC. Yellow-colored molecules were found in a screen of the NRC; and pink denotes proteins that were shown by individual publications to interact with adjacent molecules. Small boxes denote molecules that tether to PSD-95 and other members of the MAGUK family. The black box contains the AMPA receptor complex, which does not link into the NRC.

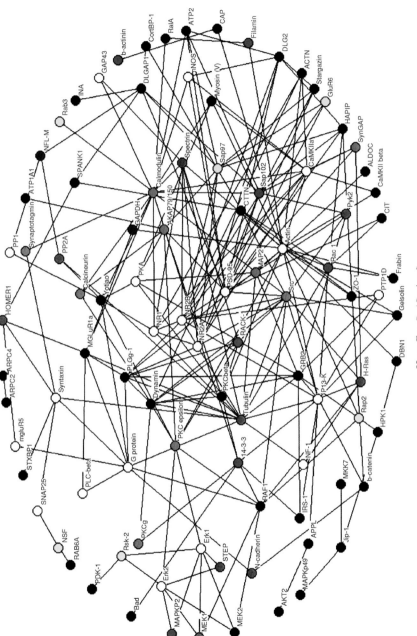

HUSI, FIG. 7. (*Continued*)

Husi, Fig. 7. Network representation of NRC proteins with phenotypic annotation. Ninety-seven NRC proteins with known direct protein interactions to other NRC proteins are plotted. The NMDA receptor subunits (NR1, NR2A, NR2B) are located in the center. The association of each protein with plasticity, rodent behavior, or human psychiatric disorders is shown in the color of the node. Key: black-no known association; red-psychiatric disorder; green-plasticity; blue-rodent behavior; yellow-psychiatric disorders and plasticity; cyan-plasticity and rodent behavior; white-all three phenotypes; and orange-psychiatric disorders and rodent behavior. The network provides a common connection or association among these disease molecules. Network simulations also show that disruption of combinations of proteins produce more severe effects on the network. This suggests that combinations of proteins (or mutant alleles) underpin the polygenic nature of a variety of disorders.

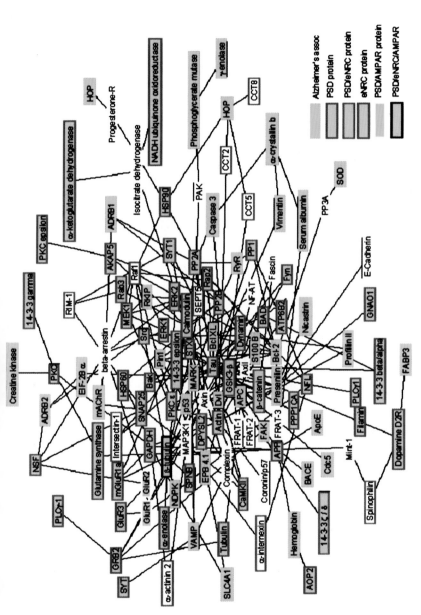

Husi, Fig. 8. Network cluster of proteins associated with Alzheimer's disease within the NRC and AMPAR complexes.

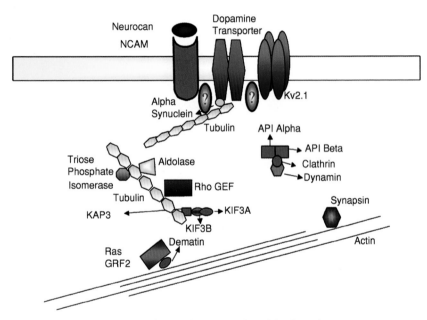

Maiya and Mayfield, Fig. 3. Schematic representation of the dopamine transporter proteome. Proteins found in the dopamine transporter complex are shown. Proteins shown in gray were not found in our studies but are known to exist in a complex with one or more proteins that were identified in our screen.

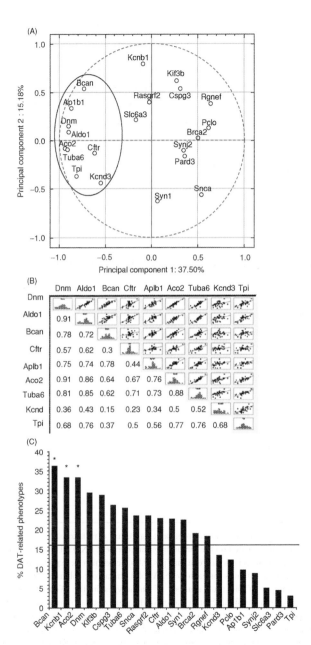

MAIYA AND MAYFIELD, FIG. 4. Results of *in silico* analysis using WebQTL database. Results of PCA on the 21 DAT-related genes are plotted on a two-dimensional diagram (A), with PC1, PC2, and PC3 loadings for each gene being shown. Nine genes with similar loading patterns are encircled. (B) Correlations among the nine genes are shown numerically (below major diagonal) and graphically

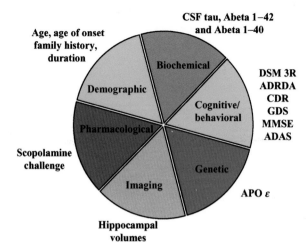

SOARES *ET AL.*, FIG. 1. Overview of clinical characteristics of NIMH dataset.

(above major diagonal). Numbers in bold represent significant correlations (r $\geq$ 0.33, p $<$ 0.05; r $\geq$ 0.42, p $<$ 0.01). Diagrams located on the major diagonal represent BXD RI strain mean distributions. (C) Proportion of significant genetic correlations (p $<$ 0.05) between gene expression and DAT-related phenotypes are shown in columns for each gene. A solid line across columns shows a proportion of DAT-related phenotypes of the total number of phenotypes in the WebQTL database (global proportion). Asterisks indicate significant deviation of the proportion of significantly correlated DAT-related phenotypes from the global proportion (by a χ^2 test). Bcan = brevican, Kcnb1 = Kv2.1, Aco2 = similar to mitochondrial aconitase, Dnm = dynamin, Kif3b = kinesin-related protein 3B, Cspg3 = neurocan, Tuba6 = tubulin, Snca = α-synuclein, Rasgrf2 = Ras GRF2, Cftr = cystic fibrosis transmembrane conductance regulator, Aldo1 = fructose bis phosphate aldolase, Syn1 = synapsin 1, Rgnef = Rho GEF, Kcnd3 = Kv4.3M, Pclo = piccolo, Ap1b1 = adaptor protein 1 beta, Synj2 = synaptojanin2, Slc6a3 = dopamine transporter, Pard3 = Par3, Tpi = triose phosphate isomerase.

A

Master gel   Alignment to master gel

B

Coefficient of variability (expressed as %) range

SOARES ET AL., FIG. 3. Gel alignments and test retest variability. (A) One master gel was created, and gels containing experimental samples were all mapped to coordinates defined by one single master gel. (B) Assessment of test retest variability as measured by coefficient of variation of individual features from aliquots of a pooled CSF sample (quality control) run multiple times. Only features that appeared on 70% of the gels were included in the analysis. Note variability changed throughout the spatial map.

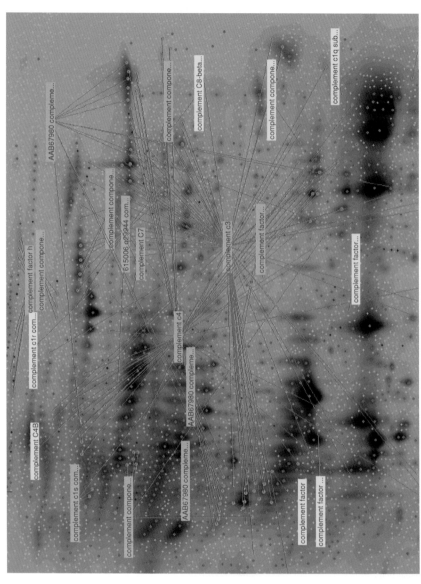

SOARES *ET AL.*, FIG. 4. The complexity of the CSF proteome as exemplified by the complement cascade.